Ophthalmic Medical Assisting
An Independent Study Course

Third Edition, Revised

Tyree Carr, MD
Executive Editor

AMERICAN ACADEMY
OF OPHTHALMOLOGY
The Eye M.D. Association

AMERICAN ACADEMY OF OPHTHALMOLOGY
The Eye M.D. Association

655 Beach Street
P.O. Box 7424
San Francisco, CA 94120-7424

The Academy provides this material for educational purposes only. It is not intended to represent the only or best method or procedure in every case, nor to replace a physician's own judgment or give specific advice for case management. Including all indications, contraindications, side effects, and alternative agents for each drug or treatment is beyond the scope of this material. All information and recommendations should be verified, prior to use, with current information included in the manufacturers' package inserts or other independent sources, and considered in light of the patient's condition and history. Reference to certain drugs, instruments, and other products in this publication is made for illustrative purposes only and is not intended to constitute an endorsement of such. Some materials may include information on applications that are not considered community standard, that reflect indications not included in approved FDA labeling, or that are approved for use only in restricted research settings. The FDA has stated that it is the responsibility of the physician to determine the FDA status of each drug or device he or she wishes to use, and to use them with appropriate patient consent in compliance with applicable law. The Academy specifically disclaims any and all liability for injury or other damages of any kind, from negligence or otherwise, for any and all claims that may arise from the use of any recommendations or other information contained herein.

The following contributors state these financial relationships:

Melvin I. Freeman, MD, FACS: Research funds—Bausch & Lomb; research funds, consultation service—Ciba Vision; royalties—Slack, Inc.; research funds, travel funds—Vistakon; research funds—Wesley Jessen.

Silvia Orengo-Nania, MD: Speakers bureau—Alcon, speakers bureau—Pharmacia Upjohn.

Each other author and contributor states that he or she has no significant financial interest or other relationship with the manufacturer of any commercial product mentioned in the text that he or she contributed to this publication or with the manufacturer of any competing commercial product.

Library of Congress Cataloging-in-Publication Data
Ophthalmic medical assisting : an independent study course / Tyree Carr, executive editor. — 3rd ed.
p. cm.
Includes bibliographical references and index.
ISBN 1-56055-041-4
1. Ophthalmic assistants—Programmed instruction. I. Carr, Tyree, 1949– .
[DNLM: 1. Ophthalmology programmed instruction. 2. Ophthalmic Assistants programmed instruction. WW 18.2 0585 1999]
RE72.5.064 1999
617.7′0233—DC21
DNLM/DLC
for Library of Congress 98-33325
CIP

Printed in China
02 03 04 5 4 3 2 1

Acknowledgments

Third Edition Reviewers/Revisers

Tyree Carr, MD (Executive Editor)
Donna Applegate, COT
F. Michael Cornell, MD
Cynthia A. Dean, COMT
Peter C. Donshik, MD
Lindreth DuBois, MEd, MMSc, COMT
Melvin I. Freeman, MD, FACS
Marcia Hinrichs, RN, MSN
Andrew G. Lee, MD
Elbert Magoon, MD
Emanuel Newmark, MD
Silvia Orengo-Nania, MD
Ralph S. Sando, MD
Diana Shamis, CO, COMT, MHSE
Paul J. Wasson, MD

Second Edition Reviewers/Revisers

Paul J. Wasson, MD (Executive Editor)
Tyree Carr, MD
Cynthia A. Dean, COMT
Craig D. Giles
Leslie France, CO
Melvin I. Freeman, MD
Darlene Miller, MA, MT (ASCP)
Silvia Orengo-Nania, MD
Carol A. Ruehl, RN
Robert L. Stamper, MD
Kenneth Woodworth, Jr, COMT

First Edition Associate Editors

The following individuals assisted in developing original course topics, course text, and examination:
Robert L. Stamper, MD (Executive Editor; Ch 1, 7)
Cesar T. Chavez, MD (Ch 3, Appendix B)
Carol A. Covell, RN, MS (Ch 11, 12)
Claude L. Cowan, MD (Ch 9)
Leslie France, CO (Ch 10)
Melvin I. Freeman, MD (Ch 14, Appendix A)
Todd A. Hostetter, BS, COMT, NCLC, CRA (Ch 8)
Joe R. McFarlane, Jr, MD (Ch 5, 6)
Paul J. Wasson, MD (Ch 2, 13)
Kenneth Woodworth, Jr, COMT (Ch 4)

First Edition Course Development Task Force

The following individuals contributed to the development of course objectives, organization, and content:
Leslie France, CO
Alice O. Gelinas, RN
Joe R. McFarlane, Jr, MD
James Randall, MD
Robert L. Stamper, MD

First Edition Text Reviewers

Richard L. Abbott, MD
Allen Beallo, MD
August Colenbrander, MD
Lindreth DuBois, MEd, CO, COMT
Peter Y. Evans, MD
Alice O. Gelinas, RN
Lani Hardage, COA
Michelle Pett Herrin, MA, CO, COMT
Robert C. Johnson, MD
Barrett Katz, MD
Michael Lambert, MD, FACS
Brian Levy, OD, MSc, FAAO
Ella Rosamont Morgan, BS, COMT
T. Otis Paul, MD
Deanna Joy Presnell, BA, COT, CST
William B. Stewart, MD
Scarlette Wilson, MD

First Edition Examination Reviewers

Kristi A. Bierly, COA
Charlotte Gardner
LaRae M. Garrigan
Beth Marasigan
Denise T. Martin
Dennis A. Riccio, COA

First Edition Writers

Mary-Jean Pramik-Holdaway, BS, BA, MS
Burton I. Wilner, PhD

Contents

Performance Boxes xii

Introduction xiii

CHAPTER 1
INTRODUCTION TO OPHTHALMIC MEDICAL ASSISTING 1

What Is Ophthalmology? 2

Who Provides Eye Care? 2

Ophthalmologist 2
Optometrist 3
Optician 3
Ophthalmic Registered Nurse 3
Orthoptist 3
Ocularist 3
Ophthalmic Photographer 3
Ophthalmic Medical Assistant 4

What Are the Certification Levels? 4

Professional Development 5

Which Rules of Ethics Apply? 5

Code of Ethics of the AAO 7

What Constitutes Professional Behavior? 7

CHAPTER 2
ANATOMY AND PHYSIOLOGY OF THE EYE 11

The Eye as an Optical System 12

The Adnexa 12

Orbit 12
Extraocular Muscles 12
Eyelids and Conjunctiva 14
Lacrimal Apparatus 16

The Eye 16

Cornea and Sclera 16
Anterior Chamber 18
Uveal Tract 18
Crystalline Lens 20
Vitreous 20
Retina 20
Visual Pathway 21

CHAPTER 3
DISEASES AND DISORDERS OF THE EYE 25

Mechanisms of Disease and Injury 26

Infectious Process 26
Inflammatory Process 26
Allergic Process 26
Ischemic Process 27
Metabolic Process 27
Congenital Process 27
Developmental Process 27
Degenerative Process 27
Neoplastic Process 27
Traumatic Process 28
Signs, Symptoms, and Syndromes 28

Abnormalities of the Adnexa 28

Orbit 28
Extraocular Muscles 29
Eyelids and Conjunctiva 29
Lacrimal Apparatus 32

Abnormalities of the Eye 33

Cornea and Sclera 33
Anterior Chamber 34
Uveal Tract 36
Crystalline Lens 36
Vitreous 36
Retina 37
Visual Pathway 37

CHAPTER 4
OPTICS AND REFRACTIVE STATES OF THE EYE 41

Principles of Optics 42

Refraction 42
Refractive Properties of Curved Lenses 43
Convergence, Divergence, and Focal Point 43
Lens Power and Focal Length 45

Refractive States of the Eye 45

Emmetropia 46
Ametropia 46
- Myopia 46
- Hyperopia 46
- Astigmatism 47
- Presbyopia 47

Types and Uses of Corrective Lenses 48

Spheres 49
Cylinders 50
Spherocylinders 50
Prisms 51

Components of Refraction 52

Retinoscopy 52
Refinement 54
Binocular Balancing 55

Interpretation of Prescriptions 55

Transposition of Prescriptions 56

Automated Refractors 56

Objective Refractors 57
Subjective Refractors 57
Objective/Subjective Refractors 57

Lensometry 57

Types of Lensmeters 57
Elements of Lensometry 58
Lensometry Technique for Multifocal Lenses 60
- Progressive-Add Multifocal Lenses 60

Lensometry Technique for Prisms 61
Placement of Optical Centers 61

Keratometry 61

CHAPTER 5
COMPREHENSIVE MEDICAL EYE EXAMINATION 69

Overview of the Examination 70
Visual Acuity Examination 70
Alignment and Motility Examination 70
Pupillary Examination 70
Visual Field Examination 70
Intraocular Pressure Measurement 70
External Examination 70
Biomicroscopy 71
Ophthalmoscopy 71

Frequency of Examination 71

Ophthalmic and Medical History 71
Chief Complaint 72
Ocular History 73
Medical History 73
Family Ocular and Medical History 74
Allergies 74
History-Taking Guidelines 74

Visual Acuity Examination 74
Distance Acuity Test 74
Pinhole Acuity Test 77
Near Acuity Test 78
Other Acuity Tests 78
Procedures Following Acuity Tests 78

Alignment and Motility Examination 79
Cover–Uncover Test 80
Prism and Alternate Cover Test 81
Worth Four-Dot Test 81
Titmus Stereopsis Test 81

Pupillary Examination 82

Visual Field Examination 83
Confrontation Field Test 84
Amsler Grid Test 84

Intraocular Pressure Measurement 84
Principles of Tonometry 85
Applanation Tonometry 86
  Tono-Pen 88
Indentation Tonometry 88
Applanation vs Indentation Tonometry 89

External Examination 89
Anterior Chamber Evaluation 89

Biomicroscopy 90
Gonioscopy 90

Ophthalmoscopy 91
Direct and Indirect Ophthalmoscopy 91

Additional Tests 92
Color Vision Tests 92
Tear Output Test 93
Evaluation of the Corneal Epithelium 93
Corneal Sensitivity Test 93
Exophthalmometry 94

CHAPTER 6
ADJUNCTIVE TESTS AND PROCEDURES 97

Vision Tests for Patients With Opacities 98
Visual Potential Tests 98
  Potential Acuity Meter 98
  Super Pinhole 98
  Interferometer 98
Contrast-Sensitivity and Glare Tests 99

Tests for Corneal Disease 99
Pachymetry 100
Specular Microscopy/Photography 101

Ophthalmic Photography 101
External Photography 101
Slit-Lamp Photography 101
Fundus Photography 101
  Fundus Camera 101
  Fluorescein Angiography 102

Ultrasonography 103
A-Scan 103
B-Scan 103

CHAPTER 7
PRINCIPLES AND TECHNIQUES OF PERIMETRY 107

Anatomic Basis of the Visual Field 108
Map of the Visual Field 108
Orientation of the Visual Field Map 110
Purposes and Types of Perimetry 111
Kinetic Perimetry 111
Tangent Screen Test 112
Goldmann Perimeter 113
Other Devices 114
Advantages and Disadvantages 114
Static Perimetry 114
Computerized Static Perimetry 115
Advantages and Disadvantages 116
Defects Shown by Perimetry 117
General Defects 117
Focal Defects 118
Hemianopic Defects 119
Other Defects 120
Conditions for Accurate Perimetry 120
Environment-Related Factors 121
Device-Related Factors 123
Patient-Related Factors 123
Examiner-Related Factors 124

CHAPTER 8
FUNDAMENTALS OF PRACTICAL OPTICIANRY 127

Types of Corrective Lenses 128
Single-Vision Lenses 128
Multifocal Lenses 128
Types of Lens Materials 129
Lens Safety Standards and Treatments 130
Lens Treatments, Tints, and Coatings 130
Measurements in Fitting Eyeglasses 131
Interpupillary Distance 131
Errors in Measuring IPD 132
Vertex Distance 134
Base Curve 135
Fitting of Eyeglass Frames 137
Effects on Patient Comfort 138
Care of Eyeglasses 138
Adjustment of Eyeglasses 139
Frame Screws 139
Optical Centers 139
Segment Heights 139

CHAPTER 9

PATIENT INTERACTION, SCREENING, AND EMERGENCIES 145

Patient–Assistant Interaction 146

Patient Greeting 146

Patient Screening 146

Triage Procedure 147

- Emergency Situation 147
- Urgent Situation 148
- Routine Situation 148

Appointment Scheduling 148

Referred Patients 149

Emergencies Encountered in the Office 149

Chemical Burns 149

Trauma 150

General Emergency Assistance 150

- Guidelines for Handling a Patient Fall 152

Hospital Admission 153

CHAPTER 10

PATIENTS WITH SPECIAL CONSIDERATIONS 157

All Patients Considered 158

Patients and Their Families 158

Office Waiting Periods 158

Disruptive Patients 159

Visually Impaired or Blind Patients 159

Patient Greeting and History-Taking 160

Patient Assistance 160

Visual Acuity Assessment 161

Infants and Young Children 161

Patient Greeting 161

Patient Positioning 162

Visual Acuity and Ability Testing 163

- Infants 163
- Toddlers and School-Age Children 164
- Charts Used to Test Children 164
- Tips for Testing Toddlers 164
- Tips for Testing School-Age Children 165

Elderly Patients 165

Age-Related Vision Changes 165

Visual Acuity Testing 166

Physically Handicapped Patients 166

Patients With Diabetes 167

Special Help for Patients With Diabetes 167

- Treatment of a Hypoglycemic Reaction 168

CHAPTER 11
BASICS OF OPHTHALMIC PHARMACOLOGY 171

Delivery Systems of Drugs 172
Topical Systems 172
Solutions 172
Suspensions 172
Ointments and Gels 172
Inserts 173
Injections 173
Oral Systems 173
Administration of Topical Drugs 173
Purposes and Actions of Drugs 173
Diagnostic Medications 173
Mydriatics 173
Cycloplegics 175
Dyes 176
Anesthetics 176
Therapeutic Medications 177
Miotics 177
Other Glaucoma Medications 177
Antimicrobials 178
Antiallergic and Anti-Inflammatory Agents 179
Nonsteroidal Anti-Inflammatory Drugs (NSAIDs) 179
Decongestants 180
Antihistamines 180
Mast Cell Stabilizers 180
Lubricants 180
Other Pharmaceuticals 180
Interpretation of a Prescription 181
First Aid for Acute Drug Reactions 182

CHAPTER 12
MICROORGANISMS AND INFECTION CONTROL 187

Types of Microorganisms 188
Bacteria 188
Viruses 189
Fungi 191
Protozoa 191
Transmission of Infectious Diseases 192
Airborne Droplets and Particles 192
Direct-Contact Transmission 192
Indirect-Contact Transmission 192
Common-Vehicle Transmission 193
Infection Control Precautions 193
Hand Washing 194
Use of Personal Protective Equipment 194
Disinfection and Sterilization 194
Moist Heat 195
Ethylene Oxide Gas 195
Aseptic Technique: Handling Sterile Medical Equipment 195
Handling and Decontaminating Contaminated Materials 196
Hygienic Practices in Potentially Infectious Situations 197
Collecting Specimens for Identification of Microorganisms 197

CHAPTER 13
MINOR SURGICAL ASSISTING IN THE OFFICE 201

Patient Preparation Before Surgery 202
Informed Consent 202
Patient Assistance 202
Patient Questions 202
Administration of Anesthetics 202
Surgical Materials and Instruments 203
Sutures and Needles 203
Forceps 205
Scissors 205
Needle Holders 205
Clamps and Curettes 205
Scalpels and Blades 206
Lacrimal Instruments 206
Cannulas 207
Common Minor Surgical Procedures 207
Chalazion Surgery 207
Other Lid-Lesion Surgery 207
Lacrimal-System Probing 208
Postsurgical Dressing and Patching 209
First Surgical Experience 209
Surgical Assisting Skills 210
Aseptic Technique and Office Surgery 210
Scrubbing, Gloving, Prepping, and Draping 210
Preparation of the Instrument Tray 211
Tasks During Surgery 212
Disposition of Instruments and Materials 212

CHAPTER 14
PRINCIPLES AND PROBLEMS OF CONTACT LENSES 217

Basic Principles 218
Contact Lenses vs Eyeglasses for Vision Correction 219
Contact Lens Specification vs Eyeglass Prescription 219
Types and Materials of Contact Lenses 219
PMMA and RGP Hard Lenses 220
Soft Lenses 220
Extended-Wear Lenses 221
Daily-Wear Lenses 221
Disposable Lenses 221
Planned-Replacement Lenses 221
Lens Designs for Special Purposes 222
Cosmetic Fashion Lenses 222
Cosmetic Restorative Lenses 222
Toric Lenses 222
Bifocal Lenses 222
Keratoconus Lenses 223
Therapeutic Lenses 223
Care of Contact Lenses 223
Cleaning 224
Disinfection 224
Lubrication 224
Storage 224
Insertion and Removal of Contact Lenses 225
Soft Lenses 225
Rigid Lenses 226
Problems With Contact Lenses 226
Allergy 227
Overwearing Syndrome 228
Improper Lens Fit 228
Irritation and Tearing 229
Corneal Problems 229
Giant Papillary Conjunctivitis 230
Solution–Lens Interaction 230
Inability to Insert or Remove Lenses 231
Lens "Lost" in Eye 231
Contraindications for Contact Lenses 231

APPENDIX A
CARE OF OPHTHALMIC LENSES AND INSTRUMENTS 235

Care of Lenses 236
Standard Care Guidelines 236
Lenses That Do Not Contact the Eye 236
Lenses That Contact the Eye 237
  Lens Sterilization 237

Care of Instruments 239
Standard Care Guidelines 239

Selected Office Instruments 240
Retinoscope 240
  Special Care and Cautions 240
Phoroptor 240
  Special Care and Cautions 240
Lensmeter 241
  Special Care and Cautions 241
Keratometer 241
  Special Care and Cautions 241
Slit Lamp 242
  Special Care and Cautions 242
Projector 242
  Special Care and Cautions 242
Applanation Tonometer 243
  Special Care and Cautions 243
Indentation Tonometer 244
  Special Care and Cautions 244
Direct Ophthalmoscope 245
Indirect Ophthalmoscope 245
Potential Acuity Meter 246
Lasers 246
  Special Care and Cautions 247

APPENDIX B
SYSTEMIC DISEASES AND OCULAR MANIFESTATIONS 249

Major Body Systems 250

Inflammatory and Autoimmune Diseases 250
Myasthenia Gravis 250
Rheumatoid Arthritis 250
Sarcoidosis 250
Sjögren's Syndrome 250
Systemic Lupus Erythematosus 251
Thyroid Disorders 251

Metabolic Disorders 252
Diabetes Mellitus 252

Vascular Diseases 252
Cerebral Vascular Accident 253
Giant Cell Arteritis 253
Migraine 253
Hypertension 253

Infectious Diseases 254
Acquired Immunodeficiency Syndrome 254
Chlamydial Infections 254
Herpes Zoster and Herpes Simplex 255
Histoplasmosis 255
Syphilis 255
Toxoplasmosis 255

Malignant Diseases 255
Metastatic Carcinoma 255
Blood Dyscrasias 256
Cerebral Neoplasms 256
Multiple Sclerosis 256

APPENDIX C
UNIVERSAL PRECAUTIONS 257

ANSWERS TO REVIEW QUESTIONS 259
GLOSSARY 269
INDEX 287

Performance Boxes

Chapter 4
Performing Basic Lensometry 58
Measuring Multifocal Power 61
Measuring Prism Power and Orientation 62
Performing Keratometry 63

Chapter 5
Performing the Distance Acuity Test 76
Performing the Pinhole Acuity Test 77
Performing the Near Acuity Test 79
Checking Direct and Consensual Pupillary Reaction 83
Performing the Confrontation Test 84
Performing the Amsler Grid Test 85
Performing Goldmann Tonometry 86
Performing the Flashlight Test 90

Chapter 8
Measuring Binocular Distance IPD 133
Measuring Monocular Distance IPD 134
Measuring Binocular Near IPD 134
Using a Distometer 136
Using a Geneva Lens Clock 136
Adjusting Frame Screws 139
Checking Optical Centers 140

Chapter 9
Irrigating the Eye 151
Assisting a Patient Who Feels Faint 152

Chapter 10
Performing a Low-Vision Test 162
Testing an Infant's Visual Ability 163

Chapter 11
Administering Eyedrops and Ointments 174
Giving First Aid 182

Chapter 12
Washing the Hands Effectively 195

Chapter 13
Applying Pressure Patches and Shields 209

Chapter 14
Inserting Soft Lenses 225
Removing Soft Lenses 226
Inserting Rigid Lenses 227
Removing Rigid Lenses 228

Appendix A
Cleaning Lenses That Do Not Contact the Eye 237
Cleaning Lenses That Contact the Eye 238
Disinfecting Lenses That Contact the Eye 238
Troubleshooting Instrument Failure 239

Introduction

PREFACE TO THE THIRD EDITION, REVISED

Several years have passed since the publication of the highly successful third edition of *Ophthalmic Medical Assisting*. Because the American Academy of Ophthalmology reviews its publications periodically, it was felt that the time was right for a review of this text, and the Academy's Allied Health Education Committee was asked to carry out the task. This revision is the result of that review.

Throughout, material has been updated as needed, particularly to take note of newer technologies and drugs. In addition, the Suggested Resources at the end of each chapter have been thoroughly updated to reflect currently available resources, including the latest editions of educational materials from the Academy and other publishers.

Finally, the Allied Health Education Committee felt it was important to note that this third edition, revised, is valuable not only as a study guide but also as an office reference. *Ophthalmic Medical Assisting* is a good, basic educational resource for the entire staff.

PREFACE TO THE THIRD EDITION

The third edition of *Ophthalmic Medical Assisting* is the outcome of an intensive review conducted by the Allied Health Education Committee of the American Academy of Ophthalmology. In deciding what text to add, remove, or revise, the committee considered both the JCAHPO criteria for Ophthalmic Medical Assistant certification and the needs of employed assistants who are expected to function effectively as part of the ophthalmologist's office staff. As with the previous two editions, the committee tried to achieve a balance between theoretical and practical information.

For this third edition, Chapter 12 was rewritten to place more appropriate emphasis on topics of true value or utility for the beginning assistant. A small number of new and revised figures were included. A new Appendix C was added that lists universal precautions. The Glossary was revised to reflect changes to the chapters, and selected pronunciations of medical and technical terms were added. All the Suggested Resources were updated to include valuable new publications and the latest editions of educational materials from the Academy and other publishers. Finally, a small number of the end-of-chapter Review Questions, the Suggested Activities, and the questions in the companion examination were revised to reflect changes to the text and provide new challenges to readers of the third edition.

TO THE OPHTHALMOLOGIST

Ophthalmic medical assistants are an important part of the eye care team. They enhance the ophthalmologist's efforts and contribute significantly to the overall quality of patient care. But just as ophthalmic medical assistants do not practice independently, neither do they gain their professional training independently. In this sense, ophthalmologists are an important part of the assistant-training team. They not only instruct but also motivate the assistants they employ.

So even though this book is subtitled *An Independent Study Course*, it has been constructed with special attention to the ophthalmologist's role in the education and professional development of assistants, particularly those just beginning in the profession. To ensure that your assistants' training is as effective as possible, consider scheduling regular meetings to review and discuss the coursework together and present practical instruction that complements the course material presented.

It is important to recognize that the assistant will most effectively learn the practical skills presented in this book when reading of the text is regularly supplemented with hands-on, supervised training. Sponsoring ophthalmologists are encouraged to make such training available to their beginning assistants.

As assistants undergo their training, it is important that other staff maintain and hone their skills as well. As an office reference, *Ophthalmic Medical Assisting* provides your entire staff with an educational resource they can turn to every day for information both clinical and technical.

Text Instructional Features

Ophthalmic Medical Assisting helps you direct your assistant's education by providing special instructional exercises and information at the end of each chapter, as described below.

Review Questions These exercises can help you gauge your assistant's progress in understanding the basic course content. Encourage your assistant to respond to these study items as each chapter is completed (answers are found at the back of the textbook). Use the exercises as a springboard for discussion with your assistant to clarify some of the more difficult concepts in ophthalmology and to discuss individual office policy.

Suggested Activities These activities help your assistant integrate the course content into daily work responsibilities in your office. They suggest practical ways to apply each chapter's information and skills under the supervision of the ophthalmologist or staff member in charge of assistant training. By overseeing these activities, you can ensure that your assistant receives the information and guidance appropriate to practice and policy in your office. You may consider reviewing each chapter and developing additional or alternative activities to assign to your assistant.

Suggested Resources These are listings of additional topic information available in print, video, and audio formats. You can help your assistant by reviewing these listings and recommending or supplying the resources that you feel are most helpful. You may consider using these suggestions in building a basic office reference library for your current and future ophthalmic medical assisting trainees.

Independent Study Course Examination

Students who work through this course textbook are encouraged to complete the companion course examination, available as a separate booklet, and submit it to the Academy for scoring. In recognition of the key role of the ophthalmologist in assistant training, the examination requires the signature of a Sponsoring Ophthalmologist. Your participation as a Sponsoring Ophthalmologist, with the educational responsibility that implies, helps ensure that students functionally comprehend the concepts and skills presented in this course and can apply them to their work. The result is a well-trained, motivated, and confident ophthalmic medical assistant who truly contributes to your patients' well-being and to the efficient operation of your practice.

TO THE STUDENT

Welcome to *Ophthalmic Medical Assisting: An Independent Study Course*. Please read this section before beginning your studies. It contains important information about the components and features of the course, with suggestions for completing the course successfully. Please also share this section and the preceding section, "To the Ophthalmologist," with the ophthalmologist in your office who will be overseeing your participation in this course.

Course Level

As a program of self-study for beginners in the field, *Ophthalmic Medical Assisting* assumes that you have at least completed high school, with some courses in basic science and mathematics, though you may have additional formal education beyond high school. The course also assumes that you have had at least 3 months' experience working in an ophthalmology office.

Course Components and Suggested Approaches

The complete course consists of this self-study textbook and the separate course examination, a booklet of 148 questions with an answer sheet. You may elect to read the textbook from cover to cover for your own education, or you may turn to selected portions as needed for professional reference on the job. Alternatively, you may choose to test your knowledge by completing the multiple-choice examination and returning it to the American Academy of Ophthalmology for scoring. Because of the complexity and diversity of the course content, you should plan to spend at least 3 months working through the textbook before attempting the course examination. Additional specific information about taking the examination based on this text and submitting it to the Academy appears later in this section and in the examination booklet itself.

Sponsoring Ophthalmologist

Just as you perform your day-to-day duties on the job under the direction of an ophthalmologist, you will be most successful in this course if a Sponsoring Ophthalmologist is available to help you direct your studies, understand the material, and apply the course information and skills to your job responsibilities. The Academy requires that the signature of a Sponsoring Ophthalmologist appear on the examination answer sheet when you submit it for scoring.

Organization and Features

This book presents a blend of fundamental medical and scientific information and basic practical skills often required of beginning ophthalmic medical assistants. Because you must frequently apply basic concepts or information from one chapter to more technically complex material in a succeeding chapter, it is strongly recommended that you read the chapters in order.

To add structure to your independent studies and gain the most from the course, use the following approach and in-text learning aids as described below.

Chapter Introductions Each chapter begins with an overview of the chapter's content and its relevance to on-the-job ophthalmic medical assisting. The introductions describe the principal topics in the order in which you will encounter them and, as such, help you determine your learning objectives for each chapter.

Performance Boxes Numbered, step-by-step instructions for performing 35 basic ophthalmologic tests or procedures appear throughout the book in shaded boxes. Share the instructions in these "performance boxes" with your ophthalmologist or other trainer, who can assist you in performing a test or procedure for the first time and tell you whether certain procedures are performed differently in your office.

In addition, it is important to obtain hands-on instruction in the procedures you are expected to carry out in your office. Actual supervised training and practice under the guidance of an ophthalmologist or an experienced technician is the most effective way to ensure that you have mastered the practical skills presented in this book.

Review Questions Answer the questions at the end of each chapter soon after you read the chapter. You will gain the most by trying to answer the questions based on your recall of information rather than looking up the answers. Then check your responses against the Answers to Review Questions grouped by chapter at the end of the book. Where definitions, descriptions, or explanations are called for, your response need not match the printed answer word for word as long as your response indicates that you understand the general concept. It is helpful to have your trainer check your responses to clarify any points you may not have understood. Make note of the questions you missed and reread the relevant portions of the text to make sure you understand the material before proceeding to the next chapter.

Suggested Activities A list of activities follows the Review Questions at the end of each chapter. The activities suggest ways for you to apply the chapter's information to the development of your practical skills. They encourage not only independent investigation but also interaction with other staff members, and they frequently involve the guidance of the ophthalmologist or experienced office staff. Be sure the person overseeing your studies is aware of these activities, because many involve the supervised use of office materials and equipment.

Suggested Resources This last part of each chapter directs you to printed publications and videotapes that you might use to further investigate the topics covered in the chapter.

Glossary A glossary of more than 500 important terms used in the text appears at the end of the book. Pronunciations of scientific and technical terms are now provided. Every term included in the glossary is also boldfaced upon its first significant appearance in the book, with its definition immediately following or appearing in nearby text. Occasionally, a term is boldfaced and defined more than once, especially if it has appeared some chapters earlier.

Independent Study Course Examination

Successful completion of the optional course examination partially fulfills the requirements for applying to take the assistant certifying examination offered by the Joint Commission on Allied Health Personnel in Ophthalmology (JCAHPO). Becoming a certified ophthalmic medical assistant through the JCAHPO process has many professional benefits, which are described in Chapter 1 of this textbook. Contact information for JCAHPO also appears there, if you wish to obtain further information about their certifying examination. Successful completion of the *Ophthalmic Medical Assisting* course examination alone does not constitute professional certification as an ophthalmic medical assistant.

The examination booklet is appropriate for use only with the third edition and third edition, revised, of *Ophthalmic Medical Assisting: An Independent Study Course*. Students using a second edition textbook can obtain a copy of the appropriate examination by contacting the American Academy of Ophthalmology. The examination booklets for the different editions are not interchangeable.

The course examination consists of a booklet with 148 multiple-choice questions and a tear-out answer sheet. Each booklet and answer sheet has its own identifying number and is intended for use by one student only. You are allowed to refer to the textbook to complete your examination. Send your completed examination answer sheet *with the required signature of your Sponsoring Ophthalmologist* to the American Academy of Ophthalmology in the addressed envelope provided with the examination booklet.

The Academy registers you for the course and records your identification number when your examination answer sheet is received, electronically scores your examination, and returns it to you, noting any questions you missed. Those receiving a passing grade also receive a letter from the Academy verifying successful completion of the course, which serves as your permanent record. If you do not receive a passing grade, you may request a blank answer sheet from the Academy and attempt the test as many times as you wish.

Detailed information about completing and submitting the examination may be found in the examination booklet itself.

1

Introduction to Ophthalmic Medical Assisting

Welcome to ophthalmic medical assisting. You have chosen to learn more about a fascinating, rewarding, and growing profession. You will assist in the effort to prevent, detect, diagnose, and manage conditions that can interfere with one of our most precious senses: sight.

To help orient you as you begin your study of ophthalmology and ophthalmic medical assisting, this chapter introduces you to the specialized branch of medicine that is ophthalmology and the various professionals who work in it. The chapter also provides an overview of your responsibilities as an ophthalmic medical assistant, including your role in the office or clinic, professional certification and continuing education, and guidelines for ethical and professional behavior.

WHAT IS OPHTHALMOLOGY?

Ophthalmology is the medical and surgical specialty that is concerned with the eye and its surrounding structures, their proper function, eye disorders, and all aspects of vision. Ophthalmology is one of the oldest specialties in medicine, dating back to the middle of the nineteenth century, when the ophthalmoscope was invented. The ophthalmoscope is used to examine the structures in the back of the eye: retina and optic nerve (Figure 1.1). This instrument provided the first opportunity for physicians to see blood vessels inside an organ without surgery. In addition, ophthalmology was the first medical specialty to develop a certification process, which is a testing procedure to assure that every certified ophthalmologist has attained a certain level of competence in the field. Now, most specialties of medicine have such certifying processes.

Ophthalmology has undergone many amazing changes since the 1960s. The ability to prevent and manage previously blinding eye diseases has improved markedly, thanks to new technology. One major medical advance of the last few decades is laser surgery for diabetic eye disease, dramatically reducing the chances of a person with diabetes becoming blind. Laser surgery and most minor eye surgery have been moved out of the hospital operating room and into the office setting (Figure 1.2). Visual rehabilitation with intraocular lens implantation after cataract surgery can restore vision to countless patients who in past decades would have had to wear thick eyeglasses or contact lenses as a means of achieving good vision. Cataract surgery is now performed as a 1-day outpatient procedure rather than a 7- to 10-day stay in the hospital as in the past. Retinal detachment, a condition in which the light-sensitive tissue at the back of the eye becomes detached, is now largely repairable through surgery, rather than consigning the patient to certain blindness. Glaucoma, a disease caused by increased pressure inside the eye, is controllable, instead of causing the patient eye pain and blindness as it did in the past. Contact lenses can be worn comfortably by millions, not just by a hardy few.

FIGURE 1.1

The ophthalmologist uses an ophthalmoscope to examine the structures in the back of the eye.

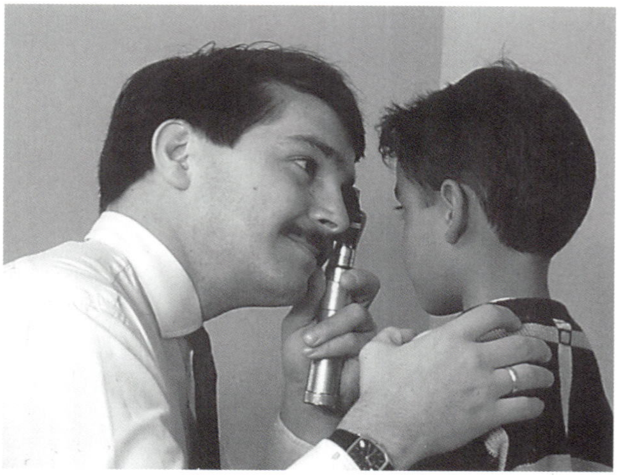

WHO PROVIDES EYE CARE?

In the United States, many different kinds of medical and nonmedical personnel participate in eye care. The multiplicity of participants may produce some confusion as to who has what responsibilities for a patient's eye health and vision. The ophthalmic medical assistant should understand who these individual health care professionals are and what their role in eye care is.

Ophthalmologist

The **ophthalmologist** (sometimes referred to as *eye physician and surgeon* or *medical eye specialist*) is a medical doctor (MD or DO) specializing in the prevention, diagnosis, and medical as well as surgical treatment of vision problems and eye diseases. The ophthalmologist has completed a 1-year *internship* after graduation from medical school and at least 3 years of specialized ophthalmologic training, called a *residency* in ophthalmology. Often, the ophthalmologist has also completed a *fellowship* (another 1 or 2 years of training) after residency in preparation for practice in a subspecialty area of ophthalmology.

An ophthalmologist may attend to such diverse problems as eyeglass prescriptions for vision difficulties; contact lens prescriptions; repair of torn eyelids; eye conditions such as dry, drooping, crossed, or lazy eyes; or eye disorders such as glaucoma, cataract, retinal detachment, diabetic retinopathy, and visual problems from brain tumors. In your reading of this book and through your experience assisting the ophthalmologist, you will learn more about these disorders as well as some of the ways to prevent or treat

FIGURE 1.2

Today laser surgery and most minor eye surgery take place in the office setting, rather than in the hospital operating room.

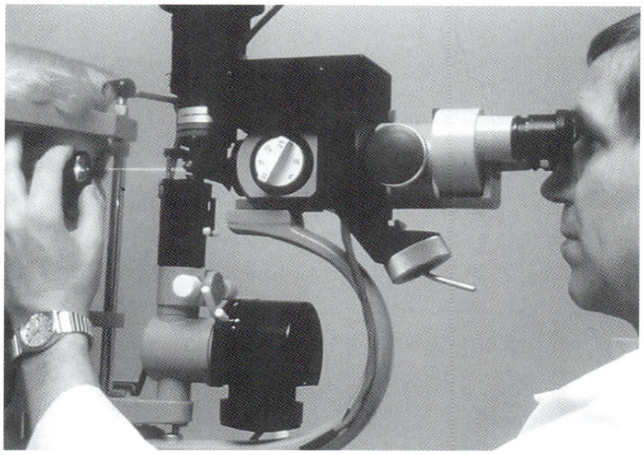

them. Ophthalmologists not only diagnose and treat eye diseases but try to preserve vision through educating the public and patients about the best way to care for their eyes.

Although the majority of ophthalmologists are capable of treating the entire spectrum of eye conditions, some concentrate on conditions related to one area of the eye only. These ophthalmologists are called *subspecialists*. Some ophthalmologic subspecialists focus their care on patients who need orbital and plastic surgery, or who have corneal and external eye disease, or who have eye disorders such as glaucoma, cataracts, and retinal or nerve problems. Doctors who treat eye and vision difficulties only in children are called *pediatric ophthalmologists*. You will learn more about these eye disorders as you progress through this course.

Optometrist

The **optometrist** is an independent practitioner who has completed a course of 4 years in optometry school after 3 or 4 years in college. Optometrists are trained in the prescription of eyeglasses and contact lenses as well as in the detection of eye disease. In some states, optometrists may diagnose and medically treat some eye diseases or perform laser surgery, although they do not have a medical degree. Optometrists do not have all of the medical training of ophthalmologists in the diagnosis and management of eye diseases.

Optician

The **optician** is an independent professional who has received 2 years of training before being licensed to make (dispense) eyeglasses and contact lenses according to prescriptions supplied by an ophthalmologist or optometrist. This vision care specialist is sometimes referred to as a *dispensing optician* or *ophthalmic dispenser*.

Ophthalmic Registered Nurse

The **ophthalmic registered nurse** is a registered nurse with special training in problems related to the eye. Ophthalmic registered nurses frequently function as surgical assistants to ophthalmologists, directors of ophthalmic surgery services, and directors of clinical services.

Orthoptist

The **orthoptist** is a specialized member of the ophthalmic medical personnel team. The orthoptist has had 2 years of postgraduate training and has passed a national certifying examination. The orthoptist's areas of expertise are in visual function testing, particularly in infants and children, and in the evaluation of eye muscle disorders. The orthoptist helps with the diagnosis, management, and nonsurgical treatment of eye muscle imbalance and related visual impairments. Orthoptists work with and under the direction of ophthalmologists.

Ocularist

The **ocularist**, another specialized member of the ophthalmic team, measures and fits patients with prostheses (artificial eyes or shells), which replace a surgically removed eye or cover an unsightly one. Ocularists usually spend several years in apprenticeship to practice their highly skilled craft and must pass a difficult examination.

Ophthalmic Photographer

The **ophthalmic photographer** photographs the eye structures for diagnosis and documentation. Many ophthalmic medical assistants do photographic work in an ophthalmologist's office. However, to become a *certified* ophthalmic photographer, a person must undergo special training and pass a rigorous examination.

Ophthalmic Medical Assistant

The **ophthalmic medical assistant** helps the ophthalmologist in a variety of diagnostic and administrative tasks. A skilled ophthalmic medical assistant can free the ophthalmologist to spend time more effectively with each patient, performing those diagnostic and treatment tasks that only the ophthalmologist can do, and to see and treat more patients. The ophthalmic medical assistant is, in effect, a multiplier of the ophthalmologist's efforts.

Some of the most common tasks the ophthalmic medical assistant is called upon to perform include

- Scheduling and greeting patients
- Helping patients to understand and comply with treatments that the doctor prescribes
- Performing certain tests and using ophthalmic instruments that provide diagnostic information
- Assisting with office surgical procedures
- Administering topical medications or diagnostic drugs as required by the ophthalmologist for testing or treatment

These tasks and others vary from office to office, depending on an individual ophthalmologist's needs and policies.

The term *ophthalmic medical assistant* is often used to describe any individual who helps the ophthalmologist with diagnostic and treatment-oriented procedures. The Joint Commission on Allied Health Personnel in Ophthalmology (JCAHPO), an organization that was founded to promote the education and utilization of allied health personnel in ophthalmology, employs the term *ophthalmic medical personnel* to denote all individuals who assist the ophthalmologist. However, JCAHPO also recognizes degrees of skill and education among such individuals by certification and designates these specific levels of experience and training with certain other terminology, which is described in the next section. Still other organizations and publications may refer informally or generically to those who help the ophthalmologist as "technical personnel," "allied health personnel," "technicians," or other similar terms. For the sake of simplicity, this text will use the terms *ophthalmic medical assistant, ophthalmic assistant*, and *assistant* interchangeably to refer to individuals at the entry level of experience.

WHAT ARE THE CERTIFICATION LEVELS?

Ophthalmic medical personnel vary in their levels of knowledge and skill. JCAHPO recognizes three official levels of certified ophthalmic medical personnel: certified ophthalmic assistant (COA), certified ophthalmic technician (COT), and certified ophthalmic medical technologist (COMT). The JCAHPO certification attests to the skills and knowledge of an individual at each of these levels after certain educational and experience prerequisites have been met and an examination has been passed. Certification assures potential employers and patients that the individual has achieved a certain level of competence. The JCAHPO credential is similar to the certification received by physicians or nurses who have completed the requirements of their chosen field.

Each successive level of ophthalmic medical assisting requires more knowledge, skill, and experience than does the previous level. The transition from ophthalmic assistant to technician can be achieved in a modular fashion. Some individuals advance directly to one of the upper levels of certification through formal schooling. The certification process is designed also to allow an individual to achieve the first level of certification without formal schooling through the use of an independent study course such as this one. This certification procedure permits the individual to advance into the succeeding stages by using a combination of reading, continuing education courses, formal instruction, and clinical experience (Figure 1.3).

Although certification as an ophthalmic medical assistant is not necessary for the successful performance of the tasks required by this position and, to date, certification has not been required by any state law, certification by JCAHPO can be an important part of a career in ophthalmic assisting. When you apply for an ophthalmic assisting position, certification assures potential employers that you have certain skills and knowledge. In addition, certification shows pride in your work and a professional attitude toward what you do.

Information about certification may be obtained directly from JCAHPO:

Joint Commission on Allied Health Personnel in Ophthalmology
2025 Woodlane Drive
St Paul, MN 55125-2995

Telephone: 800-284-3937
Fax: 651-731-0410
E-mail: jcahpo@jcahpo.org
Internet: http://www.jcahpo.org

FIGURE 1.3

The ophthalmic medical assistant grows professionally in stages by using a combination of reading, continuing education courses, formal instruction, and clinical experience.

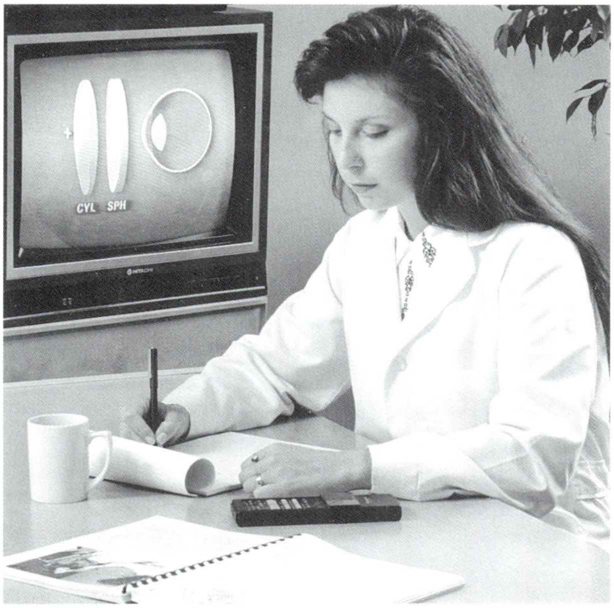

Professional Development

Certification not only implies a specific level of skill and knowledge but also signifies that the individual is interested in ongoing professional development and lifelong learning. This means a commitment to keeping your skills up to date and developing new ones through the process of continuing education. Continuing education is obtained through courses, reading, and other educational activities. Courses are available through formal ophthalmic medical assistant training programs, hospitals, and colleges and through annual and regional continuing education programs either sponsored or approved for continuing education credit by JCAHPO. These courses are listed on the JCAHPO web site and in the JCAHPO/ATPO newsletter, which you can receive simply by asking to have your name added to the mailing list.

Insight: The Journal of the American Society of Ophthalmic Registered Nurses and newsletters published by allied subspecialty organizations serve as good sources of information about new and useful educational opportunities. Further information about the offerings of the various organizations may be obtained by writing to their representatives. You may wish to ask JCAHPO for the current name and address of the individuals to contact. Organizations that may be of interest and assistance to you are

- American Orthoptic Council (AOC)
- American Society of Ocularists (ASO)
- American Society of Ophthalmic Registered Nurses (ASORN)
- Association of Technical Personnel in Ophthalmology (ATPO) (administered by JCAHPO)
- Contact Lens Association of Ophthalmologists (CLAO)
- Contact Lens Society of America (CLSA)
- Ophthalmic Photographers Society (OPS)
- Opticians Association of America (OAA)

The two societies most likely to be initially helpful for a newcomer to ophthalmic assisting are the Association of Technical Personnel in Ophthalmology and the Contact Lens Society of America.

The Joint Commission on Allied Health Personnel in Ophthalmology and most of the organizations listed above offer courses in conjunction with the annual meeting of the American Academy of Ophthalmology (AAO), the organization that represents the majority of ophthalmologists in the United States and Canada. Some continuing education courses designed specifically for ophthalmologists also can be useful for certain ophthalmic medical personnel, although such courses usually do not address the specific needs of nonophthalmologists. In addition, the AAO has a web site at http://www.eyenet.org that provides information and links to sites of related interest.

WHICH RULES OF ETHICS APPLY?

Ethics are moral principles and values that govern individual behavior. The profession of medicine has a history of well-defined ethics that dates back 2000 years. One of the principal ethical tenets is that medicine should be practiced primarily for the benefit of the patient. Upon graduating from medical school, the physician affirms to keep the patient's best interests above all other considerations. Individuals who assist the ophthalmologist likewise must observe certain generally accepted ethical principles that apply to their professional behavior.

Ophthalmic medical assistants must abide by the laws of the state in which their employer practices and must perform their services under the supervision of a licensed ophthalmologist. Attempting to work independently of an ophthalmologist constitutes practicing medicine without a license and could result in criminal charges. In some states, special rules prohibit ophthalmic assistants from performing certain tasks. You should check with your ophthalmologist to find out what the laws in your state specify.

One of the basic tenets of ethical behavior is strict honesty with both the patient and the doctor. The ophthalmic medical assistant should be forthright with the doctor. If you make a mistake, tell the ophthalmologist.

Ophthalmic medical assistants should never misrepresent themselves to a patient or family as a physician or some other type of licensed health care professional. If the patient or member of the family makes the mistake of assuming you are a doctor, do not take advantage of it but correct the assumption immediately.

To avoid any confusion about your role in the office, be sure to introduce yourself to patients specifically as the ophthalmic medical assistant. One good way to begin your interaction with a patient is to say, for example: "Hello, Ms (Mrs, Miss, Mr) ______________. My name is ______________. I am Dr ______________'s assistant." Patients often meet a bewildering array of people in a doctor's office on the first and even later visits. They will appreciate knowing where you fit in the health care system of the office or clinic; they will more likely be helpful and cooperative with you when you have to ask about their health and personal medical history.

No matter how simple or obvious the situation may be, ophthalmic medical assistants should not advise any treatment for a patient without consulting the ophthalmologist. This prohibition also applies to the patient's or your own friends and family members; even though your intent may be to help the patient, the best course of action is always to refer an individual to the ophthalmologist for advice about the condition or treatment.

Ophthalmic medical assistants should never try to interpret test results, diagnose a condition, or suggest treatments to a patient without the doctor's express instruction to do so. Even if the ophthalmic assistant is knowledgeable about the findings of a test, it is the physician who makes the **diagnosis** (determination of a condition), estimates the **prognosis** (prediction of the outcome of a condition), and prescribes the treatment after considering all the facts from the patient's medical history, the examination findings, and any special tests. Telling the patient a complete medical story based on one test is like predicting the outcome of a movie after watching only the film's first minute. Although you may be correct in your advice, you incur the considerable risk of either unnecessarily upsetting or falsely reassuring the patient. Patients have tremendous emotional investment in their eyes and vision. The practitioner should have all the facts available before discussing the meaning of tests with patients. However, explaining why and how a test is being done is important in eliciting the patient's cooperation. Patients appreciate knowing what to expect with any activity, even such commonplace ones as having eyedrops administered in the office.

Unauthorized removal of drugs, materials, or supplies from the medical office or hospital, no matter how small the amount, without specific approval of those in charge is unethical and illegal. This applies to everything from cleaning cloths to bandages, instruments to medications. Obviously, taking medications without a prescription or approval is both illegal and unwise.

One of the most important ethical considerations in medicine is the patient's right to privacy—a concept that has been handed down from the time of Hippocrates, the ancient Greek physician who is considered the father of medical science and ethics. Patients often have to entrust a medical office with information that might be embarrassing or detrimental if divulged to spouses, relatives, employers, or the community. Ophthalmic medical assistants should retain all information about the patient—including the fact that the patient visited the office at all—in complete confidence. This includes not informing even close relatives or coworkers of the patient without express permission from the patient. Letting information slip out about a patient could place you and your employer in legal difficulties. Discussing one patient in the presence of another is also strictly forbidden.

The ophthalmic medical assistant, like others in the health care system, should refrain from referring to patients by their diseases or conditions. An example of this kind of discourtesy would be to say "Check the vision on that cataract in room 2." Patients should be regarded as individuals with particular eye or vision problems. A more considerate reference to a patient would be "Check the vision of the patient with a cataract in room 2." Think of how you would like to be treated in this respect.

Code of Ethics of the AAO

The American Academy of Ophthalmology has developed a code of ethics for its members. The seven principles of ethics contained in the Academy's code are paraphrased below. The ethical guidelines they present are applicable only to ophthalmologists, but ophthalmic medical assistants who work with them will benefit from understanding the ethical goals they represent.

1. An issue of ethics in ophthalmology is resolved by the determination that the best interest of the patient is served.
2. Ophthalmologic services must be provided with compassion, respect for human dignity, honesty, and integrity.
3. An ophthalmologist must maintain competence by continued study. That competence must be supplemented with the talents of other professionals and with consultation when indicated.
4. Open communication with the patient is essential. Patient confidences must be safeguarded within the constraints of the law.
5. Fees for ophthalmologic services must not exploit patients or others who pay for the services.
6. If a member has a reasonable basis for believing that another person has deviated from professionally accepted standards in a manner that adversely affects patient care or from the Rules of Ethics, the member should attempt to prevent the continuation of this conduct by communicating with the other person or by notifying the appropriate authorities.
7. It is the responsibility of an ophthalmologist to act in the best interest of the patient.

WHAT CONSTITUTES PROFESSIONAL BEHAVIOR?

Because ophthalmic medical assistants represent the ophthalmologist-employer in much the same way diplomats represent their country, their ability to behave professionally is crucial. Patients tend to assume that the behaviors and characteristics of the office staff have been approved by the doctor and represent the standard of care they will receive. A professional office atmosphere enhances patient confidence in the doctor and helps ensure cooperation with the doctor's medical treatment or advice.

Patients who come to a doctor are often worried, frightened, or uncomfortable. They deserve sympathetic and prompt attention. An ophthalmic medical assistant who looks and acts like a professional will make the patient feel more confident and comfortable. Office staff who are helpful, courteous, and truly caring of the patient's welfare provide the kind of setting in which healing can take place. In contrast, office staff who respond in a curt, condescending, or uninterested manner will make it more difficult for the patient to be treated successfully.

All patients deserve to be treated with dignity and respect. Some people prefer to be called by their first names, but others are offended by this practice. Adult patients should be addressed by the title Mr, Mrs, or Ms and their last name, unless permission is granted by the doctor or patient to use first names.

Ophthalmic medical assistants should not only act professionally but also look professional. Clean, presentable clothes are important. Jeans, shorts, revealing clothing, and garish attire are inappropriate for office wear, especially when patients are present. If your office has a dress code, observe it. If you are required to wear a uniform, have an adequate supply to ensure that you wear a clean, well-pressed one at all times.

In addition to dressing in a professional manner, all people who work in an ophthalmologist's office should pay careful attention to personal hygiene. Body cleanliness is crucial for those who are in contact with patients. Body odor and bad breath are offensive to anyone with whom you must work closely, whether patients or coworkers, and can be especially distressing to patients who are ill. Medical office staff should use deodorants regularly and scrupulously care for their teeth and gums. In addition, the use of strong perfumes or after-shaves should be avoided when at work because they may bother some patients, and some people are actually allergic to them. Fingernails should be kept clean and trimmed.

Hair need not be elegantly styled, but it should be neat, clean, and cut short or tied back. Long hair may brush against the patient's face during certain procedures, which can be annoying, or become entangled in instruments. Heavy eye makeup may deposit on the eyepieces of optical devices and interfere with the optical quality or function of the instruments. Both hair and makeup can also spread the microorganisms that cause disease (see Chapter 12).

Patients should always be treated in a helpful, friendly manner. Certainly, ophthalmic medical assistants need not be either servile or overly familiar, but they should express an honest concern and respect for the individual patient with their face, voice, and behavior. A caring attitude, coupled with skill in your job and a professional manner and appearance, will allow you to make a significant contribution to the patient's overall well-being and total visual health.

REVIEW QUESTIONS

1. Match the types of ophthalmic health professionals with their duties.

    ____ ocularist

    ____ ophthalmologist

    ____ optometrist

    ____ orthoptist

    ____ ophthalmic medical assistant

    ____ optician

    a. Measures and fits patients with artificial eyes
    b. Helps with diagnosis, management, and nonsurgical treatment of eye muscle imbalance
    c. Dispenses eyeglasses and contact lenses from prescriptions supplied by others
    d. Prescribes and/or fits eyeglasses and contact lenses and screens for eye diseases as a nonphysician professional
    e. Prevents, diagnoses, and medically and surgically treats problems of the eye as a medical doctor
    f. Helps the doctor in a variety of clinical and administrative tasks
2. List the three levels of certified ophthalmic assisting in order of degree of training and experience.
3. Ophthalmic medical assistants may be required to do all of the following *except*
    a. Perform diagnostic tests
    b. Assist with office surgical procedures
    c. Administer certain medications to patients
    d. Diagnose patients' eye conditions
    e. Schedule and greet patients
4. Moral principles and values that govern behavior are called __________.

5. While you are performing a diagnostic test on a patient, the patient addresses you as "Doctor" and asks what you think should be done about an eye condition. As an ophthalmic medical assistant, the best initial action to take is to
   a. Tell the ophthalmologist immediately
   b. Prescribe the treatment you think is best for the patient and check your advice later with the doctor
   c. Complete the diagnostic test and tell the patient the results
   d. Tell the patient why and how the test is being done
   e. Tell the patient that you are an assistant, not the doctor, and refer the patient to the doctor for advice

SUGGESTED ACTIVITIES

1. Write to the Joint Commission on Allied Health Personnel in Ophthalmology (JCAHPO) to request further information on ophthalmic assisting as a career.
2. Discuss with the doctor in your office what tasks you might be called upon to perform.
3. Meet with an experienced assistant in one or more ophthalmology offices to discuss the career path for the ophthalmic medical assistant.
4. Find out, from other assistants, whether there is a local group of ophthalmic medical assistants in your area that you could join. Such groups offer support through study and continuing education opportunities.
5. Ask the doctor in your office if you may observe a variety of patient visits to gain firsthand knowledge about the tasks of an ophthalmic medical assistant.
6. Interview the ophthalmic medical assistants in your office or in another ophthalmology practice and ask them to describe their daily routine, what they like best about their position, and what they like least about their duties.
7. Discuss issues of dress code, hygiene, personal behavior, ethics, forms of address, and other related topics with your ophthalmologist or office manager.
8. Determine in what ways you can add to your basic and continuing education. For example, research what videotapes, audiotapes, books, and courses are available to you. Good resources to start with include the JCAHPO/ATPO newsletter *Viewpoints,* the JCAHPO web site at www.jcahpo.org, the JCAHPO certification criteria booklet, and the American Academy of Ophthalmology's annual product catalog.

SUGGESTED RESOURCES

Cassin B: *Fundamentals for Ophthalmic Technical Personnel.* Philadelphia: WB Saunders Co; 1995.

Code of Ethics. San Francisco: American Academy of Ophthalmology. Revised 1995. (Available on www.aao.org and from Fax-on-Demand, #104.

DuBois LG: *Fundamentalsof Ophthalmic Medical Assisting.* Clinical Skills videotape. San Francisco: American Academy of Ophthalmology; 1999.

Herrin MP: *Ophthalmic Examination and Basic Skills.* Ophthalmic Technical Skills Series. Thorofare, NJ: Slack; 1990.

Introducing Ophthalmology: A Primer for Office Staff. San Francisco: American Academy of Ophthalmology; 2002.

Stein HA, Slatt BJ, Stein RM: *The Ophthalmic Assistant: A Guide for Ophthalmic Medical Personnel.* 7th ed. St Louis: Mosby; 2000.

Stein HA, Slatt BJ, Stein RM: *Ophthalmic Terminology: Speller and Vocabulary Builder.* 3rd ed. St Louis: Mosby; 1992.

Stein HA, Slatt BJ, Stein RM: *A Primer in Ophthalmology: A Textbook for Students.* St Louis: Mosby-Year Book; 1992.

Vaughn D, Asbury T: *General Ophthalmology.* 13th ed. Stamford, CT: Appleton & Lange; 1992.

2

Anatomy and Physiology of the Eye

The ability to see is produced by the actions of various parts of the eye, nerve cells, and the brain. Structures surrounding the eye, such as the lids and lashes, protect and assist this organ in its visual function. If any component of the visual system fails to operate properly, sight may be impaired. The ophthalmic medical assistant plays an important role in helping the ophthalmologist to detect, treat, and prevent disorders that may affect vision. To provide such help, the assistant must be able to describe and recognize the parts of the visual system and understand how they operate. The assistant should be acquainted with the normal appearance of these structures and with deviations from normal.

This chapter introduces you to the eye as the primary organ of vision and to its surrounding structures. The chapter considers in detail the anatomy (structure) and physiology (function and operation) of the various parts of the visual system. The relationship of the eye to the brain in the visual process is also discussed. This chapter includes indented text between rules to introduce you to major diseases and disorders affecting the part of the eye under discussion. These conditions are discussed in depth in Chapter 3.

THE EYE AS AN OPTICAL SYSTEM

When a person looks at an object, light rays are reflected from that object to the eye. As the rays pass through the optical system of the **globe**, or **eyeball**, they are bent to produce an upside-down image of the object at the back of the inner eyeball. Here the image is converted to electric impulses that are carried to the brain, where the image is translated so that the object is perceived in its upright position.

The first part of the eye's optical system is the clear, round membrane at the front of the globe, called the **cornea**. This transparent membrane begins the process of focusing light the eye receives. Behind the cornea is a colored circle of tissue called the **iris**. The iris controls the amount of light entering the eye by enlarging or reducing the size of the opening in its center, called the **pupil**.

Immediately behind the iris is the **crystalline lens** (or, more simply, the **lens**), the second part of the optical focusing system of the eye. The large space behind the crystalline lens is filled with a clear, jelly-like substance called the **vitreous**, or **vitreous body**. Because the vitreous is optically transparent, light rays focused by the cornea and lens can pass through it unaffected to produce an image on the inner back surface of the eye, the **retina**. The light-sensitive cells of the retina convert the image to electric impulses that are carried to the brain by the **optic nerve**. The electric impulses are integrated in the brain's visual cortex to produce the sensation of sight. Figure 2.1 shows the principal structures involved in the eye as an optical system.

The parts of the eye and their anatomy and physiology are considered in greater detail later in this chapter, following a discussion of the tissues that surround the eye.

THE ADNEXA

The tissues and structures surrounding the eye are called the **adnexa**. They include the orbit, the extraocular muscles, the eyelids, and the tear-producing and tear-draining lacrimal apparatus. These structures serve to protect and support the globe.

Orbit

The **orbit** is the bony cavity in the skull that houses the globe, the extraocular muscles, the blood vessels, and the nerves, all of which are cushioned by layers of fat. The globe is situated within the bony orbit in such a way that it is protected from major injury by a rim of bone (Figure 2.2).

Extraocular Muscles

The muscles that control the movement of the globe are called **extraocular muscles** to distinguish them from muscles inside the eyeball. The six extraocular muscles are named by their positions in relation to the globe. These positions determine the direction of movement of the eyeball when the muscles contract (Figure 2.3):

FIGURE 2.1

The eye as an optical system.

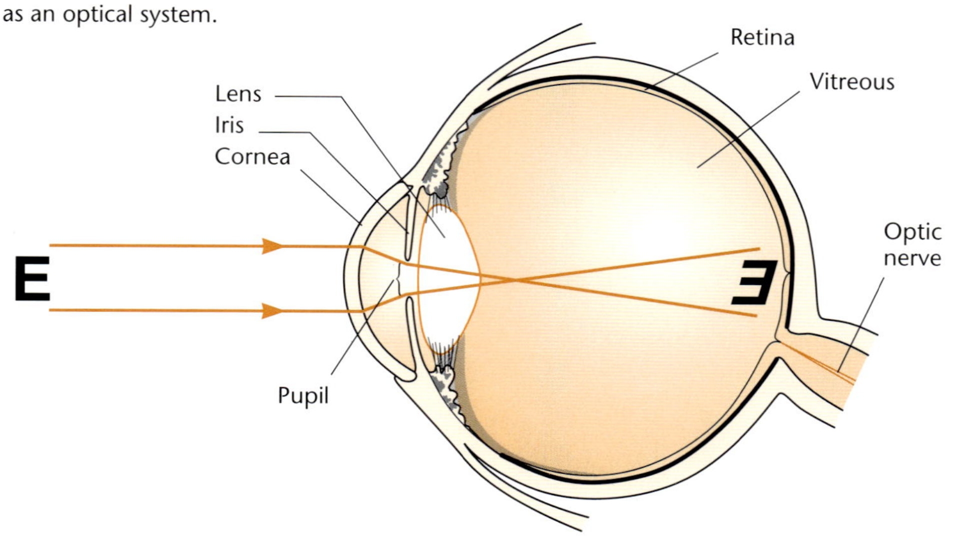

FIGURE 2.2

The orbit.

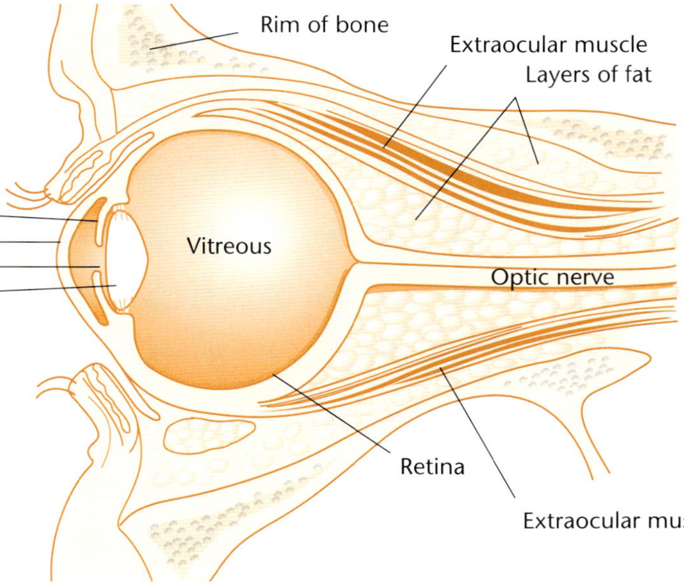

FIGURE 2.3

The extraocular muscles.

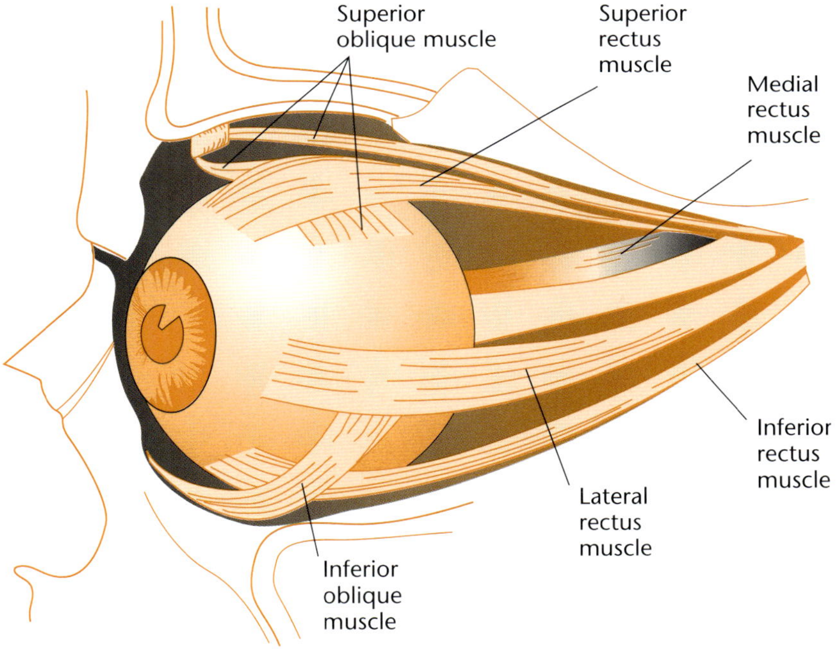

1. The **medial rectus muscle** rotates the eye inward toward the nose, a movement called **adduction**.
2. The **lateral rectus muscle** rotates the eye outward toward the temple, a movement called **abduction**.
3. The **superior rectus muscle** is the primary muscle responsible for turning the eye upward.
4. The **inferior rectus muscle** is the primary muscle responsible for turning the eye downward.
5. The **superior oblique muscle** rotates the eye both downward and inward toward the nose in primary position.
6. The **inferior oblique muscle** rotates the eye upward and outward toward the temple.

Movement of the eye in most directions usually requires the coordinated contraction and/or relaxation of two or more muscles. For example, when a person looks directly upward, the superior rectus acts together with the inferior oblique to raise the eye, while the inferior rectus and superior oblique relax. When a person looks toward the nose, the medial rectus contracts while the lateral rectus relaxes.

In addition to the coordinated action of muscles in one eye, proper vision requires coordination of the contraction of muscles in the two eyes. The extraocular muscles must rotate each globe so that both eyes are directed toward the same target; that is, both eyes must be in visual alignment. Movement of the two eyes in visual alignment generally requires the coordinated action of different muscles for the left and right eyes. For example, when a person looks to the right, the medial rectus of the left eye contracts at the same time as the lateral rectus of the right eye. Conversely, when a person looks to the left, the lateral rectus of the left eye contracts in coordination with the medial rectus of the right eye.

The eyes are kept in visual alignment by the coordinated contraction and relaxation of the six pairs of external ocular muscles. When the eyes are directed toward a single target and are perfectly aligned, **binocular vision** results. The brain blends the separate images received by the two eyes so that the person perceives a single view, a process called **fusion**.

Weakness, paralysis, or other restriction of an extraocular muscle in one eye may prevent coordinated movement of that eye in relation to the other. If the extraocular muscles do not work in a coordinated manner, the eyes become misaligned and vision may be disturbed, a condition called **strabismus**. If the misalignment is significant, the brain may be unable to fuse the two images. The result is double vision or suppression of vision in one eye.

Eyelids and Conjunctiva

The **eyelids** are the moving folds of skin that cover the outer portion of the eyeball. They help protect the eye from injury and exclude light. They also aid in the lubrication of the ocular surface. A film of tears is normally present on the outer surface of the eye, and the blinking action of the upper lid spreads this tear film evenly over the ocular surface to provide a clear layer that does not interfere with vision.

The almond-shaped opening between the upper and lower lids is called the **palpebral fissure**. The point where the lids meet on the nasal (inner) side of the palpebral fissure is called the **medial canthus**. The temporal (outer) junction of the lids is called the **lateral canthus**.

The margin, or edge, of the eyelid contains several structures. On the **anterior** (front) edge are rows of hair follicles for the eyelashes. The eyelashes, technically known as **cilia**, help protect the surface of the eye by sweeping away airborne dust particles and other foreign matter when the eyelids blink.

The eyelashes normally curl upward on the upper lid and downward on the lower eyelid. Occasionally, an eyelash may grow in the wrong direction and rub against the surface of the eye, irritating the cornea. This eyelid abnormality is called **trichiasis**. Under other conditions, a lash follicle may become inflamed and produce a reddened, sore lump near the outer edge of the lid, known as a **stye** or **external hordeolum**.

On the **posterior** (back) margin of the eyelid (the edge closest to the globe) is a row of tiny holes, the openings of oil-secreting glands that are hidden in the tissue of the eyelids. These glands are called the **meibomian glands**. The oil they secrete becomes part of the tear film that lubricates the outer surface of the eyeball. Figure 2.4 depicts the external eyelids and associated structures.

As with the lash follicles, a meibomian gland may become inflamed and infected, in this case producing a swelling on the inner eyelid called an **internal hordeolum**. Over time, this inflammation may produce a lump called a **chalazion** on the outer lid. Yet another lid condition is **blepharitis**, a common inflammation that produces reddened and crusted lid margins.

The eyelids themselves are composed of three layers: an outer layer of skin, a middle layer of fibrous tissue and muscle, and an inner layer of tissue called the *conjunctiva*. Within the middle layer of the upper and lower eyelids is a dense, plate-like framework, the **tarsus** or **tarsal plate**, that gives the eyelids their firmness and shape. Also located in the middle layer is the **orbicularis oculi**, a circular muscle that closes the eye when it contracts, as in winking. A second muscle, the **levator palpebrae** superioris, is attached to the upper tarsal plate. When it contracts, it raises the upper lid.

FIGURE 2.4

The external eyelids.

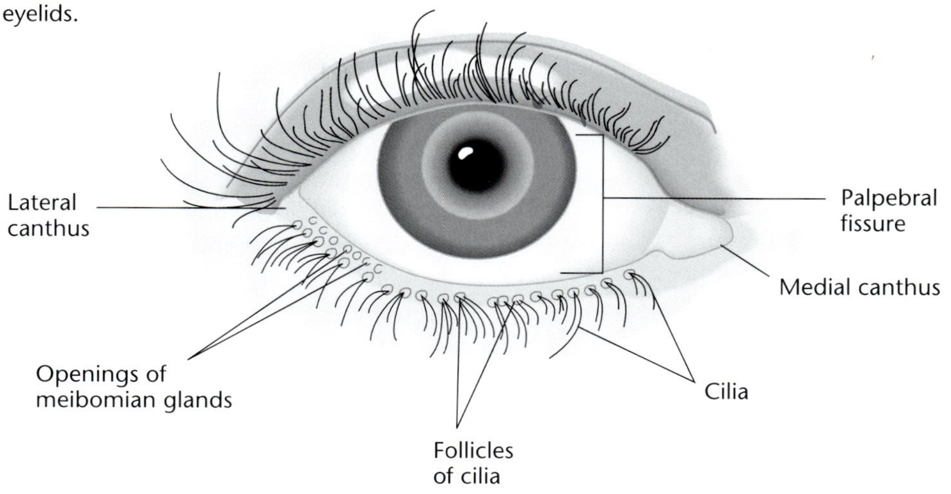

FIGURE 2.5

Cross section of the eyelid.

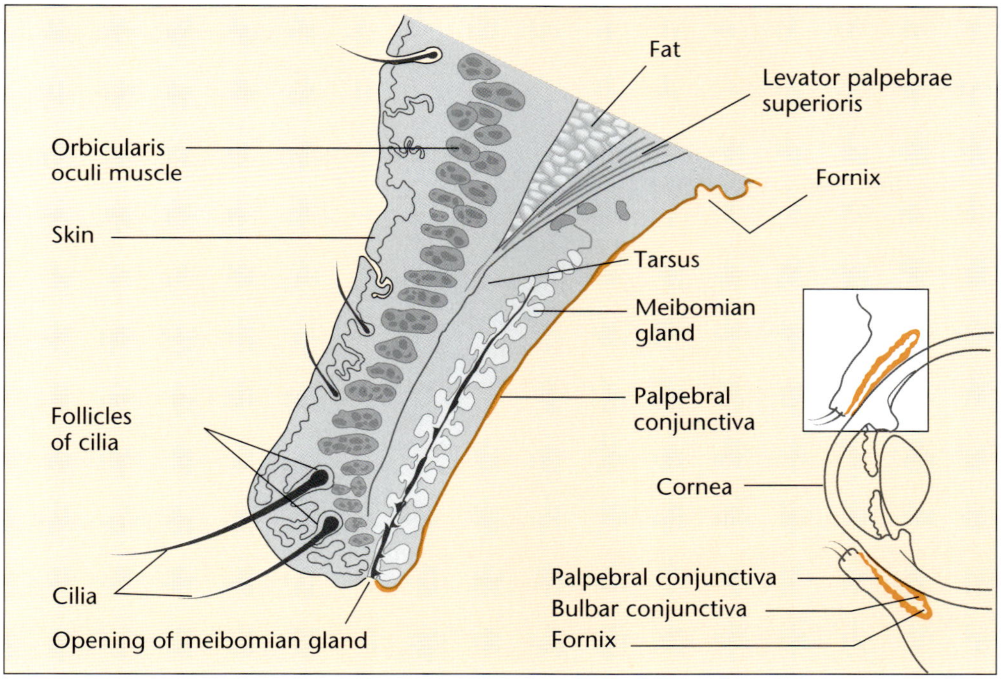

If the levator muscle loses its ability to function, the upper lid droops and cannot be raised properly. This condition is called **ptosis**. Malformation of the eyelid tissues or damage to them may cause the lower lid margin to fall or pull away from the eye, a condition called **ectropion**. Conversely, the upper or lower lid margins may be turned inward, a condition called **entropion**. Either condition produces continuous irritation and possible damage to the cornea.

The third layer of the eyelids, the **conjunctiva**, is a thin, translucent mucous membrane that lines the inner surface of the lids and the outer front surface of the eyeball, except for the cornea. The portion of this tissue lining the eyelids is called the **palpebral conjunctiva**; the section covering the outer eyeball is called the **bulbar conjunctiva**. The area where the palpebral and bulbar portions of the conjunctiva meet beneath the upper and lower lids is actually a loose pocket of conjunctival tissue, called the **fornix** or **cul-de-sac**. Figure 2.5 shows the eyelid and the conjunctiva.

The slippery nature of the conjunctival tissue helps the eyelids to slide easily against the outer surface of the eyeball. Coursing through the conjunctiva is an elaborate network of fine blood vessels that help nourish the underlying tissue of the eyelids and the surface of the eyeball.

Irritation, allergy, or infection may cause the small conjunctival blood vessels to swell, making the conjunctiva appear red, a condition called **conjunctivitis** or "pink eye." Occasionally, one of the conjunctival blood vessels may rupture, allowing blood to flow under the tissue. These **subconjunctival hemorrhages** may occur after violent coughing or often without explanation. They usually resolve in a few weeks without treatment and are not a threat to the health of the eye. However, recurring subconjunctival hemorrhages could indicate a potentially serious medical problem.

Lacrimal Apparatus

The **lacrimal apparatus** consists of the orbital structures that produce tears and the ducts that drain the excess fluid from the front of the eyes into the nose. A small amount of tears is produced continuously during the waking hours, not just when the eye is irritated or when a person cries. The tears become part of a three-layered coating called the **tear film** that covers the anterior surface of the globe. This film helps provide ocular comfort and clear vision, and gives moisture and nourishment to the eye.

The outer layer of the tear film is formed from the oily substance secreted by the meibomian glands of the eyelid. This layer helps prevent evaporation of moisture from the middle layer. The tear fluid that makes up the middle aqueous layer supplies moisture, oxygen, and nutrients to nourish the cornea. Tears are produced by the **lacrimal gland**, located in the lateral part of the upper lid (the side away from the nose) just under the upper orbital rim. Other small, accessory lacrimal glands are distributed throughout the upper fornix. The innermost tear-film layer is composed of a **mucinous** (sticky) fluid produced by specific cells in the conjunctiva called **goblet cells**. This layer promotes an even spread of the tear film over the cornea.

Dry eyes are a common complaint, especially among elderly people. Patients with dry eyes complain of irritation and a feeling of grittiness, described medically as a **foreign-body sensation**.

The tear film is evenly spread over the surface of the eye when the lids close during a blink. The excess tears then form a "tear lake" along the lower lid margin before passing through tiny openings, the **upper punctum** and **lower punctum**. These **puncta** (plural of *punctum*) are located on the upper and lower eyelid margins near the nose.

The puncta are entrances to tubes called the **upper canaliculus** and **lower canaliculus**. These **canaliculi** (plural of *canaliculus*) join together and connect with the **lacrimal sac**. Tears entering the puncta pass through the canaliculi and into the lacrimal sac. The lacrimal sac empties by means of the **nasolacrimal duct** into the nasal cavity, where the tears become part of the fluid that moistens the mucous membrane of the nose. Passage of excess tears through this system is the reason you have to blow your nose after crying and the reason patients have a "funny taste" in their mouth after using eyedrops. Figure 2.6 summarizes the structures of the lacrimal apparatus.

Inflammation of the lacrimal sac is called **dacryocystitis**. This relatively common condition usually occurs as a result of obstruction of the nasolacrimal duct. Such obstruction results in chronic tearing. If the blockage is severe, surgery may be required.

THE EYE

The globe is an almost perfect sphere that houses the optical structures directly involved in the visual process. The globe is often divided anatomically into two parts. The front of the eye, or **anterior segment**, includes the structures between the front surface of the cornea and the vitreous. The remainder of the eyeball, the **posterior segment**, is composed of the vitreous and the retina.

Cornea and Sclera

The outermost, front part of the globe is the **cornea**, which appears as a bulge. The cornea is a thin, tough, crystal-clear membrane, often referred to as the "win-

FIGURE 2.6

The lacrimal apparatus.

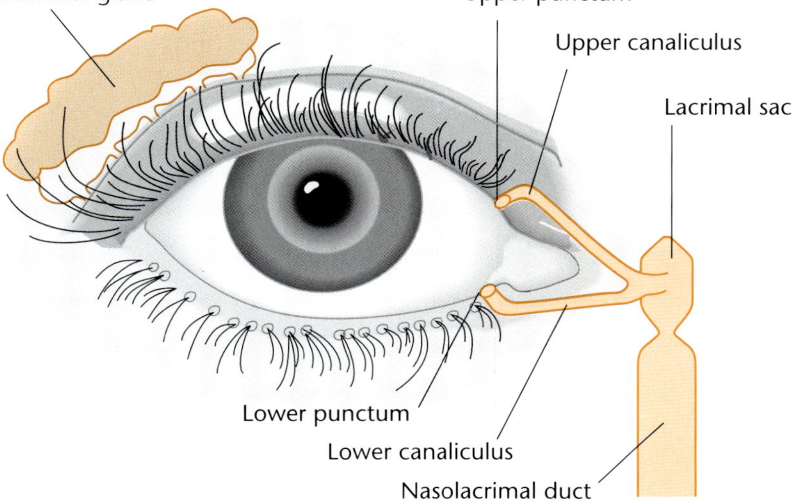

FIGURE 2.7

The five layers of the cornea.

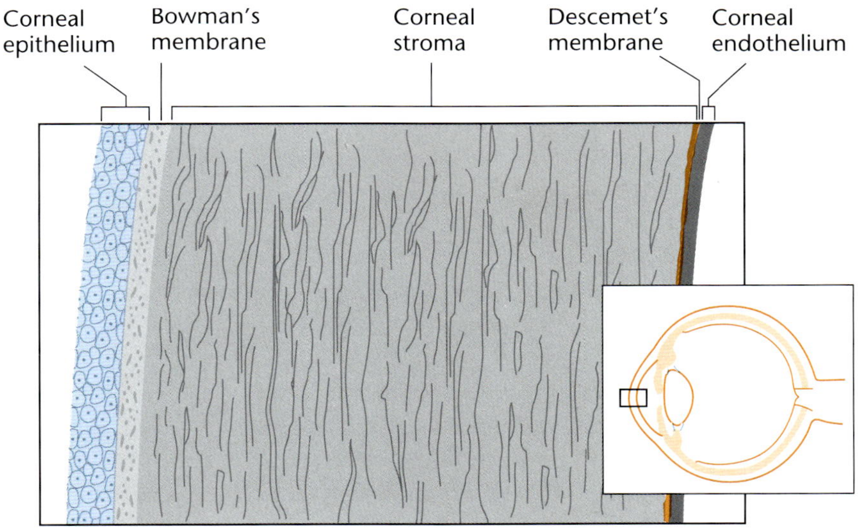

dow of the eye." Transparency of the cornea results from its highly ordered cell structure and from its lack of blood vessels, a characteristic that distinguishes it from other tissues. The cornea receives its nourishment from the tear film that covers it and from a specialized fluid called *aqueous humor* that flows beneath it.

The curvature of the cornea and its transparency permit it to perform its principal function, which is to focus light rays reflected to the eye. The cornea contributes about two thirds of the focusing power of the eye. The tear film aids in this process by providing a smooth surface over the cornea.

The cornea is made up of five layers (Figure 2.7), listed from the outside surface in:

1. Corneal epithelium
2. Bowman's membrane
3. Corneal stroma
4. Descemet's membrane
5. Corneal endothelium

The nerves that supply the cornea lie immediately beneath the **corneal epithelium**, the cornea's first line of defense against infection and injury.

Bowman's membrane acts as an anchor for the epithelial layer. The **corneal stroma** is the main body of the cornea. This layer and **Descemet's membrane** contribute rigidity to the cornea. The cells of the **corneal endothelium** serve as pumps to maintain a proper fluid balance within the cornea.

When the corneal epithelium is injured, a **corneal abrasion**, or scratch, results. Even a small scratch can be very uncomfortable because of the nerves beneath the epithelial layer. These injuries are very common, but they heal rapidly if they do not become infected. A **corneal ulcer** may result if an injury to the corneal epithelium becomes infected. When inflammation spreads and clouds the normally transparent cornea, loss of vision can result.

The white tissue surrounding the cornea is a continuation of the fibrous outer layer that forms the main structural component of the globe, protecting the intraocular contents. This tissue is called the **sclera**. The exposed part of the sclera is covered with the thin, translucent bulbar conjunctiva. What appears as the "white of the eye," therefore, is actually two layers of tissue: the sclera and the almost invisible conjunctiva that covers it. The junction between the sclera and the cornea is called the **limbus**. The limbus is also the point where the bulbar conjunctiva terminates, since it does not cover the cornea.

Anterior Chamber

Between the cornea and the iris is a small compartment, called the **anterior chamber**, filled with a clear, transparent fluid called **aqueous humor**. The aqueous humor is produced by secretory tissue located behind the iris. As the fluid is secreted, it flows across the back of the iris, through the pupil, and into the anterior chamber.

The aqueous fluid leaves the eye at the junction of the cornea and the iris, called the **anterior chamber angle**, or **filtration angle**. From there it passes through the **trabecular meshwork**, a spongy structure that filters the aqueous fluid and controls its rate of flow out of the eye. After passing through the trabecular meshwork, aqueous humor drains through a conduit in the sclera called the **canal of Schlemm**, then into other, tiny conduits, and finally into small blood vessels on the surface of the eye. The balance between the outflow and the production of aqueous fluid maintains the intraocular pressure and is extremely important to the proper function of the eye. Figure 2.8 depicts the anterior chamber angle and the direction of aqueous flow.

FIGURE 2.8

The anterior chamber angle and the flow of aqueous fluid.

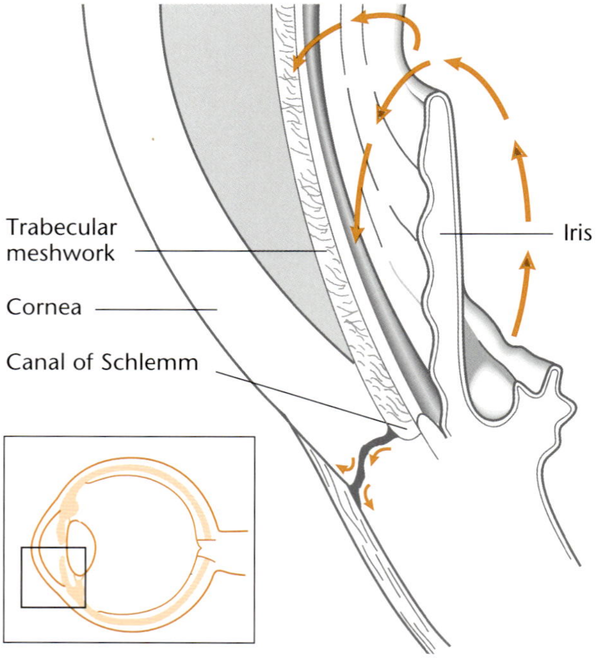

If drainage of aqueous fluid is impaired, pressure inside the eye rises, producing **glaucoma**, which can damage the eye and lead to blindness.

Uveal Tract

The iris, ciliary body, and choroid together form the **uveal tract**, or **uvea**.

The iris is a colored diaphragm of tissue that is stretched across the rear of the anterior chamber behind the cornea. By varying the size of the pupil, the circular opening in its center, the iris controls the amount of light entering the inner part of the eye. Fibers of the **dilator muscle** stretching from the pupil to the boundaries of the iris contract to widen (dilate) the pupil in reduced light conditions. The **sphincter muscle** that encircles the pupil contracts to make the pupil smaller in response to bright light. The pupil itself appears black because the interior of the eye is dark.

The iris varies in color from one individual to another and may also change color in the same person with age. In newborn infants, the iris often appears blue due to an absence of pigment in the transparent tissue. As the eye develops, the more permanent iris color becomes apparent.

FIGURE 2.9

The uveal tract. (A) The iris, ciliary body, and choroid in relation to other structures of the eye. (B) Details of the uveal structure.

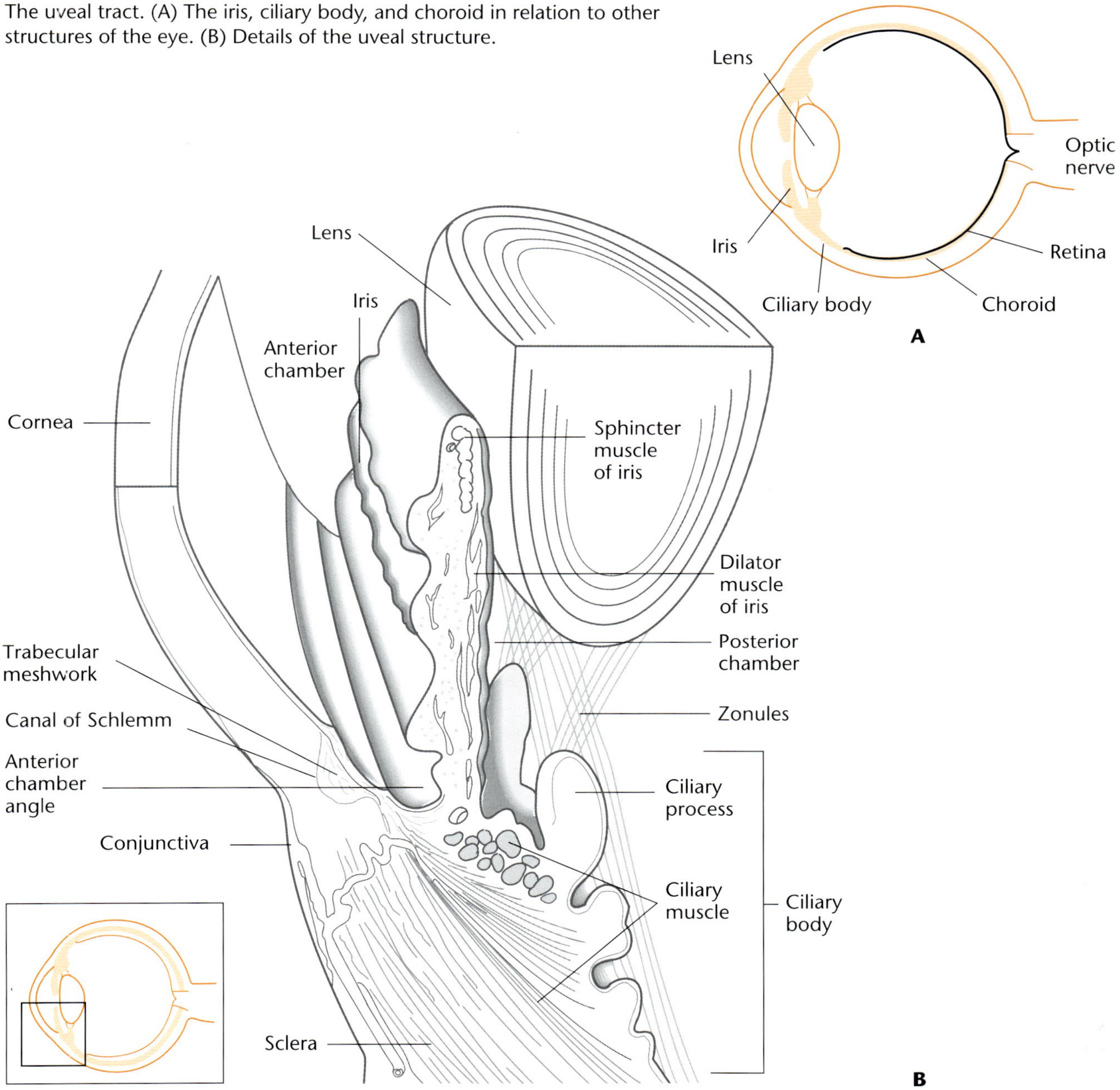

The space between the back of the iris and the front of the vitreous is called the **posterior chamber**. This space is filled, like the anterior chamber, with aqueous fluid.

The **ciliary body** is a band-like structure made of muscle and secretory tissue that extends from the edge of the iris and encircles the inside of the sclera toward the front of the eye. The inner surface of the ciliary body is arranged in folds, rows, or ridges called **ciliary processes**. These structures secrete the aqueous humor that fills the anterior and posterior chambers. The muscle fibers in the ciliary body form the **ciliary muscle**. The ciliary body supports another structure in the eye, the crystalline lens, by means of connecting fibers.

The third part of the uveal tract, the **choroid**, is a continuation of the ciliary body in the form of a layer of tissue that lies between the sclera and the retina, the innermost surface of the posterior segment of the eyeball. The choroid is made up largely of blood vessels, which supply nourishing blood to the outer layers of the retina. Figure 2.9 shows the structures of the uveal tract.

Crystalline Lens

The transparent structure located immediately behind the iris, suspended in the posterior chamber, is the **crystalline lens**. The lens is suspended by transparent fibers called **zonules** that radiate from the lens and attach to the ciliary body. The lens itself consists of an elastic capsule filled with a clear, paste-like protein.

The lens completes the process of focusing light rays reflected to the eye, a process begun by the cornea. In contrast to the cornea, the curvature of the lens can change in order to focus images of objects that are closer to the eye. This action, called **accommodation**, occurs with the help of muscles of the ciliary body. When the ciliary muscle contracts, the zonules relax, permitting the lens to become rounder and increasing its focusing power.

Elasticity of the crystalline lens decreases as part of the normal aging process. By the age of 45, a significant amount of the lens' ability to increase its curvature is lost and the individual is no longer able to focus on very near objects, a condition called **presbyopia**. For this reason, many people over the age of 45 wear reading glasses. Also with aging, proteins of the lens deteriorate, leading to **opacification** (clouding) of the lens, called a **cataract**. When the cloudiness progresses to the point that it interferes with the patient's daily routine or totally blocks vision, the cataract can be surgically removed. The lost optical power must be replaced by an appropriate lens (spectacles, contact lenses, or intraocular lenses).

Vitreous

The vitreous is a clear, jelly-like substance that fills the intraocular cavity behind the lens. This substance acts as a shock absorber and maintains the spherical shape of the globe. Normally, the vitreous is optically transparent, so that light rays bent by the cornea and the lens can pass unimpeded to focus an image on the retina.

The vitreous may liquefy as part of the normal aging process, occasionally producing small clumps or strands of concentrated gel floating in the now-fluid vitreous. These particles, called **floaters**, cast shadows on the retina and appear to the patient as moving spots.

FIGURE 2.10

The macular area and the optic disc.

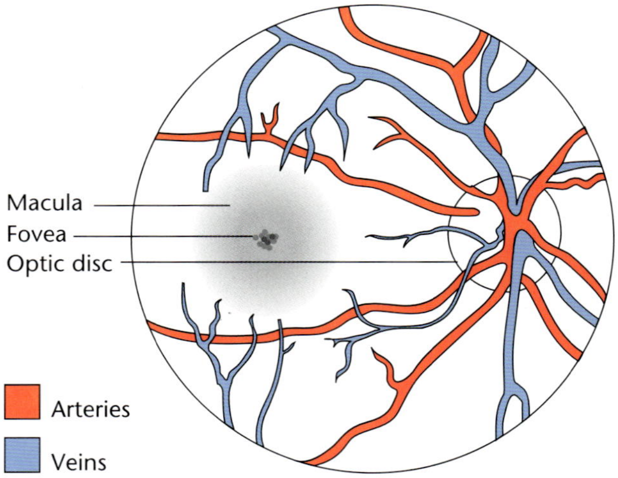

Retina

The retina is a transparent layer of tissue that forms the innermost lining of the globe. The layer consists mainly of nerve cells and is actually an extension of the brain. The posterior two thirds of the retina is called the "visual portion" because it is the surface on which images are focused by the cornea and lens.

The retina is composed of an inner layer of nerve cells and an outer **pigment epithelium** that lies against the choroid. The base of the nerve cell layer contains two types of **photoreceptor** (light-sensitive) cells, the **rods** and the **cones**, each with a different function in the visual process. The rods are largely responsible for vision in reduced light ("night vision") and for peripheral (side) vision. The cones provide sharp central vision and the perception of color.

The retina is nourished by blood vessels on its surface and by the vessels in the choroid underneath. The central retinal artery enters and the central retinal vein exits at a location in the retina known as the **optic disc**, or **optic nerve head**. Close to the center of the retina is a specialized area known as the **macula**. The center of the macula is called the **fovea** (Figure 2.10). Because most of the cone cells are concentrated in the macula, proper function of this area is crucial to the finely detailed central vision needed for reading and other detailed visual tasks.

FIGURE 2.11

The retina at its junction with the optic disc.

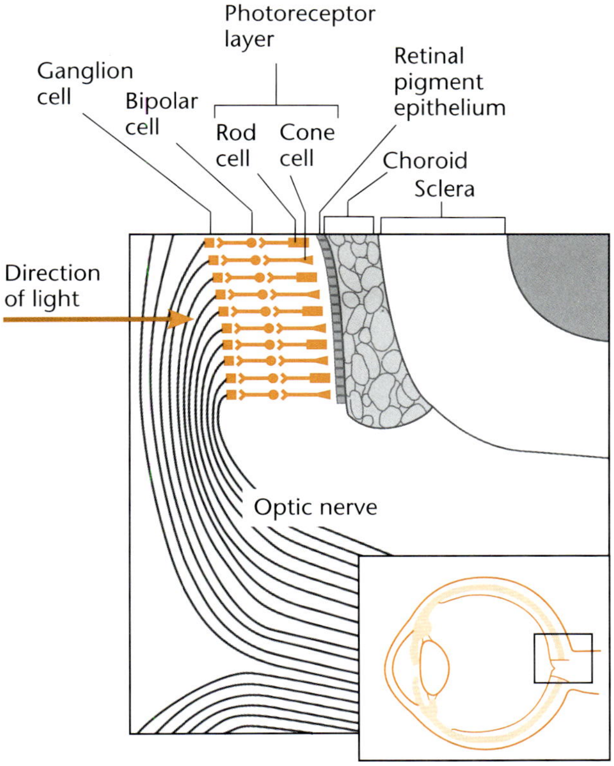

Injury to the macula or degeneration of this part of the retina due to age reduces visual acuity (sharpness). In extreme cases, the eye may be left with only peripheral vision. If other areas of the retina are damaged, blind spots will occur in corresponding parts of the visual field.

When light stimulates the rods and the cones in the retinal photoreceptor layer, electric (nerve) impulses are generated in these cells and relayed to **bipolar cells**, which lie above the rods and cones. The nerve impulses then pass to **ganglion cells** at the top, or innermost surface, of the retina. The ganglion cells possess long, fiber-like **axons**, which course over the surface of the retina and converge at the optic disc, at the back of the eye. The axons from the ganglion cells form the optic nerve. The optic nerve thus resembles a cable of uninterrupted axon strands or nerve fibers, each carrying a visual message, as the nerve exits the globe. Because no rods or cones are present at the optic disc, this small area is sightless and is called the **physiologic blind spot** in the field of vision. Figure 2.11 summarizes the structures at the junction of the retina and the optic disc.

Visual Pathway

The route taken by light-generated nerve impulses after they leave the eye is called the **visual pathway** or **retrobulbar visual pathway**. The initial portion of this pathway consists of the optic nerve from each eye. The two optic nerves merge at a point behind the eyes in the brain called the **optic chiasm**. Here axon fibers from the nasal retina of each eye cross to the opposite side of the chiasm, while axons from the temporal retina of each eye continue on their respective sides of the chiasm. The realigned axons emerge from the chiasm as the left and right **optic tracts** and end in the left and right **lateral geniculate bodies**. At these midbrain "way stations," the axons of the optic tracts **synapse** (connect) to nerve cells called **optic radiations**, which travel to the right and left halves of the **visual cortex** at the back of the brain. Figure 2.12 depicts the visual pathway and its principal structures.

The purpose of the apparently complex crossing of nerve fibers from the nasal retina of the two eyes becomes clear in the context of the visual messages they carry. The image received by the nasal retina of the left eye is essentially the same as the image focused on the temporal retina of the right eye. Conversely, the image on the nasal retina of the right eye is closely similar to the image on the temporal retina of the left eye. Although the left and right optic tracts emerge from the chiasm with nerve fibers from *both* eyes, the visual message each optic tract carries is of an image from one direction, or field of vision.

The visual messages transmitted in the form of nerve impulses from the two eyes are integrated in the visual cortex of the brain to create the sensation of sight. The object originally viewed by both eyes is perceived as a single image, seen upright and from the correct perspective.

Disorders affecting different parts of the visual pathway produce characteristic changes in the field of vision. The nature of visual field disturbances, therefore, can help in determining which part of the visual pathway is affected.

FIGURE 2.12

The visual pathway.

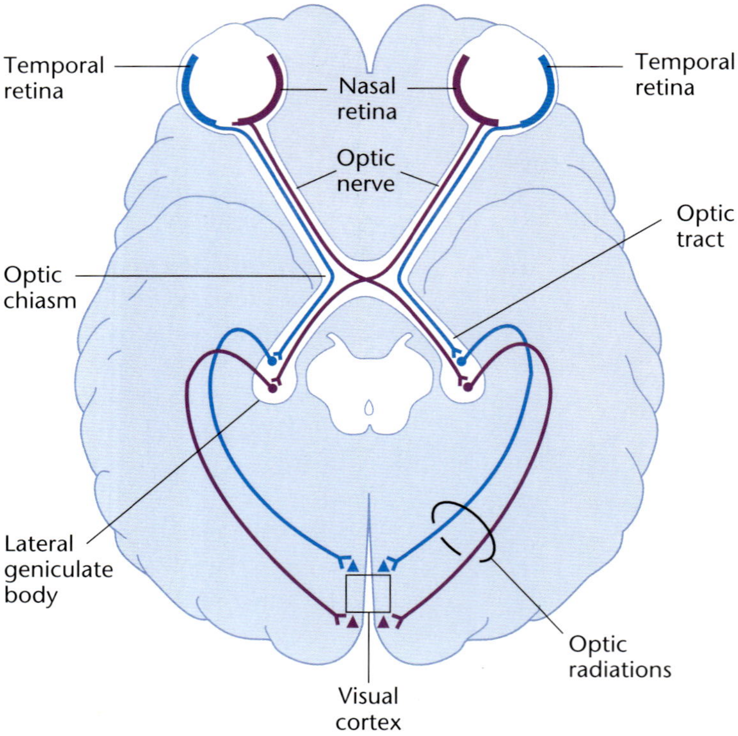

REVIEW QUESTIONS

1. Briefly describe how the eye converts light rays to a perceived image, naming the principal structures involved in the process.
2. Name the four primary structures included in the adnexa.
3. Describe the structure and function of the orbit.
4. Match the six extraocular muscles with their functions.

____ medial rectus

____ lateral rectus

____ superior rectus

____ inferior rectus

____ superior oblique

____ inferior oblique

a. Outward rotation
b. Upward rotation
c. Downward rotation
d. Inward rotation
e. Upward and outward rotation
f. Downward and inward rotation

5. What are the three functions of the eyelids?
6. Name the three layers of the eyelid.
7. What are the two principal functions of the lacrimal apparatus?
8. Give two reasons why tears are important to the functioning of the eye.
9. What is the relationship between the lacrimal gland, lacrimal sac, and nasolacrimal duct?
10. Name the three layers of tear film and their functions.
11. On the cutaway view of the eye, identify the following structures: cornea, sclera, lens, vitreous, retina, cilia, conjunctiva.

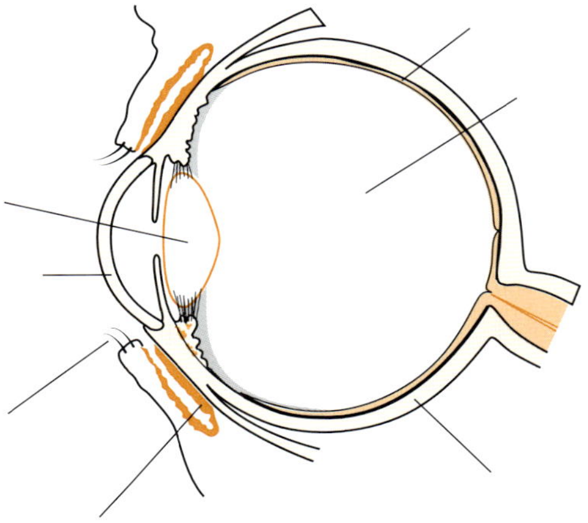

12. What is the principal function of the cornea?
13. Match the five layers of the corneal tissue with their functions. (Two of the layers perform the same function.)

    ____ endothelium

    ____ epithelium

    ____ Bowman's membrane

    ____ Descemet's membrane

    ____ stroma

    a. Serves as first line of defense against infection and injury
    b. Contributes rigidity
    c. Acts as anchor for epithelium
    d. Maintains proper fluid balance
14. What is the main function of the sclera?
15. Why is a balance between the inflow and outflow of aqueous humor important?
16. Describe the course of aqueous humor into and out of the eye, naming the principal ocular structures involved.
17. Name the three main structures that make up the uveal tract.
18. Describe how the pupil dilates and contracts, naming the muscles involved.

19. What is the function of the ciliary processes?
20. What is the main function of the choroid?
21. Which structure besides the cornea provides the eye's focusing power?
22. What is the physiologic process and purpose of accommodation?
23. The lens is attached to the ciliary body by transparent fibers called ________.
24. What is the main function of the vitreous?
25. Briefly describe how the retina works to produce sight.
26. The retina includes a photoreceptor layer containing two types of cells: ________ and ________.
27. How are the functions of these two types of retinal photoreceptor cells different?
28. The macula contains most of the ________ cells.
29. Describe the route of nerve impulses through the retrobulbar visual pathway.

SUGGESTED ACTIVITIES

1. Obtain a commercial model eye. Under supervision of your ophthalmologist or other trainer, disassemble it, and reassemble it, naming the various structures as you do so.
2. Cover the labels on a poster of the anatomy of the eye with a sheet of paper or strips of masking tape and write in the labels. Then compare your labels with those on the poster to see how accurate you were.

SUGGESTED RESOURCES

Cassin B: *Fundamentals for Ophthalmic Technical Personnel.* Philadelphia: WB Saunders Co; 1995; chaps 1–3.

Cassin B, Rubin ML, eds: *Dictionary of Eye Terminology.* 4th ed. Gainesville, FL: Triad; 2001.

Goldberg S: *Ophthalmology Made Ridiculously Simple.* Miami: MedMaster; 1996.

Marieb E: *Human Anatomy and Physiology.* 5th ed. San Francisco: Benjamin Cummings; 2001.

Stein HA, Slatt BJ, Stein RM: *The Ophthalmic Assistant: A Guide for Ophthalmic Medical Personnel.* 7th ed. St Louis: Mosby; 2000.

3 Diseases and Disorders of the Eye

Various disorders may interfere with the normal function of the eye and ocular adnexa and thereby affect sight. To help the ophthalmologist correct or prevent damage to the visual system, the ophthalmic medical assistant must be able to recognize common eye problems and understand how and why they developed. It is also important for the assistant to know the medical terms used to describe these disorders and the disease mechanisms that produced them. In addition, the assistant should have a general knowledge of the kind of treatment needed to manage or correct the problem.

This chapter introduces you to the general concepts of disease and to the processes by which diseases evolve. The specific disorders that may occur in various parts of the eye and ocular adnexa are discussed in detail. You will learn the causes of these disorders, their effects on vision, and the procedures used to treat them. Such information will help you to understand and perform diagnostic tests and other responsibilities of ophthalmic medical assisting.

MECHANISMS OF DISEASE AND INJURY

The term **disease** means a specific process in which **pathologic** (abnormal) changes result in malfunction of a particular part or system of the body. A variety of biologic or other mechanisms can cause disease. However, because none of the body's parts or systems exists in isolation, pathologic changes in one part of the body frequently affect the operation of another part. Thus, the process that is the **etiology** (cause) of one disease may itself be a disease process or the result of another disease. The term **injury** is often associated with disease because the processes that produce, or are, disease may damage and destroy cells, the microscopic units that compose a tissue, organ, or system.

The mechanisms of disease and injury can be divided into 10 general types:

1. Infectious
2. Inflammatory
3. Allergic
4. Ischemic
5. Metabolic
6. Congenital
7. Developmental
8. Degenerative
9. Neoplastic
10. Traumatic

Infectious Process

Humans share this planet with many kinds of animals and plants, including unnumbered varieties of very small organisms invisible to the unassisted eye. These **microorganisms** are present in the air we breathe, in the food we eat, and on the objects we touch. They are even present inside our bodies. In many cases, we live in harmony with these **bacteria, fungi**, and **viruses** and even benefit from some of them. For example, bacteria present in the intestine feed on waste matter and produce a vitamin that promotes blood clotting. However, penetration of some microorganisms through the body's natural defenses and into the tissues can have very damaging results. Invasion and multiplication of these harmful microorganisms, called **infection**, can injure cells by competing for nutrients and producing toxic substances or simply by interfering with the cells' normal activities and reproduction.

Bacterial and fungal infections frequently begin in the tissues immediately surrounding the microorganism's point of entry. Such infections are described as *local*. If they are unchecked, the infections may spread to surrounding tissues and become *diffuse*. In some cases, infections can get into the bloodstream and cause trouble at sites quite remote from the point of entry.

Inflammatory Process

The body generally reacts to infection first by a local protective tissue response called **inflammation**. Specialized cells move to the affected area and act to destroy the injurious agent, while other cells release fluids to dilute any toxic substances produced by the infectious agent. Still other cells then proceed to wall off both the offender and the damaged tissue. Inflammation generally produces pain, heat, redness, and swelling in the region affected. Although inflammation develops in response to infection, it may also occur following any injury or damage to tissue. Inflammation is often the body's response to foreign substances, such as bacteria or chemicals. The body releases its army of scavenger cells to try to neutralize the invading organism or substance. The medical term for inflammation of a tissue or organ is obtained by adding the suffix *-itis* to the name of the tissue or organ. Thus, inflammation of the iris is known as *iritis*, inflammation of the retina *retinitis*, and so forth.

Inflammation that flares up quickly and remains for only a short period is called **acute** inflammation. If the condition persists for a long period, it is called **chronic** inflammation. The terms *acute* and *chronic* are also applied to infection and other disease processes, depending on whether they are brief or persistent. Although the purpose of inflammation starts out as protective, the changes it produces can result in a loss of function of the tissue or organ involved. Inflammation thus can itself act as a disease process.

Allergic Process

The body's initial inflammatory response to infection is generally followed by a wider and more complex **immune reaction**. Part of this response is the development of **antibodies** to proteins present in the specific infecting microorganism. If a person is later re-exposed to the same invader, the antibodies will serve to neutralize the microorganism and may prevent recurrence of the infection. Even if reinfection is prevented, however, inflammation may still occur.

Many people have an overactive immune system that produces antibodies not only to infecting microorganisms, but to foods they eat, to plant pollens in the air they breathe, and to medications they take. Re-exposure to these substances causes these people to have **allergic reactions**. Generally, the reactions are no more serious than a runny nose, watery eyes, and an occasional skin reaction, but in some people they produce difficulties in breathing, such as asthma, or even death. Allergy, therefore, is an important disease mechanism. As with microbial infection, allergic reactions may be accompanied by inflammation.

Ischemic Process

Ischemia is the term given to a severe reduction in the blood supply to any part of the body. The cells of most body structures depend on the blood carried by nearby vessels for nutrients and oxygen and as a means to remove waste products. Interruption of the blood flow to a particular body part can occur if the vessels become **occluded** (blocked)—for example, by a blood clot—or if the vessels break as the result of injury or high blood pressure. Even a relatively short period of ischemia and the resulting **hypoxia** (loss of oxygen) can lead to damage or death of the cells the vessels serve.

Metabolic Process

Metabolism refers to the combination of all the physical and chemical processes by which the body converts food into the building blocks of the body's tissues and into the energy the body uses. An extraordinary number of individual processes are involved to both build and repair the machine that is the body and to keep it running. In addition to food and water, the metabolic processes require various chemicals and materials to assist the chemical reactions. Examples include minerals, vitamins, substances called *enzymes*, which speed the processes, and *hormones*, which regulate them.

Most of the enzymes and hormones needed are produced by special tissues or organs in the normal individual. In some people, a defect may cause enzyme or hormone production to increase, decrease, or stop altogether, causing a whole series of problems in other body functions and leading to damage in other organs, sometimes including the eye. Examples of overproduction of a hormone include increased thyroid in the disease hyperthyroidism and increased cortisol levels in Cushing's disease. A familiar example of decreased hormone production is the disease **diabetes mellitus**. People with this condition are unable to produce enough of the hormone **insulin** required for the metabolism of sugar. Sugar then accumulates in the blood and urine, upsetting other body systems and damaging tissues, including the eye.

Congenital Process

Various disease processes develop in the child or adult because of an outside influence, such as infection or injury, or for no known reason. In some individuals, these processes or their effects may be present from the time of birth; that is, they are **congenital**. Congenital disease, as well as congenital malformations or malfunctions of the eye and other body structures, may be **genetic** (inherited), or they may be acquired during development of the fetus or during delivery.

Developmental Process

Development of the body tissues and structures begins at conception and continues throughout gestation. Growth and development continue after birth and through puberty until a person reaches adulthood. In some fetuses, babies, and young people, one or another organ, body structure, or body system may not develop properly or at all, due to genetic factors, infection, trauma, or unknown causes. Faulty development of these structures or systems results in their inability to function properly.

Degenerative Process

Automobile parts tend to wear out with age. This is also the case with parts of the eye and other organs of the body. Gradual deterioration in the structure or function of body tissues is called a **degenerative** disease process, and such diseases often occur in old people. Age is not the only cause, however; genetic factors may be responsible for degenerative pathology in young people and even children, as well as in the elderly. Injury, infection, and inflammation may also lead to degenerative disease.

Neoplastic Process

A **neoplasm** is a new growth of different or abnormal tissue, such as a tumor or a wart. The growth may be **benign**—that is, not dangerous to the well-being of the individual—or it may be **malignant** (cancerous). The cells in malignant tissue are deformed and multiply at an extraordinary rate. These cells may also **metastasize**—move to other parts of the body—and begin to produce new tumors, eventually overwhelming the normal function of the body structures and draining them of their food and oxygen. While generally more inconvenient than dangerous, benign neoplasms can cause problems by physically interfering with the operation of other structures.

Traumatic Process

Trauma is a sudden wound or injury to the eye or other part of the body, often from outside the person. The injury may be a cut or a blow or a fragment of wood or metal penetrating the eye. These are examples of physical or mechanical trauma, but the body is vulnerable to other kinds of assault. **Toxins** (poisons) may be a serious cause of trauma, whether they are received by mouth, contact with the skin, inhalation, or from a snake or insect bite. **Thermal trauma** is the term for burns or freezing of tissues. **Chemical trauma** is a major concern of the ophthalmologist because of the serious and rapid damage caused by such chemicals as acid or alkali entering the eye. By its nature, the traumatic disease process often requires emergency care and treatment.

Signs, Symptoms, and Syndromes

All of the disease processes described can affect the vision of individuals and prompt them to seek the help of an ophthalmologist. The changes in vision they experience and the pain or other effects they feel are called **symptoms**. Abnormal changes observed by the physician on examination of the patient are called **signs**. Some signs and symptoms may be the same in a particular condition. However, distinction between the two terms is useful because symptoms tend to be more *subjective* or personal, while signs are usually *objective*. Obviously, both signs and symptoms are important in the diagnosis of disease. **Syndrome** is the term given to a set of signs or symptoms that is characteristic of a specific condition or disease.

ABNORMALITIES OF THE ADNEXA

Many disease processes can affect the ocular adnexa. Infections and inflammation of the orbit, lids, and lacrimal system are among conditions commonly seen in the ophthalmology office. Disorders of the extraocular muscles that affect functional vision are often seen in pediatric ophthalmology practices.

FIGURE 3.1

Proptosis (exophthalmos).

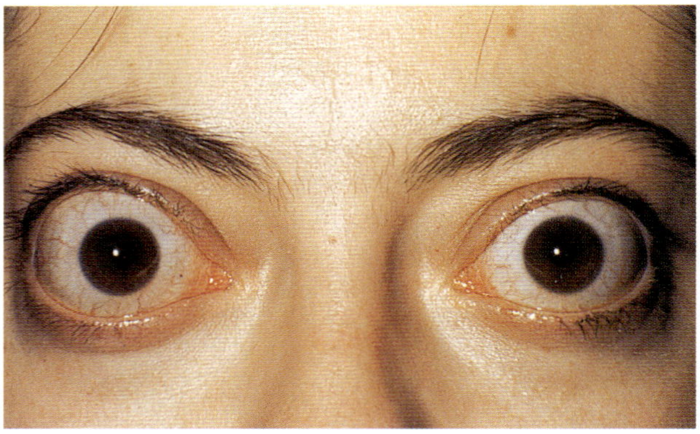

Orbit

Because the orbit is made of solid bone and is open only at the front, any increase in volume of the orbital contents will push the eyeball forward—a condition called **proptosis** or **exophthalmos** (Figure 3.1). Exophthalmos often occurs in **Graves' disease**, a condition of unknown origin that involves the thyroid gland next to the throat and causes the soft tissues surrounding the eyeball to swell. Studies to determine thyroid function should be made on any patient with exophthalmos.

Exophthalmos in only one eye may indicate an orbital tumor. A decrease in vision or abnormal results of specialized tests of the orbit are further evidence of a tumor. **Hemorrhage** (accumulation of blood from a broken vessel) or **edema** (swelling from large amounts of fluid) that results from inflammation or infection in the orbit may also result in exophthalmos. The blood or fluid may spontaneously resorb.

Diffuse infection of tissues in the orbit is called **orbital cellulitis**. This condition may also produce grossly swollen eyelids and red eyes, sometimes without exophthalmos. Symptoms of orbital cellulitis include decreased vision and ocular pain that is made worse with eye movement. Because of its nearness to the brain, orbital cellulitis can be a life-threatening disease. Treatment often includes antibiotics taken by mouth or by injection, and hospitalization may be necessary.

Trauma to the eye or orbit with a blunt object, like a ball or a fist, can break the bony orbital floor or walls and push the eyeball and other contents into the **sinuses** (bony caverns of the skull). This **blowout fracture** may require surgery to reconstruct the orbit and to correct any damage to the ocular structures.

Extraocular Muscles

When the tissue bulk in the orbit is greater than normal (for example, with Graves' disease or an orbital tumor), the extraocular muscles may not be free to move normally. The eyes may go out of alignment, a condition called **strabismus**. In strabismus, the fovea of one eye may not be directed at the same object as the fovea of the other eye. As a result, the patient may complain of **diplopia** (double vision). Treatment is generally directed to the primary (underlying) disease.

Strabismus may also result when one or more muscles lose their elasticity from scarring. Muscle scarring may occur after any long-term inflammation, but most commonly in Graves' disease. Surgical repair or tightening of the damaged muscles may restore alignment.

Trauma or other disease processes may cause strabismus as the result of complete or partial **palsy** (paralysis) of muscle function due to nerve damage. Treatment in this case is generally directed to the primary disease.

Strabismus can also result from a congenital weakness of one or more extraocular muscles. In this case, the normal, stronger member of a pair of muscles will tend to pull the eye in a direction away from the weak muscle. The tendency of the eyes to deviate in some cases is prevented by the brain's effort to fuse the images. Deviation in this condition, called **phoria**, occurs only when a cover is placed over one eye. If the deviation is present even when the eyes are uncovered, the condition is called **tropia**. Outward deviation of the eye is called **exo deviation** (**exophoria** and **exotropia**); inward deviation is called **eso deviation** (**esophoria** and **esotropia**). Figure 3.2 shows two of these deviations. The eyes may also deviate in an upward, downward, or other direction, depending on which pairs of extraocular muscles are mismatched in strength.

Treatment of congenital strabismus generally consists of prescription eyeglasses, patching one eye, and surgically tightening the weak muscles. This is usually done at an early age because delays can risk permanent loss of binocular vision and **stereopsis** (three-dimensional visual perception). To circumvent the confusion produced by the diplopia of misaligned eyes, the brain of a child tends to suppress the image from the deviating eye—a condition known as **strabismic amblyopia**. This is particularly the case in children under 6 years of age because of their greater neural adaptability. If a child has suppressed the vision from one eye over a long period of time, the unconscious habit may continue even after surgery has produced normal alignment of the two eyes. The condition can often be corrected by retraining the nonworking ("lazy") eye if started in childhood. This is accomplished by placing a patch over the dominant eye for long periods, even months. Once amblyopia has been present past the age of 7 or 8, it is often permanent. Therefore, it is important that diagnosis and treatment occur before that age.

FIGURE 3.2

Strabismus. Esotropia (left) and exotropia.

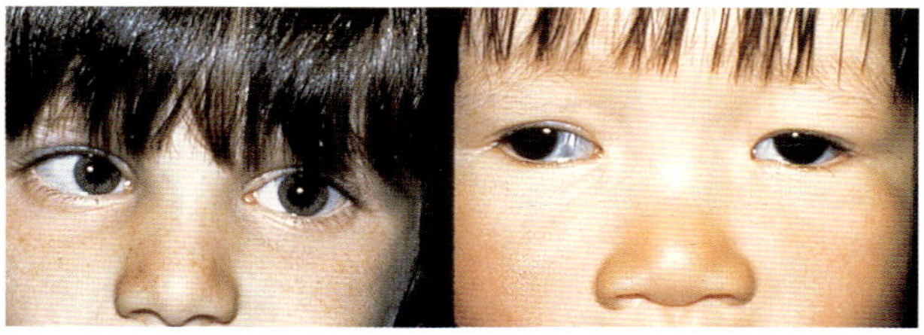

Suppression of vision from one eye (amblyopia) can also occur when problems with the cornea, lens, or retina produce blurred or obscured vision in a child. Diagnosis and treatment of these conditions are discussed later in this chapter.

Nystagmus is a condition in which the eyes continually shift in a side-to-side or up-and-down rhythmic motion and then snap back to a normal position. Both eyes may move together or in different directions. The cause of this defect lies in parts of the brain rather than in the extraocular muscles themselves and is not generally correctable.

Eyelids and Conjunctiva

Bacterial infection of a gland surrounding an eyelash follicle produces a localized **abscess** known as a **stye** or **external hordeolum** (Figure 3.3A). Treatment consists of hot moist packs and antibiotic drops. Occasionally, the abscess must be **incised** (lanced) and drained. Infection of a meibomian gland results in an abscess on the inside of the eyelid called an **internal hordeolum** (Figure 3.3B). Inflammation accompanies these infections and, in the case of the meibomian gland, may remain long after recovery from infection in the form of a nontender **granulomatous** (solid) lump called a **chalazion** (Figure 3.3C). The lump may eventually be absorbed without treatment or it can be removed surgically.

Blepharitis is a common, low-grade, chronic infection with inflammation of the lid margins, generally produced by bacteria (Figure 3.3D). The lid margins appear slightly red with crusts along the lash line. Treatment includes careful lid cleaning and topical antibiotic–steriod treatment, with oral antibiotics needed in special situations, often for many weeks. The condition frequently recurs.

Several disease processes can alter the normal position of the eyelids and thus directly or indirectly affect vision. **Ptosis** is an abnormality in which the upper eyelid droops, due to muscle or nerve damage or to mechanical causes (Figure 3.3E). Congenital ptosis may be caused by partial paralysis of the **oculomotor nerve**, which activates the levator palpebrae muscle. Treatment is surgical. Acquired ptosis is caused by any disease process affecting the nerve supply to the upper levator palpebrae muscle or by degenerative changes in one levator palpebrae tendon. Examples include injuries, diabetes, myasthenia gravis, or tumors that press on the nerve. Treatment of acquired ptosis is directed against the primary disease, but surgical correction of the ptosis may be required.

Ectropion is a turning of the lid margin outward and away from the eye (Figure 3.3F). Excessive drying of the cornea and exposed eye results, causing irritation and tearing. The condition is generally caused by abnormal muscle tone of the orbicularis oculi muscle or by scarring. Treatment is surgical and directed to the specific cause.

In **entropion** (Figure 3.3G), the lid margins are turned inward, causing **trichiasis**, in which the eyelashes rub against the eyeball and produce tearing, discomfort, and possible scratching of the cornea. The condition may be caused by excessive action of the orbicularis oculi muscle or by scarring and is treated surgically.

Lagophthalmos is a condition in which the globe is not completely covered when the eyelids are closed. It may be caused by facial-nerve paralysis, trauma, or by an enlarged or protruding eye. Treatment is directed to the primary disease.

Benign tumors are very common on the skin surface of the eyelids. Surgical removal may be necessary, especially if vision is disturbed. **Basal cell carcinoma** is the most common malignant lid tumor (Figure 3.3H). The tumor has a characteristic appearance of a pit surrounded by raised "pearly" edges. Surgical removal cures if it is performed early.

The conjunctiva that lines the inner surface of the eyelids folds on itself to cover the outer surface of the globe except for the cornea, as already described. Diseases that affect the palpebral conjunctiva almost always involve the bulbar portion of this tissue as well. The bulbar conjunctiva is the eye's first line of defense after the eyelids. As such, it is exposed to dust, pollens, and other foreign matter. **Conjunctivitis** (inflammation of the conjunctiva) is a very common disease, often due to infection with bacteria or viruses, or to allergy. Inflammation causes the small blood vessels in the palpebral and bulbar conjunctiva to swell (or "become injected" in clinical terminology), making the conjunctiva appear pink, hence the common term "pink eye" (Figure 3.4A on page 32).

Bacterial conjunctivitis is recognized by a **mucopurulent** discharge, that is, a thick fluid containing mucus and pus—products of the mucous membranes, dead cells, bacteria, and white blood cells of the immune system. Recovery generally occurs within 2 weeks without treatment, but antibiotic drops and ointment in the eye can speed the process.

Viral conjunctivitis produces a watery discharge and changes in the follicles of the palpebral conjunctiva. The conjunctiva appears to be covered with hundreds of tiny bumps. The infection generally runs its course in 1 to 3 weeks. Some forms of viral conjunctivitis require treatment, although the treatment is often nonspecific, providing only symptomatic relief.

Allergic or vernal (springtime) conjunctivitis causes tearing and itching. Redness and swelling are also present. **Topical** (surface) **application** of medication usually controls the disease.

Ophthalmia neonatorum is conjunctivitis occurring in the newborn. The disease may be produced by various bacteria or viruses to which the infant is exposed during passage through an infected birth canal. Silver nitrate solution, administered to newborns to prevent eye infection, may itself produce conjunctivitis. Laboratory studies are required to determine the specific cause or responsible microorganism and to select treatment. The disease is rare in modern medical practice.

FIGURE 3.3

Eyelid disorders. (A) Stye (external hordeolum). (B) Internal hordeolum. (C) Chalazion. (D) Blepharitis. (E) Ptosis. (F) Ectropion. (G) Entropion. (H) Basal cell carcinoma.

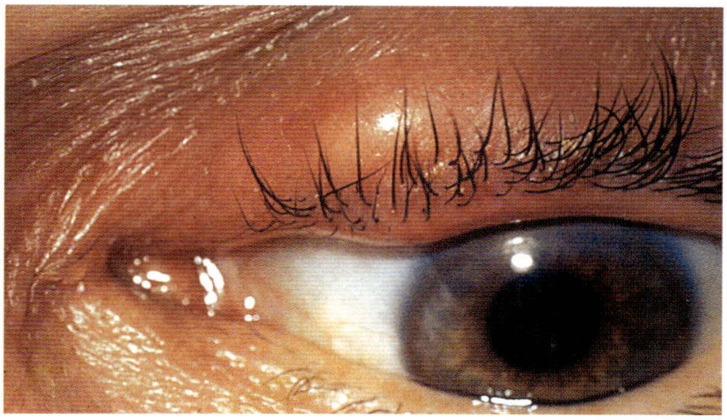

A Stye (external hordeolum).

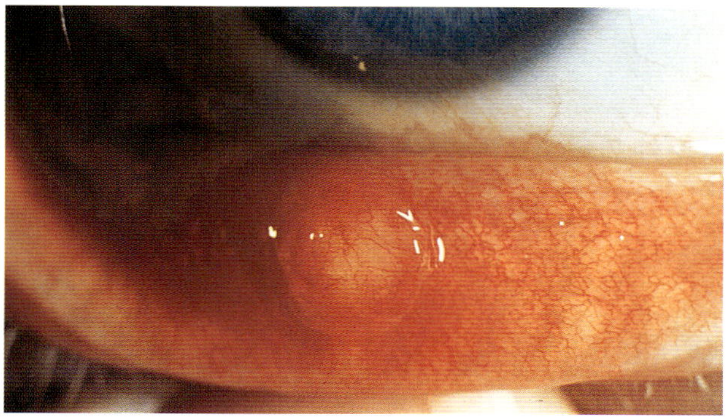

B Internal hordeolum.

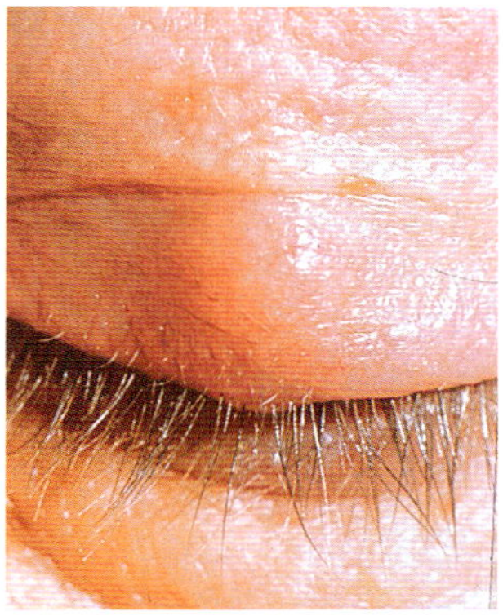

C Chalazion.

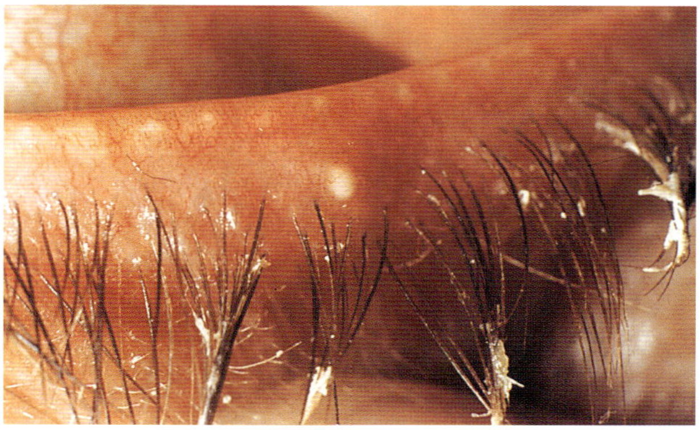

D Blepharitis.

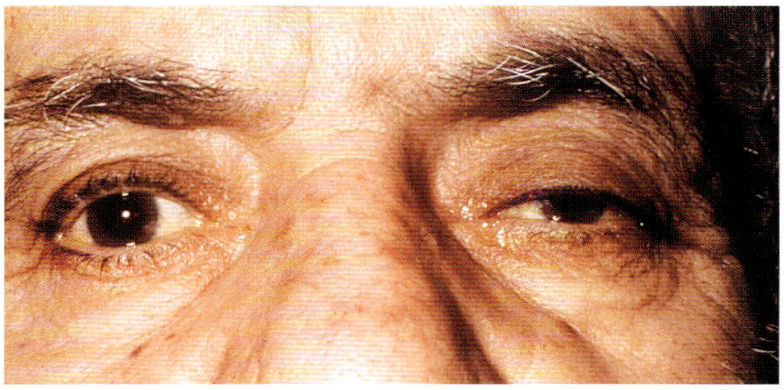

E Ptosis.

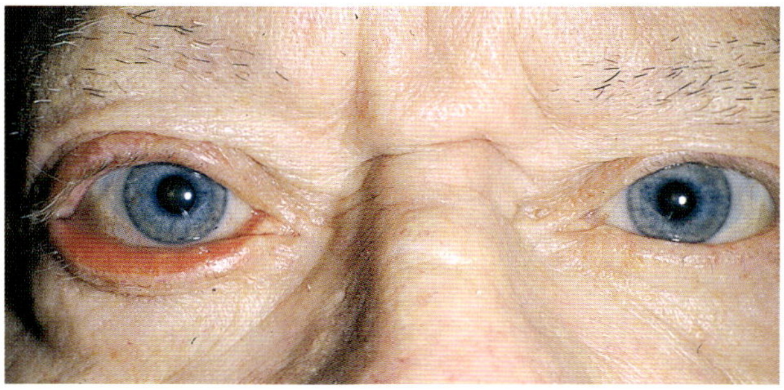

F Ectropion.

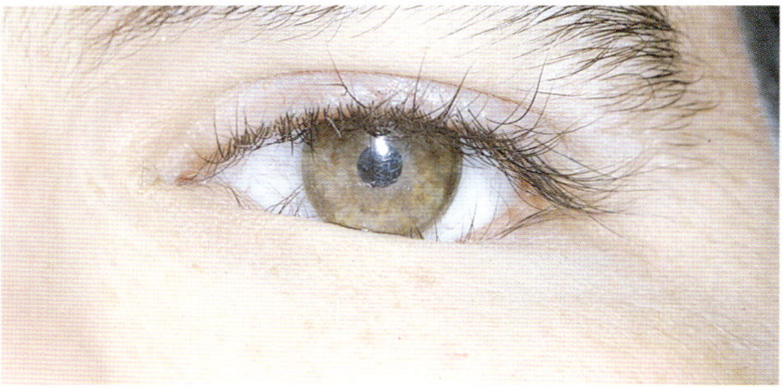

G Entropion.

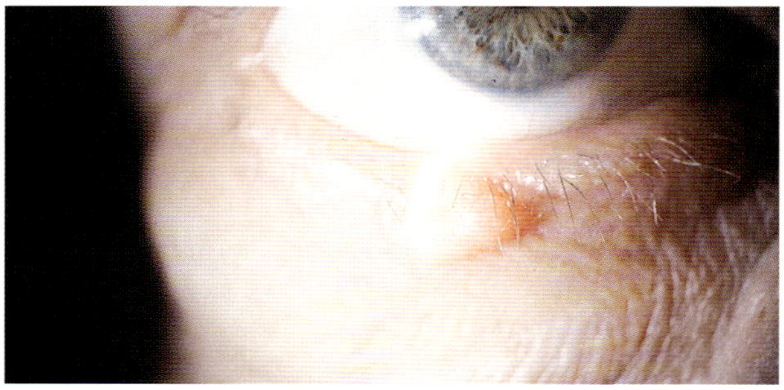

H Basal cell carcinoma.

FIGURE 3.4

Conjunctival disorders. (A) Conjunctivitis. (B) Subconjunctival hemorrhage. (C) Pinguecula. (D) Pterygium.

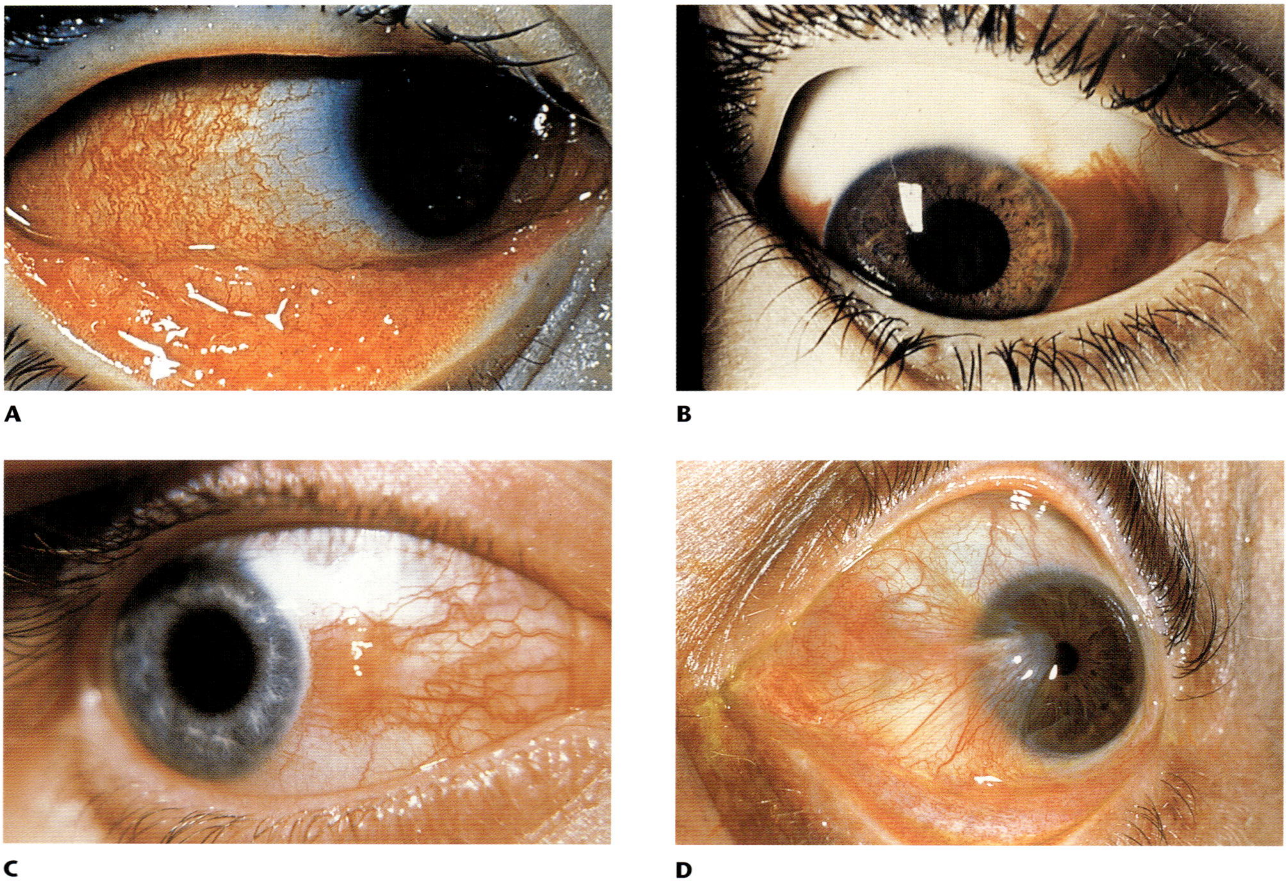

Occasionally, one of the tiny blood vessels that course through the conjunctiva may rupture, allowing blood to flow under the tissue. These **subconjunctival hemorrhages** (Figure 3.4B) occur after violent sneezing or coughing, rubbing of the eyes, or often without explanation. They have no symptoms, but the appearance of a bright-red flat area on the conjunctiva may frighten a patient. The condition resolves in a few weeks, and no treatment is required.

A **pinguecula** is a small, benign, yellow-white mass of degenerated tissue beneath the bulbar conjunctiva (Figure 3.4C). The mass may be located on either side of, but not on, the cornea and may be present in both eyes. Pingueculae do not threaten vision but can cause minor eye irritation. A **pterygium** is a wedge-shaped growth on the bulbar conjunctiva, probably the result of sun irritation (Figure 3.4D). Unlike a pinguecula, the abnormal tissue gradually grows over the cornea and may cause irritation, chronic redness, foreign-body sensation, and sensitivity to light. The growth can be surgically removed but may recur. Both pingueculae and pterygia are probably caused by ultraviolet light damage to the conjunctival surface.

Nevi (freckles) are very common tumors involving the bulbar conjunctiva. They appear as yellowish pink or brown areas on the conjunctiva. Nevi are considered benign, but a small percentage become malignant. They are easily removed by surgery.

Lacrimal Apparatus

The tear-producing lacrimal gland is generally free of disease, although tear production may decline with age. **Dacryocystitis** (inflammation of the lacrimal sac) in the drainage portion of the lacrimal system occurs occasionally (Figure 3.5). Dacryocystitis is usually caused by blockage of the nasolacrimal duct.

FIGURE 3.5

Dacryocystitis.

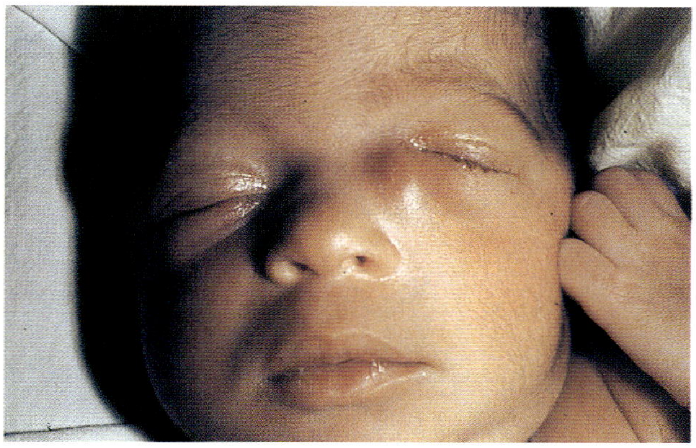

FIGURE 3.6

Hypopyon with corneal ulcer.

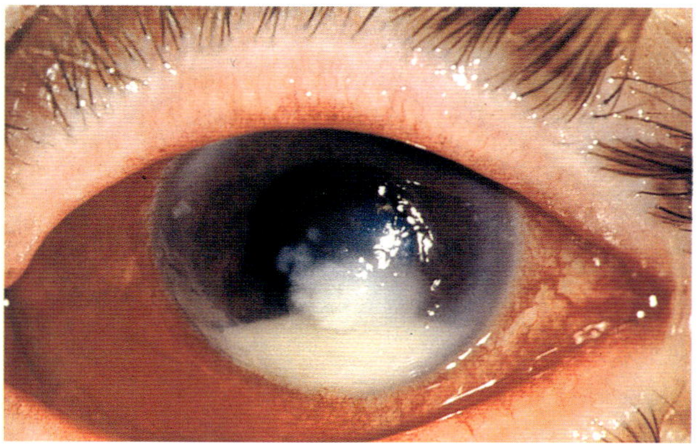

Major signs and symptoms include tearing with pain, swelling, and tenderness. In infants under 1 year of age, the condition generally results from a congenitally narrow nasolacrimal duct. The duct often widens spontaneously by 1 year of life, but it may be probed open if the narrowing persists. Dacryocystitis occurs in adults as a result of chronic lacrimal sac infection, facial injury, or tumor. Antibiotics are helpful if bacterial infection is the cause of the condition. Surgery may also be required if the blockage is severe.

Keratoconjunctivitis sicca (dry eyes) is a common complaint in the general population, particularly among elderly people and individuals with certain systemic diseases. Patients with dry eyes complain of irritation and a foreign-body sensation. This condition is caused by a decrease in the quality or quantity of the tear film. Breaks in the oily outer layer of the tear film permit more rapid evaporation of the middle aqueous layer. Rapid tear breakup time causes dry spots in the tear film over the cornea, with some patients experiencing blurred vision. Present treatment is the use of artificial tears in the form of eyedrops. In severe cases, closure of the lacrimal puncta may be necessary.

ABNORMALITIES OF THE EYE

Although the eye is a small organ, its complexity makes it susceptible to a variety of disease processes. Whether they result from infection, inflammation, trauma, systemic disease, or other disease processes, many eye disorders have the capacity to threaten vision. Fortunately, many diseases that may have led to blindness in the past are capable of being treated successfully today.

Cornea and Sclera

Inflammation of the cornea is referred to as **keratitis**. The cornea may lose its luster and even its transparency. Trauma to the cornea may produce **abrasion** (scratch) and **laceration** (tear) of the protective epithelial layer. The doctor can observe these **lesions** (breaks in the tissue) by staining the epithelium with special dyes. If the lesions do not become infected and the cause of the inflammation is removed, the corneal epithelium will regenerate and heal itself without treatment. On the other hand, bacterial or fungal infection of the lesions can produce a **corneal ulcer**. The corneal epithelium becomes eroded, and the cornea loses its transparency and develops a gray-white opacity that can obscure vision. With an infected cornea, pus often accumulates in the anterior chamber, a condition called **hypopyon** (Figure 3.6). The bulbar conjunctiva appears quite red. Symptoms include moderate to severe pain, sensitivity to light, and excessive flow of tears. Laboratory studies are necessary to determine the specific causative microorganism. Treatment includes antibiotics administered topically (by drops), subconjunctivally, and systemically (by mouth and/or injection). Most ulcers respond to treatment but usually leave a scar on the cornea and possibly decreased vision.

Herpes simplex virus, the virus that produces cold sores, can also lead to keratitis and corneal ulcer. An ocular herpes simplex infection produces symp-

FIGURE 3.7

Dendritic appearance of a corneal ulcer caused by herpes simplex virus.

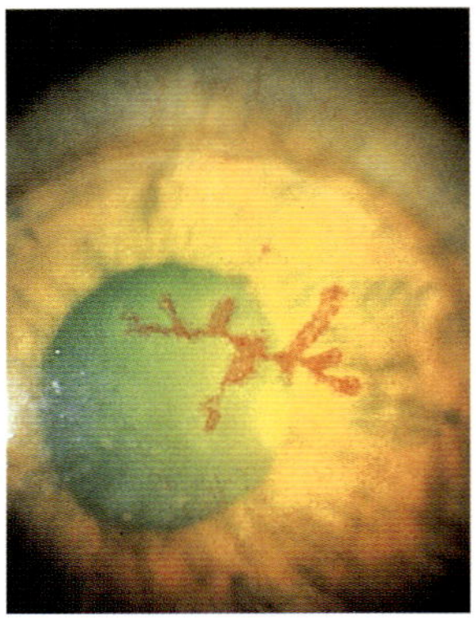

FIGURE 3.8

Hyphema.

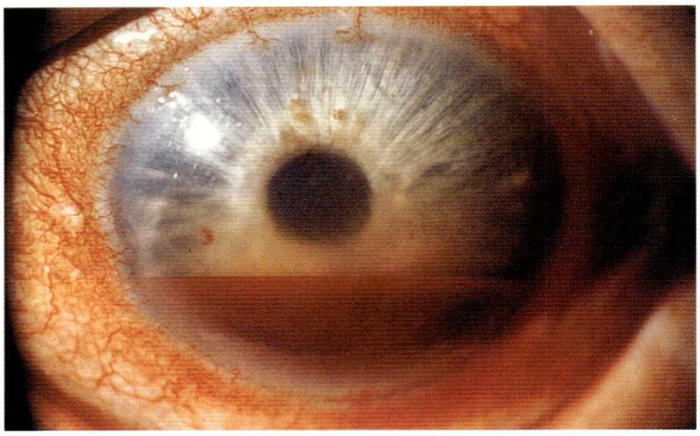

toms similar to but less severe than those associated with bacterial or fungal ulcers. The doctor may observe a dense corneal opacity and, through the use of a special fluorescent dye, a **dendritic** (branch-shaped) figure on the corneal surface (Figure 3.7). Treatment starts with antiviral medication applied to the eye. If unsuccessful, simple scraping of the corneal epithelium often helps heal the ulcer. Herpes simplex ulcers tend to recur. Repeated attacks can lead to severe corneal scarring or thinning, which in turn may require a corneal transplant.

Arcus senilis is a common degenerative change of the cornea affecting persons over the age of 50. The outer edge of the cornea gradually becomes opaque, generally in both eyes. Vision is unaffected and there are no other symptoms. No treatment is needed.

Keratoconus is a degenerative corneal disease of genetic origin. The cornea thins and assumes the shape of a cone, seriously affecting vision. Mild or moderate cones permit treatment with contact lenses, but more severe cones require corneal transplant surgery to restore useful vision.

Inflammation of the sclera, known as **scleritis**, may occur in patients having the systemic condition rheumatoid arthritis. **Episcleritis**, inflammation of the layer overlying the sclera, may result from allergy, although the exact cause is uncertain.

Anterior Chamber

Infection or inflammation within the eye may cause a pool of pus (**hypopyon**) to layer at the bottom of the anterior chamber. Blood may also pool in the anterior chamber (**hyphema**) as the result of trauma or certain diseases (Figure 3.8). Treatment is generally directed to the primary disease.

Malformation and malfunction of structures within the anterior chamber are responsible for a very common and potentially blinding condition called **glaucoma**. Glaucoma exists when the **intraocular pressure** is too high for continued normal function of the eye. The abnormally high pressure can damage the optic nerve, causing an irreversible loss of vision. As explained in Chapter 2, the intraocular pressure is maintained by a balance between the steady secretion of aqueous humor from the ciliary body behind the iris and the steady outflow of the fluid through the trabecular meshwork in the anterior chamber angle. If drainage of aqueous humor out of the eye is hindered in any way, the intraocular pressure rises, producing glaucoma. Such interference with drainage of the aqueous humor and the resulting glaucoma may have multiple causes.

Many forms of glaucoma have no symptoms, even while they gradually cause irreversible destruction of vision. However, if glaucoma is detected early and intraocular pressure is reduced to normal or tolerable levels by medication or laser or incisional surgery, the progression to blindness can be retarded or halted completely. Early diagnosis of glaucoma depends largely on the measurement of intraocular pressure with a **tonometer**, examination of the optic nerve head with an **ophthalmoscope**, and evaluation of the patient's **visual field**, that is, the height and breadth of space seen by the eye when it looks straight ahead. Measuring intraocular pressure by itself is

FIGURE 3.9

Primary open-angle glaucoma.

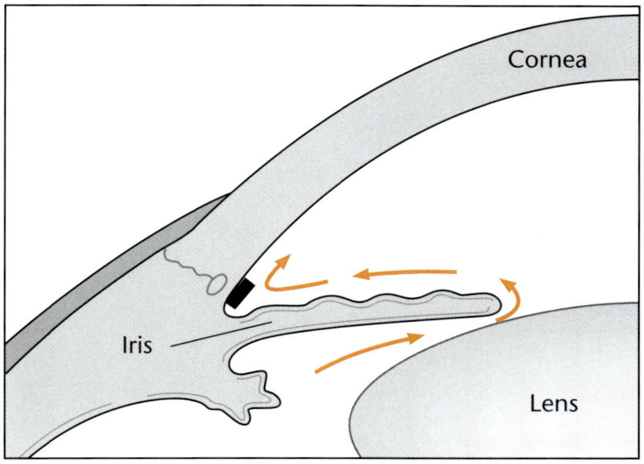

FIGURE 3.10

Primary angle-closure glaucoma.

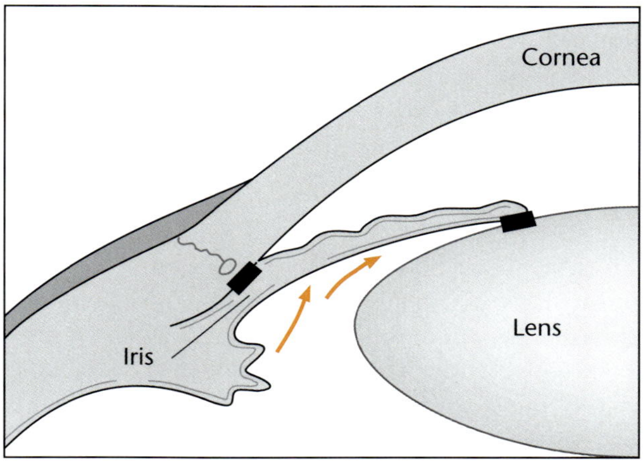

not enough to assure the absence of glaucoma. Intraocular pressure can vary throughout the day and might be normal in a patient with early glaucoma at the time of the examination.

Four main types of glaucoma have been identified, primarily on the basis of etiology:

1. Primary open-angle glaucoma (or chronic open-angle glaucoma)
2. Primary angle-closure glaucoma (or primary closed-angle glaucoma)
3. Secondary glaucoma
4. Congenital glaucoma (developmental glaucoma)

Primary open-angle glaucoma accounts for 60% to 90% of all adult glaucomas. In this form of glaucoma, the anterior chamber angle appears in its normal open position. Resistance to aqueous drainage occurs in the outflow channels between the trabecular meshwork and the uveoscleral blood vessels of the body's circulation (Figure 3.9). The intraocular pressure usually rises slowly over a long period of time, even years. Most patients are without symptoms, although some may complain of mild discomfort in the eyes, tearing, and halos around lights. Loss of vision starts at the periphery (outer edges) of the visual field and often is not noticed by the patient until it has nearly reached the center. By this time, the optic nerve has lost most of its function permanently.

Detection of open-angle glaucoma depends heavily on visual field studies and on examination of the optic nerve head. Treatment of this type of glaucoma consists mainly of medication to lower intraocular pressure. If medication fails to control the pressure, laser or incisional surgery may be used to reduce aqueous production or to provide new channels for aqueous outflow.

Primary angle-closure glaucoma results from a structural abnormality of the eye. It generally occurs in people over the age of 60 and accounts for about 10% of all glaucomas. A small percentage of people have a shorter distance between the iris and cornea than normal. As these people age, the natural increase in the size of the lens, located immediately behind the iris, blocks the flow of aqueous humor through the pupil, gradually bowing the iris forward until its outer edge blocks the aqueous outflow channels in the anterior chamber angle (Figure 3.10). Intraocular pressure rises rapidly the moment the blockage occurs, producing a sudden glaucoma. Patients report eye pain and redness, blurred vision, rainbow-colored halos around lights, headache, and sometimes nausea and vomiting. An angle-closure attack requires emergency treatment with pressure-reducing medication, usually followed by laser surgery **(iridotomy)** to open the anterior chamber angle.

Various ocular and other diseases can reduce drainage, thus causing the intraocular pressure to rise. These disease processes include inflammation, tumors, blood vessel blockage, eye trauma, diabetes mellitus, and certain medications taken for other disease conditions. The resulting glaucoma is called **secondary glaucoma** because it occurs secondary to another disease. Treatment is directed both at the primary disease condition and at reduction of intraocular pressure with medications.

Congenital glaucoma is a rare disease in infants due to a malformation of the anterior chamber angle. These patients often have other ocular deformities. Treatment is primarily surgical.

Uveal Tract

The iris, ciliary body, and choroid together form the uvea or uveal tract. Inflammation, infection, and tumors that affect one part of the uveal tract often eventually involve the other parts. **Iritis** (inflammation of the iris) causes pain and blurred vision. This condition must be differentiated from glaucoma by the measurement of intraocular pressure because treatment includes use of medications to dilate the pupil, agents that could be dangerous in glaucoma. Topical steroids are also used in iritis, and these medications may also be harmful in glaucoma. The progression of iritis may itself produce secondary glaucoma.

Several systemic diseases, particularly diabetes, may cause **neovascularization** (the abnormal growth of new blood vessels) on the surface of the iris. The iris may develop a reddish color. This condition, called **rubeosis iridis**, may cause blood to leak into the anterior chamber or may obstruct the anterior chamber angle. Treatment is directed to the primary disease and to the conditions produced by the rubeosis. Tumors, cysts, nodules, and nevi may also develop on the iris. If they produce symptoms, surgical removal may be tried.

Dysfunction of the muscles within the iris, usually due to a fault in the nerves that supply them, may cause the pupils to be of unequal size, a condition called **anisocoria**. Treatment depends on the cause of faulty nerve function. Iris muscle or nerve damage or disease in other parts of the visual pathway may prevent the pupils from dilating or contracting normally in response to light. Treatment generally consists of surgical repair of the damage or is directed to the primary disease.

Crystalline Lens

The inner core of the lens begins to dry at birth, and elasticity of the structure decreases gradually as part of the normal aging process. Sometime between about age 40 and age 45, ability of the lens to accommodate for near vision has deteriorated to the point that many people require reading glasses. This condition is called **presbyopia**.

FIGURE 3.11

Cataract.

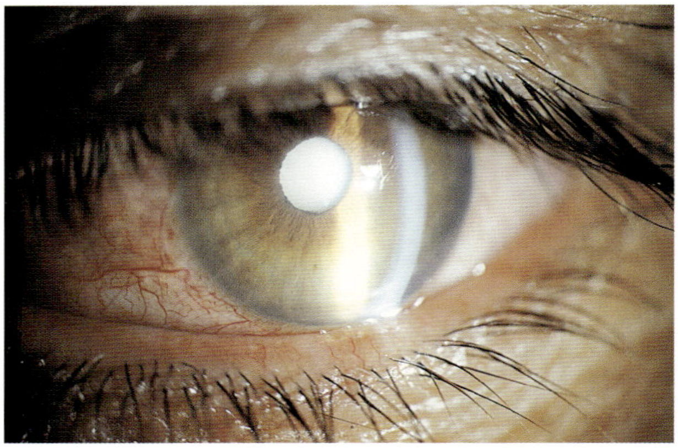

Another effect of aging is the natural deterioration of the proteins of the lens with a progressive loss of transparency. Such opacification of the lens is called a **cataract** (Figure 3.11). When the cloudiness is sufficient to interfere with the patient's daily routine or totally blocks vision, the cataract can be surgically removed. Absence of the crystalline lens, usually because of cataract extraction, is called **aphakia**. The lost optical power of the lens must be replaced by a contact lens, intraocular lens, or eyeglasses for more normal vision (**aphakic correction**). Correction with an intraocular lens is called **pseudophakia**. Today, intraocular lens implantation is the most common method of replacing the lost optical power after cataract removal.

Cataracts can also result from injury or disease, or may be congenital. Congenital cataracts may be genetic in origin or secondary to maternal infections. Cataracts of genetic origin may also develop in children or adults. In all cases, treatment consists of surgical removal of the opacified lens.

Vitreous

Small particles of dead cells and other debris appear in the vitreous, and degeneration of the vitreous occurs—all as part of the normal aging process. The particles and vitreous collagen fibers, called **floaters**, are seen by the patient as spots or cobwebs. No treatment is required, and they are of no concern unless they suddenly increase in number. In that event, they may indicate a detachment of part of the vitreous from the retina. Vitreous detachment is also a normal part of aging.

Infection of the vitreous and adjacent tissues by bacteria accidentally introduced through injury or surgery is an emergency situation. This condition, called **endophthalmitis**, can destroy an eye within days. Treatment consists of massive doses of antibiotics given locally and systemically. Surgical removal of the infected vitreous may also be required.

Abnormal retinal vessels may produce a hemorrhage into the vitreous that interferes with vision. The blood is usually absorbed over time without treatment. If blood or resulting fibrous tissue remains, the vitreous may have to be removed surgically.

Retina

Retinal detachment (separation of the sensory and pigment layers of the retina) is a vision-threatening emergency requiring surgical repair. The condition may occur as the result of injury, from unknown causes, or, in rare cases, from vitreous detachment. The patient notices stars or flashes of light at one corner of the eye, followed several hours later by a sensation of a curtain moving across the eye and a painless loss of vision. Treatment consists of reattachment by **cryopexy** (freezing by surgical means), **photocoagulation** ("welding" with light from a laser), **pneumatoretinopexy** (injection of gas into the eye), **scleral buckle** (placing a block of silicone or other material on the eye to indent the wall), or some combination of these.

Long-standing diabetes mellitus produces a progression of pathologic changes in the retina called **diabetic retinopathy**. Hemorrhages may occur in the retinal blood vessels, in some cases followed by the development of new vessels and fibrous tissue. Retinal detachment can result from severe disease. The blinding form of diabetic retinopathy can often be prevented or delayed by laser surgery of the retina.

Acquired immunodeficiency syndrome (AIDS) results from infection with the **human immunodeficiency virus (HIV)**. AIDS patients have a deficient immune system and, as a result, are susceptible to a variety of bacterial, fungal, and parasitic infections of various tissues including the retina. Treatment consists of intraocular and systemic antibiotics, selected on the basis of the infecting microorganism.

Age-related macular degeneration, as its name describes, is a degenerative disease affecting older people. Sensory cells of the macula degenerate with a loss of central vision. Occasionally, the process can be halted by laser surgery, but for most people no good treatment exists.

Retinitis pigmentosa is a hereditary, progressive retinal degeneration that affects both eyes, usually in children. It begins with loss of vision in dim light, followed by loss of peripheral vision, progressing after years to blindness. There is no treatment. Occlusion of blood vessels that serve the retina or optic nerve—due to trauma, heredity, or other diseases—results in hypoxia and death of the retinal and optic nerve cells. There is no treatment, and blindness frequently results.

Chronic increased intraocular pressure (glaucoma) may produce a tiny hemorrhage of optic nerve blood vessels and destruction of the nerve fibers in the optic disc.

Increased pressure within the skull can produce **papilledema**, swelling of the optic disc with engorged blood vessels. The normal physiologic blind spot is enlarged in the visual field, but the rest of the vision is normal. Treatment is directed to the primary cause of increased pressure.

The condition **optic neuritis** (inflammation of the optic nerve) can produce a sudden, but reversible, loss of sight. Treatment may consist of large doses of steroids given orally or by injection.

Visual Pathway

Damage of nerve fibers in the retrobulbar (behind the eye) visual pathway may occur as the result of pressure due to a tumor in the surrounding tissues, stroke (ischemia or hemorrhage within the brain), or trauma. Inflammation or disease may also affect the function of the nerve cells. The location of the damage in the retrobulbar visual pathway causes characteristic changes in the visual field. The position of the visual field loss, in turn, may indicate the site of neural damage in the retrobulbar visual pathway. Treatment is directed to the cause of the neural damage. Pathologic conditions of the visual pathway and changes in the field of vision are discussed in detail in Chapter 7, "Principles and Techniques of Perimetry."

REVIEW QUESTIONS

1. Name the 10 general types of disease/injury processes.
2. Distinguish between a sign, symptom, and syndrome.
3. When the orbital volume increases, the resulting protrusion of the eyeball is called __________ or ___________.
4. What alterations in the appearance of the eye may be caused by orbital cellulitis?
5. Define *strabismus* and state three possible causes.
6. Match the names of the conditions with their descriptions.

   ____ external hordeolum

   ____ chalazion

   ____ blepharitis

   ____ ectropion

   ____ internal hordeolum

   ____ trichiasis

   ____ ptosis

   ____ entropion

   ____ lagophthalmos

   a. Abscess caused by infection of a gland surrounding a lash follicle
   b. Abscess caused by infection of meibomian gland
   c. Nontender solid lump under lid
   d. Red and encrusted lid margins
   e. Inward turning of lid margin
   f. Globe is not completely covered when lids are closed
   g. Outward turning of lid margin
   h. Irritation caused by eyelash rubbing against eyeball
   i. Droopy upper lid
7. Define *keratoconjunctivitis sicca* and name the usual treatment.
8. Name the condition resulting from inflammation of the lacrimal sac.
9. Distinguish between the signs and symptoms of bacterial, viral, and allergic conjunctivitis.
10. Describe a subconjunctival hemorrhage and its probable cause.
11. Distinguish between a pinguecula and a pterygium with respect to appearance and symptoms.
12. Name the symptoms and treatment of a bacterial or fungal corneal ulcer.
13. Describe how a corneal ulcer caused by the herpes simplex virus differs from a bacterial or fungal corneal ulcer.

14. Describe the condition known as *keratoconus*.
15. Describe what happens when drainage of aqueous humor is hindered, and name the resulting pathologic condition.
16. Match the four main types of glaucoma with their descriptions.

    ____ primary open-angle

    ____ primary angle-closure

    ____ secondary

    ____ congenital

    a. Malformation of anterior chamber angle along with other ocular deformities
    b. Reduced aqueous drainage resulting from another disease
    c. Reduced aqueous drainage in outflow channels between trabecular meshwork and blood vessels
    d. Blocked drainage because the iris is bowed forward due to a swollen lens
17. What principal change occurs in a lens affected by a cataract?
18. Name four possible causes of cataracts.
19. What are floaters?
20. What is the name of an infection of the vitreous and adjacent tissues?
21. What is a retinal detachment?
22. What symptoms do patients experience with a retinal detachment?
23. How is eye function altered as a result of age-related macular degeneration?
24. What is papilledema?
25. Name four possible causes of damage to the nerve cells of the visual pathway.

SUGGESTED ACTIVITIES

1. Ask your ophthalmologist to allow you to observe patients who have any of the diseases or disorders described in this chapter. Note any variations in the signs described, and ask the physician to explain the apparent differences. It is important to remember that an individual rarely shows all the possible signs or symptoms of a condition.
2. Select one structure of the adnexa or the eye and list as many disorders and diseases as you can, including their possible causes, signs, symptoms, and treatments.

SUGGESTED RESOURCES

Bradford CA, ed: *Basic Ophthalmology for Medical Students and Primary Care Residents.* 7th ed. San Francisco: American Academy of Ophthalmology; 1999.

Cassin B: *Fundamentals for Ophthalmic Technical Personnel.* Philadelphia: WB Saunders Co; 1995; chaps 27–28.

Goldberg S: *Ophthalmology Made Ridiculously Simple.* Miami: MedMaster; 1996.

Stein HA, Slatt BJ, Stein RM: *The Ophthalmic Assistant: A Guide for Ophthalmic Medical Personnel.* 7th ed. St Louis: Mosby; 2000.

Von Noorden GK, Campos EC: *Binocular Vision and Ocular Motility: Theory and Management of Strabismus.* 6th ed. St Louis: Mosby; 2002.

4 Optics and Refractive States of the Eye

As the primary organ of vision, the eye operates much like a camera. Light rays reflected from objects pass through the optical system of the eye, the cornea, and lens and are focused to form images of the objects on the light-sensitive retina. Various disease conditions of the eye and the visual pathway can interfere with vision or even totally destroy sight. However, nonpathologic deficiencies in the optical system of an essentially healthy eye may also produce less than satisfactory vision. In this case, the "camera" isn't broken; it just produces pictures that are out of focus or distorted. Such nonpathologic deficiencies in the eye's optical system, known as refractive errors, can be corrected by the use of supplementary lenses in the form of eyeglasses or contact lenses or by refractive surgery.

Ophthalmic medical assistants may participate in the determination of the patient's refractive state and the measurement of refractive errors that may be present. Such assistance requires a basic knowledge of optics—a science that studies the properties and behavior of light—especially as it pertains to lenses used to correct refractive errors. In addition to optics, lenses, and the nature of refractive errors, this chapter discusses the basic principles and elements of procedures used to discover, measure, and correct refractive errors. It includes instructions for performing and recording the results of two major related tests: lensometry and keratometry.

FIGURE 4.1

The spectrum of electromagnetic radiation. Note the narrow band of visible light.

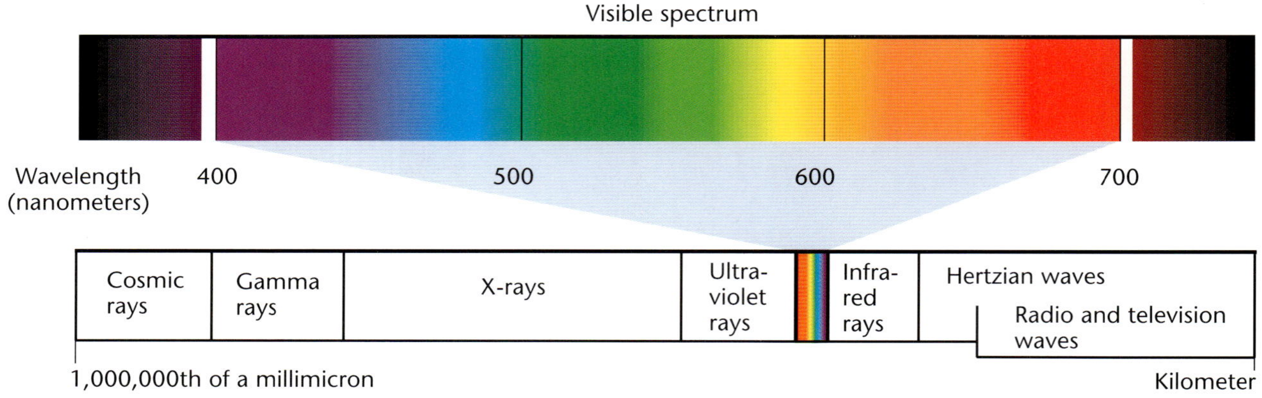

PRINCIPLES OF OPTICS

Optics is the branch of physical science that deals with the properties of light and vision. To simplify study of this complex subject, the science of optics has been divided into different areas. Two principal areas that most concern ophthalmology are **physical optics**, which describes the nature of light in terms of its wave properties, and **geometric optics**, which deals with the transmission of light as rays and is concerned with the effect of lenses on light and the production of images.

What is commonly referred to as light is the very small *visible* portion of a wide spectrum of **electromagnetic radiation** (Figure 4.1). The spectrum ranges from invisible cosmic, gamma, and x-rays, through visible light waves, to invisible radio and television signals. All these forms of energy travel through space and various substances as waves, each wave having a crest and a trough just as ocean waves do.

One way of differentiating the types of electromagnetic energy is by wavelength—the distance between crests of the wave. X-rays, for example, have a wavelength of about one billionth of a centimeter, while, at the opposite end of the spectrum, radio waves have a wavelength that is measured in kilometers. The wavelengths of light visible to the human eye lie roughly in the middle of the spectrum of electromagnetic radiation, ranging from about 400 to 750 *billionths* of a meter. These wavelengths comprise light with the colors violet, blue, green, yellow, orange, and red. Violet light has the shortest wavelength; red, the longest.

As with all forms of energy in the electromagnetic spectrum, light can travel through certain substances but may be blocked by others. Substances that completely block light are called **opaque**; those that transmit light but significantly interfere with its passage are referred to as **translucent**; substances that permit the passage of light without significant disruption are referred to as **transparent**. It is the behavior of light rays as they pass through transparent objects that most affects the correction of refractive errors.

Refraction

Light rays are **refracted** (bent) when they pass at an angle from one transparent medium, such as air, into another transparent medium, such as water, glass, or plastic, and are refracted once again when they exit the second medium. A simple illustration of refraction can be obtained by poking a straw into a glass of water (Figure 4.2). If you look at the straw from directly above, you will see it continue straight into the water; but if you look at it from an angle, the straw appears to bend at the point where it enters the water. This phenomenon is due to the differences in the speed at which light travels through various substances.

Light travels through a vacuum at a speed of 300,000 kilometers per second (about 186,000 miles

FIGURE 4.2

Refraction. Viewed at an angle, a straw appears to bend when it enters the water in a glass.

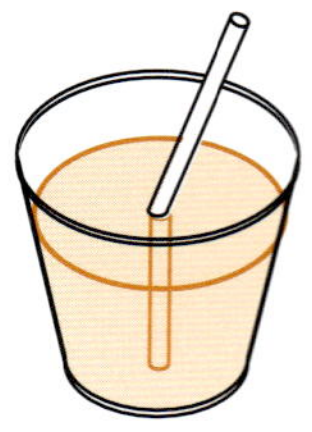

Table 4.1 Index of Refraction for Substances of Interest in Ophthalmology

Substance	*Index*
Air	1.00
Water	1.33
Aqueous humor	1.34
Cornea	1.37
Crystalline lens	1.39
PMMA plastic	1.49
Crown glass	1.52
Flint glass	1.65

per second). On passage through other transparent media or substances, light slows down somewhat, depending on the **density** (compactness) of the particular substance. The ratio of the speed of light in a vacuum to its speed in a specific substance is called the **refractive index** of that substance:

$$\text{refractive index} = \frac{\text{speed of light in a vacuum}}{\text{speed of light in a specific substance}}$$

The more dense the substance, the slower the speed of light and the higher the refractive index. Refractive indices of some common substances are presented in Table 4.1. Because the speed of light in air is close to that in a vacuum, the refractive index of air is 1.00. The refractive indices of other, more dense substances are all greater than 1.00. The refractive index of transparent substances such as glass or plastic (that is, the extent to which these substances bend light) is a useful property considered in the manufacture of lenses.

Refractive Properties of Curved Lenses

Lenses are transparent optical devices shaped in ways that can alter normal vision (such as with microscopes and telescopes) and improve poor vision (such as with eyeglasses and contact lenses). An understanding of how curved lenses are formed and how they refract light to achieve various optical effects may be gained by considering the refractive properties of prisms.

FIGURE 4.3

Passage of light through prisms. (A) Prism deviates light toward its base. (B) Light rays passing through two prisms placed base to base converge. (C) Light rays passing through two prisms placed apex to apex diverge.

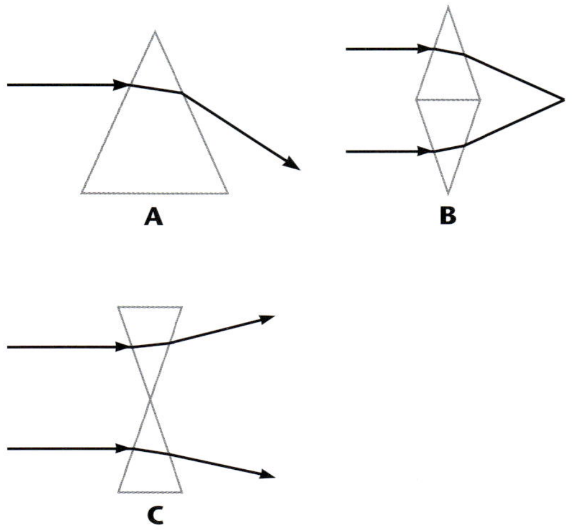

A **prism** is a triangular piece of glass or plastic with **plane** (flat) sides, an **apex** (top), and a **base** (bottom). When a light ray passes through a prism, the emerging light ray bends in a direction toward the *base* of the prism (Figure 4.3A). If two prisms are placed together base to base, light rays passing through the glass or plastic will be refracted to **converge** (come together) at some point on the other side of the prisms (Figure 4.3B). If, on the other hand, two prisms are placed together apex to apex, the light rays will **diverge** (spread apart) on the other side of the prisms (Figure 4.3C).

Smoothing the sharp angles of adjacent prisms into curves where they meet yields the two basic forms of lenses. The first type is called a **convex lens** (Figure 4.4A). This lens is a piece of glass or plastic in which one or both surfaces are curved outward. In the second type, the **concave lens** (Figure 4.4B), one or both surfaces are curved inward. These simple forms retain the same light-converging or light-diverging properties of the pair of prisms from which they are derived.

Convergence, Divergence, and Focal Point

The effects of lenses on light are generally considered in terms of light rays that emanate or are reflected from a distant object. These rays are said to be **parallel** to one another; that is, they travel side by side in the same direction.

FIGURE 4.4

A pair of prisms smoothed to form (A) a convex lens and (B) a concave lens, and the subsequent matching refractive characteristics of the lenses.

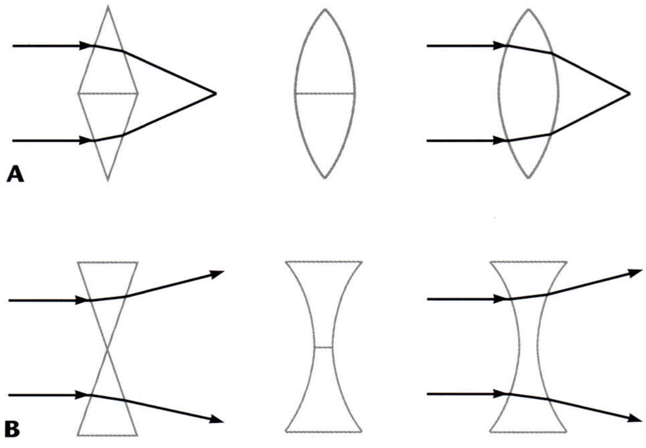

FIGURE 4.5

Passage of light rays through a convex (converging) lens. C = center of lens. F = focal point on principal axis behind lens.

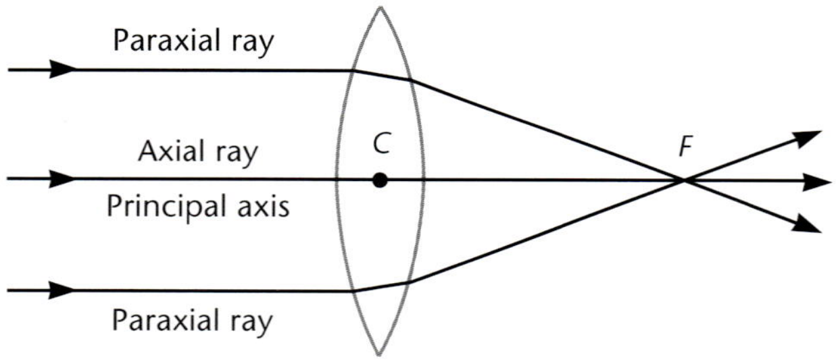

FIGURE 4.6

A real, inverted image of the light source is seen when a screen is placed at the focal point of the convex lens.

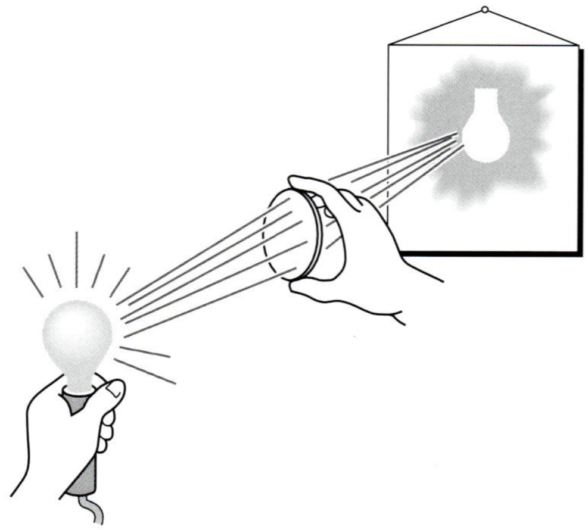

FIGURE 4.7

Passage of light rays through a concave (diverging) lens. C = center of lens. F' = virtual focal point on principal axis in front of lens.

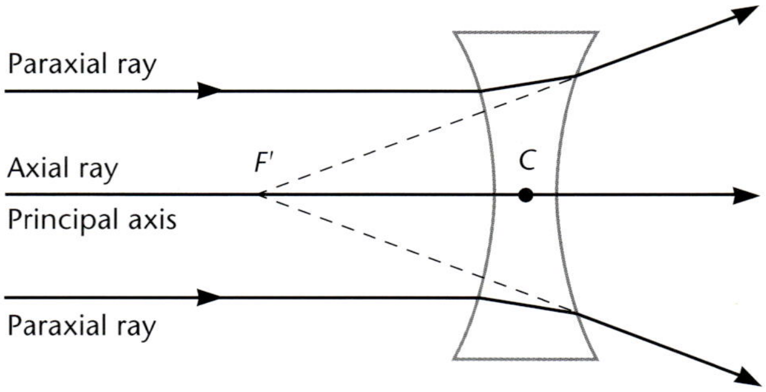

A light ray that strikes the center of a lens of any shape passes undeviated through the lens material, regardless of the lens' index of refraction. This pathway is known as the **principal axis** of the lens, and the light ray is called the **axial** or **principal ray**. Parallel light rays from a distant source that enter the lens at any point other than the center are called **paraxial rays**.

With convex lenses, the paraxial rays from a distant source are refracted by the lens material and *converge* at a point somewhere along the principal axis *behind* the lens, that is, on the side of the lens opposite from the object (Figure 4.5). This point is known as the **focal point** of the lens. If you placed a piece of paper or a screen at the exact focal point, you would see a clear, real image of the object from which the light rays originally emanated, although the image would be inverted (upside down) and reversed (Figure 4.6). Convex lenses are called **positive** or **plus lenses**.

With concave lenses, the paraxial rays from a distant source are refracted by the lens material and *diverge* as they emerge from the lens (Figure 4.7). As a result, they cannot be focused behind the lens, and they produce no real image. However, if the direction of the diverging light rays is extended backward in a drawing, an imaginary or "virtual" focal point can be found in *front* of the lens where the lines meet the principal axis, that is, on the same side of the lens as the object. A **virtual image** of the light source can be seen at this point, but it cannot be focused on a screen. Concave lenses are called **negative** or **minus lenses**.

FIGURE 4.8

The relationship of lens power to focal length. (A) Three plus, or convex (converging), lenses. (B) Three minus, or concave (diverging), lenses.

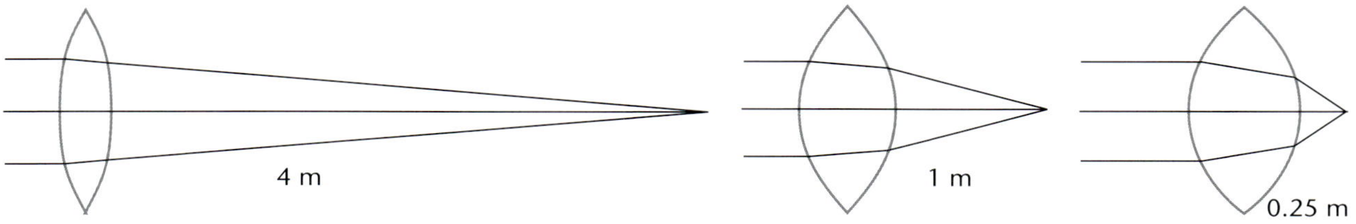

A

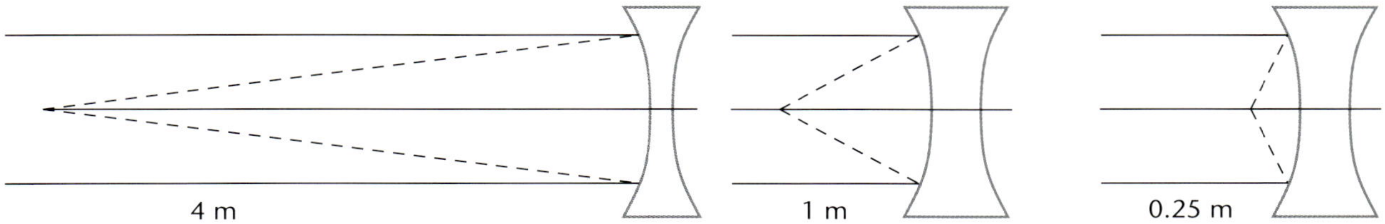

B

Lens Power and Focal Length

The **vergence power**, or simply **power**, of a lens is a measure of its ability to converge or diverge light rays. This ability depends on the refractive index of the lens material and on the shape of the lens. "Fat" convex lenses of a given material produce greater convergence than do "thin" convex lenses of the same substance and so are more powerful. Similarly, concave lenses with greater curvature cause more divergence than do concave lenses with less curvature and thus are more powerful.

The greater the convergence or divergence of light rays by a lens, the closer the focal point will be to the lens along its principal axis (Figure 4.8). In other words, the distance between the focal point and the lens, the **focal length**, is related *inversely* to the power of the lens (that is, the stronger the lens, the shorter its focal length). Lens power is considered in terms of focal length, as follows: the power of a lens is equal to the *reciprocal* of the focal length measured in meters and is expressed in units called **diopters**:

$$D = 1/F$$

where D = lens power in diopters and F = focal length in meters. For example, a convex lens with a focal length of 2 meters has a power of 1/2, or 0.50 D; a convex lens with a focal length of 0.25 meter has a power of 1/0.25, or 4.00 D.

As described earlier, concave (minus) lenses cause light rays from a distant source to diverge, producing a virtual image in front of the lens. For this reason, the power of a minus lens is expressed in negative diopters. For example, a concave lens with a focal length of 2 meters has a power of –1/2, or –0.50 D; a concave lens with a focal length of –0.25 meter has a power of –1/0.25, or –4.00 D. Understanding the basis and methods of expressing lens power is important in measuring and correcting refractive errors of the eye.

REFRACTIVE STATES OF THE EYE

The principles of optics and the properties of lenses discussed above apply equally to the optical system of the human eye. The eye is a plus-power system consisting of the convex cornea and crystalline lens, which refract light rays reflected from objects and focus them to produce real images on the retina. The overall converging power of the eye is approximately 60 diopters, 40 of which are attributed to the cornea and 20 to the crystalline lens. Because the normal lens can change its curvature and thus its power, it serves

FIGURE 4.9

The emmetropic eye: parallel rays of light focus sharply on the retina.

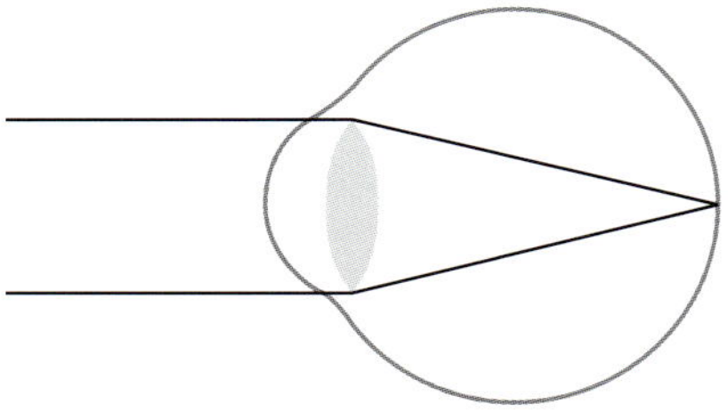

FIGURE 4.10

The myopic eye: parallel rays of light are brought to a focus in front of the retina.

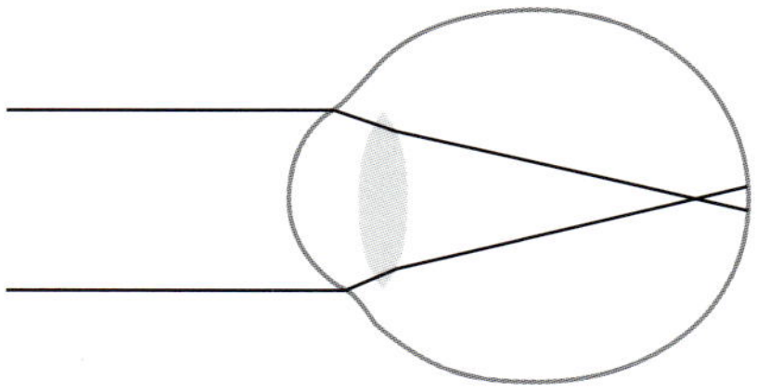

FIGURE 4.11

The hyperopic eye: parallel rays of light would come to a focus behind the retina in the unaccommodated eye.

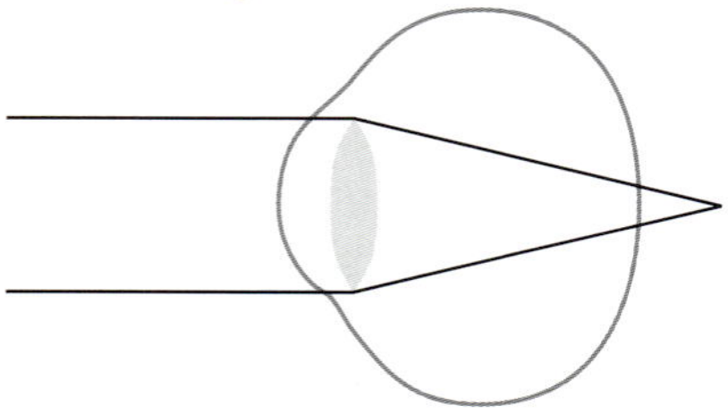

as the fine adjustment of focus. This capability, called *accommodation*, is important because although the screen (retina) on which images are focused is fixed in its distance from the refractive elements of the eye, the objects on which gaze is directed are not.

The term **refractive state** refers to the relative ability of the refractive components of the eye (the cornea and lens) to bring objects into focus on the retina. The two principal refractive states are emmetropia, an ability to focus correctly, and ametropia, an inability to focus correctly due to various refractive errors.

Emmetropia

In the normal eye, light rays from a distant object are focused sharply on the retina by the relaxed lens without the need of any accommodative effort. This condition is called **emmetropia** (Figure 4.9).

Ametropia

When the relaxed, or nonaccommodating, eye is unable to bring light rays from a distant object into focus, the condition is called **ametropia**. Three basic conditions may produce this refractive error: (1) myopia, (2) hyperopia, or hypermetropia, and (3) astigmatism. A fourth abnormality, presbyopia, is a condition of diminished power of accommodation that primarily affects near vision and is a normal condition of aging.

Myopia

Myopia (nearsightedness) is a condition in which the cornea and lens of the nonaccommodating eye have too much plus power for the length of the eye. As a result, images of distant objects are focused in front of the retina and thus appear blurred (Figure 4.10). Various causes have been suggested to explain the development of myopia, ranging from excessive close work and reading to improper diet. However, research efforts to confirm the causes of myopia have been inconclusive. Most authorities agree that some myopia is genetic in origin and is the result of an eyeball inherently longer than normal. Near vision in people with myopia is almost always good. Because of the greater relative plus power of their optical system, myopic individuals not wearing corrective lenses require less accommodation for near vision than do people with normal eyes.

Hyperopia

Hyperopia (farsightedness) is a condition in which the cornea and lens have too little plus power for the length of the nonaccommodating eye. As a result, light rays from a distant object come to a focus at a point theoretically behind the retina and the image appears blurred (Figure 4.11). For many individuals, accommodation by the lens can supply the needed additional converging power and bring the distant light rays into focus on the retina. The problem, of course, is that the lens may not have sufficient *addi-*

FIGURE 4.12

Classes of regular astigmatism. (A) Simple hyperopic astigmatism: one meridian focuses light on the retina, the other theoretically behind the retina. (B) Simple myopic astigmatism: one meridian focuses light in front of the retina, the other on the retina. (C) Compound hyperopic astigmatism: both meridians focus light theoretically behind the retina. (D) Compound myopic astigmatism: both meridians focus light in front of the retina. (E) Mixed astigmatism: one meridian focuses light in front of the retina, the other behind the retina.

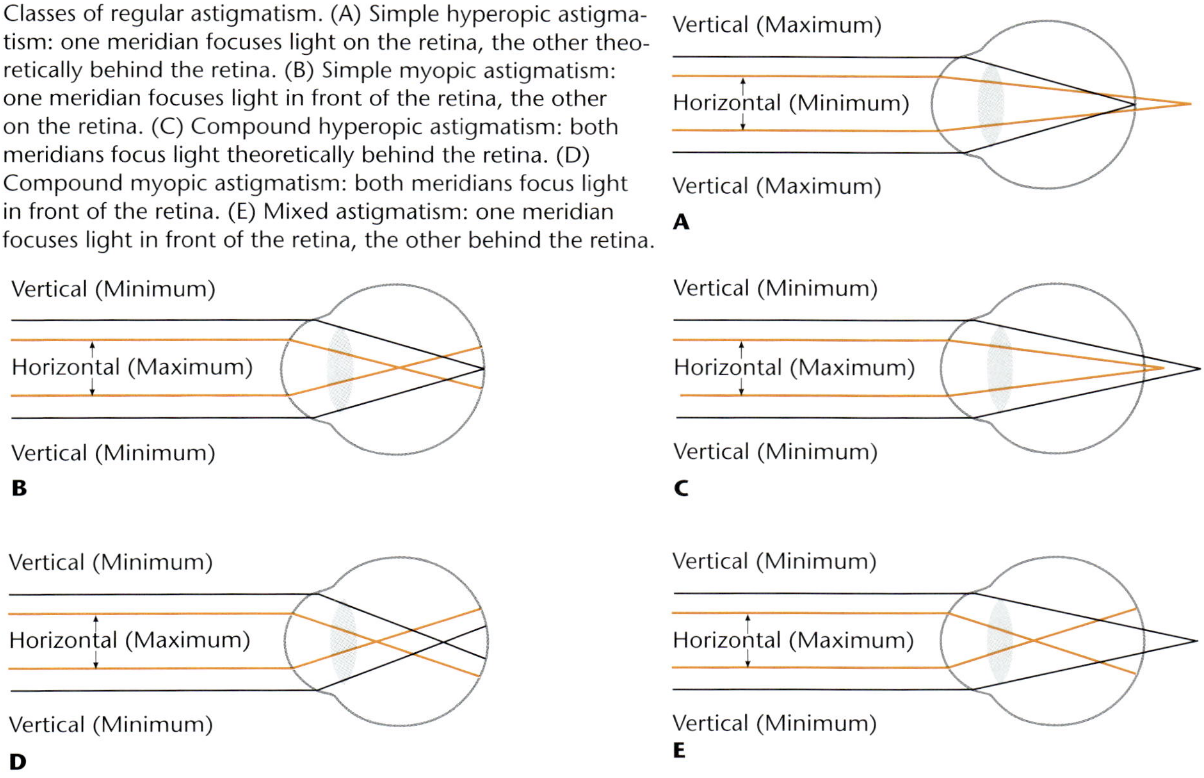

tional accommodative power to focus light rays for near vision. Healthy children have an ample reserve of accommodation and, if hyperopic, can unconsciously accommodate for both distant and near objects. As accommodative ability gradually declines with maturity, these hyperopic individuals will notice a loss of clear near vision.

Almost all infants are hyperopic at birth, but generally the eye lengthens and approaches normal size as the infant matures. The chief cause of hyperopia is an eye that remains shorter than normal. In other cases, the cornea and/or lens has less curvature than normal.

Astigmatism

The cornea of the normal eye and of most myopic and hyperopic individuals has a uniform curvature, with resulting equal refracting power over its entire surface; this is the **spherical cornea**. In some individuals, however, the cornea is not uniform—the **toric cornea**—and the curvature is greater in one **meridian** (plane) than another, much like a football. The result is different levels of myopia or hyperopia in different optical planes. Light rays refracted by the toric cornea are not brought to a single point focus, and retinal images from objects both distant and near are blurred and may appear broadened or elongated. This refractive error is called **astigmatism**.

The **principal meridians**—the meridians of maximum and minimum corneal curvature—are usually at right angles to each other in astigmatism and are usually (but not necessarily) in the vertical and horizontal planes. In **regular astigmatism**, which is the more common form, the cornea would resemble a football standing on one end or on its side or, less often, tipped to one side. In **irregular astigmatism**, which is less common, the corneal "football" would have an irregular or bumpy shape. Various types of regular astigmatism have been identified on the basis of the refractive power and position of the principal meridians, as illustrated and described in Figure 4.12.

Presbyopia

Presbyopia is a progressive loss of the accommodative ability of the crystalline lens due to the natural processes of aging. To understand presbyopia, consider the mechanism of accommodation (Figure 4.13). An emmetropic eye can focus light rays from

FIGURE 4.13

Accommodation in the emmetropic eye. (A) No accommodation is necessary to focus light rays from a distant object, but (B) rays from a near object are focused behind the retina, unless (C) accommodation is brought into play.

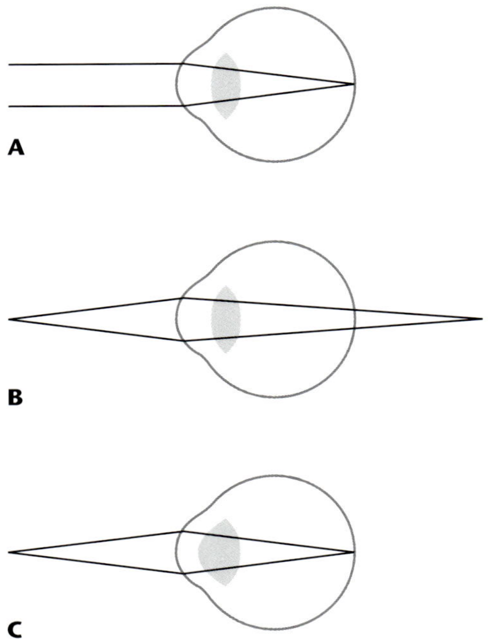

distant objects on the retina without the aid of accommodation. However, light rays from near objects (those closer than 20 feet, or 6 meters, which is generally considered to be "optical infinity") would normally focus behind the retina unless accommodation —an increase in the curvature and thus the plus power of the crystalline lens—occurred. This accommodative mechanism is particularly strong in children but gradually diminishes with age as the lens loses its elasticity. The normal hardening of the lens begins at birth but generally does not cause a problem until about the age of 40 or 45 years. When the loss of accommodation interferes with, or prevents, clear near vision, the result is presbyopia.

Presbyopia may occur in the presence of emmetropia, myopia, and hyperopia, as well as astigmatism. Its onset results in increasing difficulty with near visual work, such as reading small print (especially in dim light), sewing, and the like. However, this effect and the age at which a myopic or hyperopic individual might first perceive this difficulty can vary according to the type and extent of the refractive error and whether an individual wears corrective lenses or contact lenses.

TYPES AND USES OF CORRECTIVE LENSES

The principal refractive errors of the eye can be corrected by the use of ophthalmic lenses in the form of eyeglasses or contact lenses, refractive surgery, or surgical implantation of an artificial lens (intraocular lens implants).

There are several types of refractive surgery, including radial keratotomy (RK), photorefractive keratectomy (PRK), and laser-assisted in situ keratomileusis (LASIK). In RK, the ophthalmologist uses a surgeon's knife to make tiny radial cuts around the visual axis (primary line of sight) of the cornea to correct nearsightedness. In PRK and LASIK, which are newer techniques, the excimer laser is used to reshape the cornea to correct nearsightedness, farsightedness, and astigmatism. After these procedures, most people become much less dependent on their eyeglasses or contact lenses. However, the vast majority of people with refractive errors today still use glasses or contact lenses. A more detailed discussion of refractive surgery is beyond the scope of this text.

Lenses used to correct refractive errors are generally made of glass or plastic and, like all lenses, refract light rays as described earlier in this chapter. In various forms, corrective lenses can supply needed additional convergence (as in hyperopia), compensate for excess convergence (as in myopia), correct refractive errors that are not uniform in all meridians of the eye (as in astigmatism), and provide near vision that has been reduced due to presbyopia.

Table 4.2 lists the principal ophthalmic lens types, shapes, and corrective uses. The basic types of ophthalmic lenses used to test for and correct refrac-

Table 4.2 Properties and Uses of Ophthalmic Corrective Lenses

Lens Type	*Lens Shape and Power*	*Corrective Use*
Sphere	Convex (+)	Hyperopia
	Concave (–)	Myopia
Cylinder	Spherocylindrical (+ or –)	Astigmatism
Prism	Plane, with at least two nonparallel surfaces	Double vision

FIGURE 4.14

Refraction by a spherical lens (in this case, a planoconvex sphere). Because its radii of curvature (*a, b*) are equal, a sphere brings light rays to a single point focus (*F*).

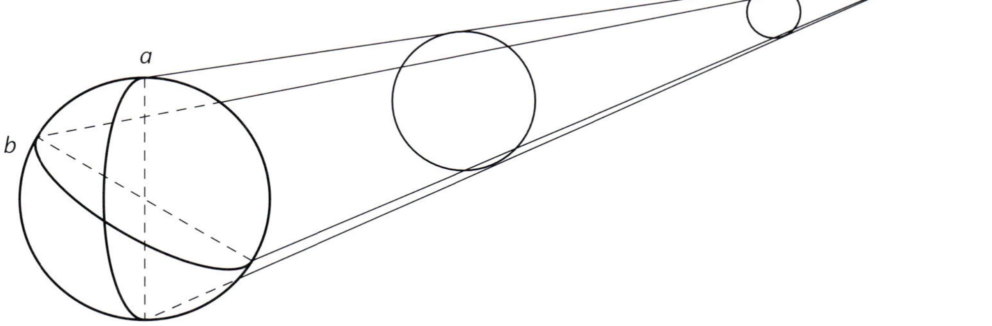

tive errors are spheres, cylinders, and a combination of the two (spherocylinders). Although they are not lenses in the traditional sense, prisms are sometimes categorized as such because they are incorporated into eyeglasses to correct visual misalignments. Ophthalmic medical assistants require an understanding of the specific properties and uses of these lenses in order to take measurements used in arriving at a patient's corrective eyeglass or contact lens prescription and to measure certain qualities of existing corrective lenses. These procedures are discussed later in this chapter.

FIGURE 4.15

Segmented multifocal lenses. (A) Bifocal. (B) Trifocal.

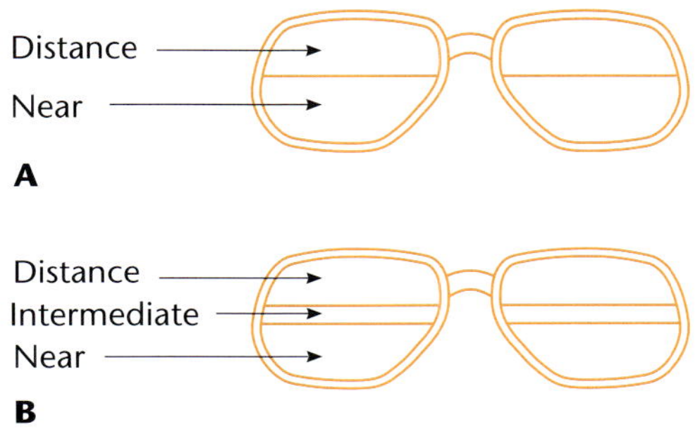

Spheres

A lens that has the same curvature over its entire surface and, thus, the same refractive power in all directions, or meridians, is referred to as a **spherical lens** or **sphere**. Spherical lenses may be convex or concave and of any dioptric power. The term *sphere* or *spherical lens* was adopted because the lens may be thought of as having been cut from a sphere of glass or plastic. Because of its uniform curvature and refractive ability, a spherical lens is able to focus light rays at a single point (Figure 4.14).

Spherical plus-power (convex) lenses are used to provide clear near vision for hyperopic individuals. Plus-power spherical lenses also provide near vision to emmetropic individuals with presbyopia; corrective eyeglasses for this purpose are sometimes referred to as reading glasses, since wearers use them only for reading and other near work. Spherical minus-power (concave) lenses are used to provide distance vision for those with myopia. Because near vision is often good with myopia, myopic individuals who develop presbyopia may need only remove their glasses to read and do close work.

For some patients, segmented two- or three-part eyeglass lenses—**bifocals** and **trifocals**—may be prescribed (Figure 4.15). In these eyeglasses, commonly referred to as **multifocal lenses**, the uppermost portion carries the minus or plus sphere correction (and cylinder if needed) for distance vision, while the power of the lowermost segment is adjusted for near vision (14 to 16 inches). The lower segment is always plus power added to the distance correction. The difference between the power of the upper segment and that of the lower segment is known as the **add**. In the case of myopia, the adjustment is a less negative (or more positive) correction, while a hyperopic individual receives plus power in addition to that required for distance vision. The middle segment in trifocals corrects vision for an intermediate distance (2 to 4 feet). The types and specific uses of these and other multifocal lenses are discussed in depth in Chapter 8, "Fundamentals of Practical Opticianry."

FIGURE 4.16

The axis of a cylinder is located 90° from its meridian with curvature.

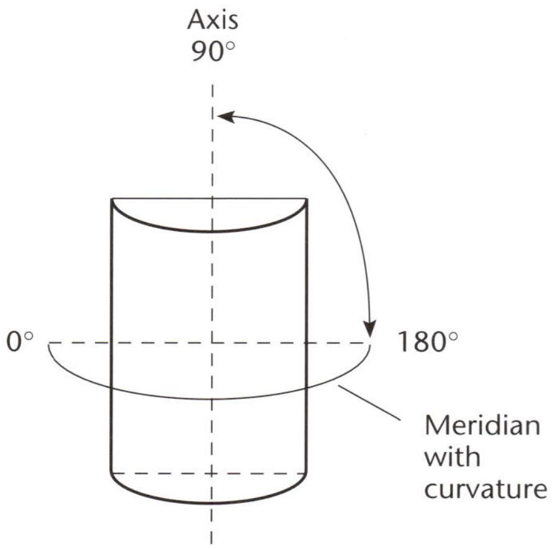

FIGURE 4.17

Refraction by a cylinder. Because a cylinder has refracting power in only one meridian (perpendicular to its axis), it focuses light to a focal line.

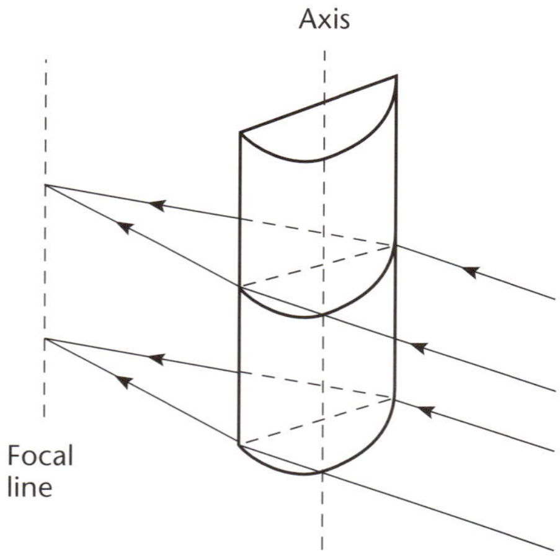

Cylinders

Pure **cylindrical lenses**, or **cylinders**, differ from spheres in that they have curvature, and thus refractive power, in only *one* meridian. They may be convex or concave and of any dioptric power. The meridian perpendicular to (90° from) the meridian with curvature is called the **axis** of the cylinder (Figure 4.16). By convention, the orientation (position in space) of the cylinder is indicated by the axis, which ranges from 0° (horizontal) through 90° (vertical), and back to 180° (the same as 0°). In contrast to a spherical lens, a cylinder focuses light rays to a **focal line** rather than to a point (Figure 4.17).

FIGURE 4.18

(A) A toric (spherocylindrical) football has different curvatures in each of two principal meridians. (B) A spherical basketball possesses the same curvature over its entire surface.

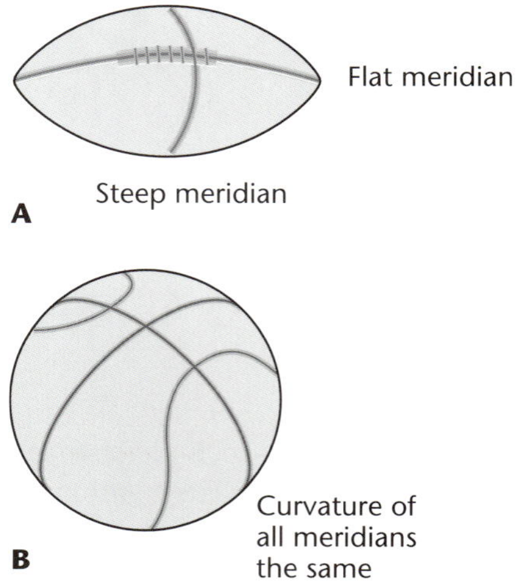

Pure cylindrical lenses are used in ophthalmology only for testing purposes. Theoretically, a pure cylindrical lens—one that possesses power in only one meridian—might be used to correct astigmatism. However, most astigmatic individuals are hyperopic or myopic as well and require correction in more than one meridian. To provide the correction they need, a lens formed from the combination of cylinder and sphere is generally required.

Spherocylinders

A **spherocylinder**, as its name suggests, is a combination of a sphere and a cylinder. It is sometimes also called a **toric lens**, but in practice is often referred to as a **cylinder** for the sake of simplicity.

If a spherical lens may be imagined as cut from an object shaped like a basketball, a spherocylindrical lens can be thought of as cut from an object shaped like a football. Unlike the spherical "basketball," which has the same curvature over its entire surface, the spherocylindrical "football" has different curvatures in each of two perpendicular meridians (Figure 4.18). The meridian along the length of the football is termed the "flat" meridian, and the one at the football's fat center is termed the "steep" meridian.

Because the perpendicular radii of its curvature are not equal, a spherocylinder does not focus light to a single focal point, as does a sphere. Rather, it refracts light along each of its two meridians to two

FIGURE 4.19

Refraction by a spherocylinder. Because its perpendicular radii of curvature (*x, y*) are not equal, a spherocylinder does not focus light to a point, but to two lines (*y* focal line, *x* focal line) in different places. The clearest image is formed at the circle of least confusion.

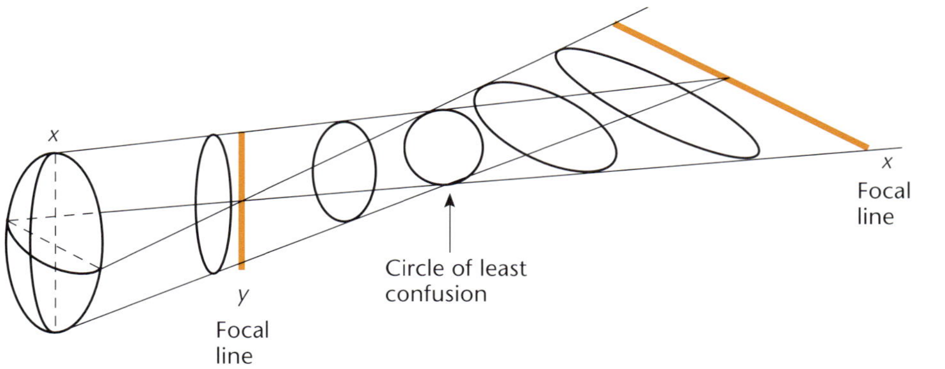

different focal lines (Figure 4.19). The clearest image is formed at a point between these two focal lines, which is given the geometric term *circle of least confusion*. The ability of a spherocylindrical lens to refract light along each of two meridians makes it ideal to correct myopia or hyperopia that is combined with astigmatism. The spherocylinder can supply varying amounts of plus and/or minus correction to each of the two principal meridians of the astigmatic eye.

Two qualities of a spherocylinder must be recorded in order to prescribe the appropriate correcting lens for an astigmatic individual or to measure a patient's existing corrective lens: (1) the amount (in dioptric power) and the type of correction (plus or minus) in each of the two principal meridians; and (2) the position of the astigmatic axis. The latter must be known because although the meridians are usually perpendicular to each other, they may not be in strict vertical (90°) and horizontal (180°) position. The technique of measuring these qualities of spherocylindrical lenses, as well as specific qualities of other types of lenses, is called **lensometry**. The purpose and methods of performing lensometry are discussed later in this chapter.

Prisms

Because of its shape, a prism deviates (refracts) light rays toward its base. This effect causes objects viewed through prisms to appear displaced toward the prism apex (Figure 4.20). Depending on the refractive power and orientation of a prism, an object can be seen to appear in various locations other than its actual position. Because of this unique refracting property, prisms are employed in a number of ophthalmic instruments. Prisms are used to measure visual misalignments, and they can be incorporated into eyeglass lenses to correct diplopia.

FIGURE 4.20

(A) Because of its shape, a prism refracts light rays toward its base. (B) If an object is viewed through a prism, the object appears displaced toward the prism apex.

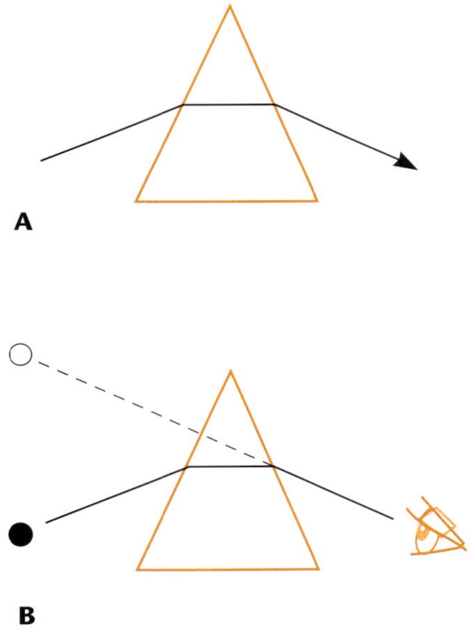

The refractive power of a prism depends on its composition and the size of its apex angle. This power is measured in terms of the prism's ability to deviate a ray of light and is expressed in prism diopters (Figure 4.21). A prism measuring 1 prism diopter (1^{Δ}) deviates parallel rays of light 1 centimeter at a distance of 100 centimeters (1 meter) from the prism. A prism that deviates rays 1 centimeter at a distance of 2 meters measures 0.5^{Δ}; a prism that deviates rays 1 centimeter from a distance of ½ meter (0.5 m)

FIGURE 4.21

Prism refractive power. A prism measuring 1 prism diopter deflects a light ray 1 centimeter at a distance of 1 meter.

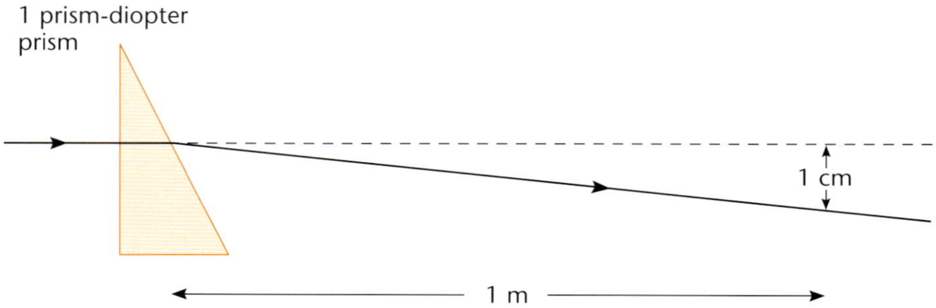

measures 2^{Δ}. Knowledge of this measurement convention is important in understanding the power and orientation of a prism needed to test for visual misalignments and correct double vision.

COMPONENTS OF REFRACTION

The physicist defines **refraction** as the bending of light rays as they pass through substances of different densities. In eye care, the term **refraction** is used to describe the process of measuring a patient's refractive error and determining the optical correction needed to focus light rays from distant objects onto the retina and provide the patient with clear vision.

The process of refraction comprises two main components: **refractometry**, a multifaceted measurement of refractive errors with a variety of specific instruments and techniques, and clinical judgment, which is required to prescribe appropriate optical correction. Ophthalmic medical assistants are often responsible for many of the measurements involved in refractometry; the ophthalmologist alone provides the clinical judgment needed to verify the refractometric results, assess related needs of the patient, and prescribe appropriate correction. Because considerable skill and experience are required to perform the complex steps of refractometry well, this section provides only general descriptions and principles of these processes.

Refractometry may be divided into three separate steps:

1. Retinoscopy
2. Refinement
3. Binocular balancing

These steps may be performed manually with a variety of instruments and materials or partly with automated refractors. The automated units can be moderately accurate and very efficient, but their utility will depend on their ability to produce the specific kinds of information the ophthalmologist needs to determine the appropriate correction. Performance of manual refractometry is an important skill for ophthalmic medical assistants. Even in practices where automated refractors are used, knowledge of the principles and methods of manual refractometry is required to use the equipment properly.

Whether manual or automatic, refractometry may be performed either with or without the use of cycloplegic drops, solutions of drugs that temporarily paralyze the ciliary muscle and thus block accommodation. Known as **cycloplegic refraction**, this method is useful in measuring refractive errors in patients under 20 years old, whose powerful accommodative ability may contribute to false measurements and lead to inadequate correction of their refractive problem. When performed without cycloplegic drugs, as is the case with most other patients, the method of measurement is referred to as a **manifest refraction**.

The ophthalmologist usually determines whether manifest or cycloplegic refractometry is more appropriate for a given patient. Specific information about the uses, actions, and administration of cycloplegic drops appears in Chapter 11, "Basics of Ophthalmic Pharmacology."

Retinoscopy

Retinoscopy is the initial step in refractometry. It is used to determine the approximate nature and extent of a refractive error and to estimate the type and power of the lens needed to correct that error. Retinoscopy is sometimes referred to as **objective refractometry** because it requires no participation or

FIGURE 4.22

A retinoscope.

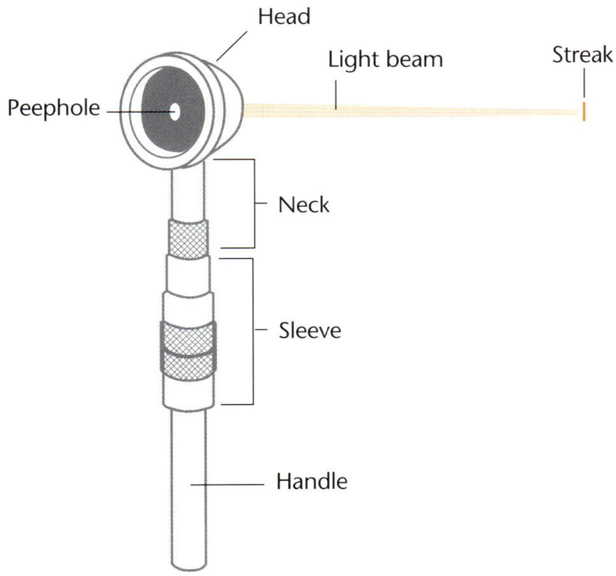

FIGURE 4.23

Reflexes produced by the streak retinoscope. (A) Normal. (B) "With" motion: the reflex moves in the same direction as the streak of light, indicating a hyperopic eye. (C) "Against" motion: the reflex moves in the direction opposite to that of the streak, indicating a myopic eye. (D) Neutralization point: there is no apparent movement of the reflex, and the pupil is filled with a red glow.

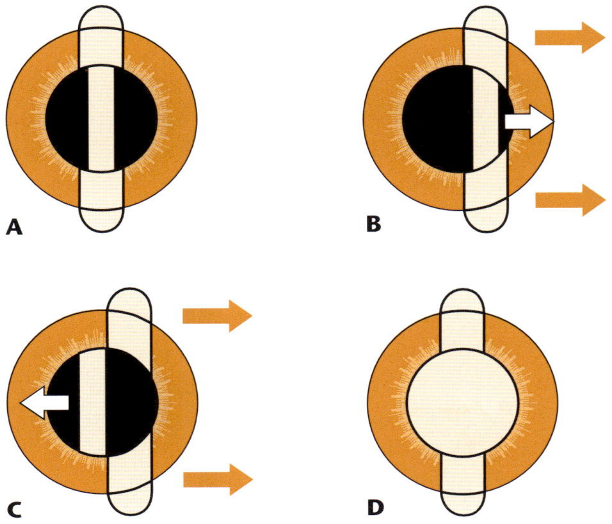

response from the patient. For some patients, such as children, retarded individuals, and others unable to communicate well, retinoscopy is the only way to determine the refractive error.

In performing retinoscopy, the examiner uses a **retinoscope**, an instrument consisting of a light source and a viewing component (Figure 4.22). A mirror in the retinoscope directs an adjustable beam of light at the patient's eye, while the examiner observes the eye through the viewer. Two basic types of retinoscopes are available: one produces a spot of light; the other, a streak. The discussion here is limited to the more commonly used streak retinoscope, as spot retinoscopes are essentially obsolete.

One eye is examined at a time in retinoscopy. If the patient's accommodation has not been blocked by cycloplegic drops, the patient is instructed or otherwise guided to **fixate** (gaze steadily at) a distant object. The examiner projects the streak of light from the retinoscope directly into the patient's eye. The light beam passes through the optical system of the eye and is reflected back by the patient's retina, appearing as a "retinoscopic reflex" in the patient's pupil.

The examiner, who sees the reflex as a red-orange glowing line (Figure 4.23A), watches its movement while sweeping the light across the pupil. As the light sweeps across the pupil, the different types of refractive errors of the eye produce characteristic movements of the reflex.

The direction in which these reflexes move is affected by the retinoscopic lighting effect chosen by the examiner. Retinoscopes allow the user to select either one of two lighting effects by raising or lowering a sleeve on the instrument handle to change the instrument's optical system. The **plano** (flat) **mirror effect** produces slightly divergent rays. The **concave mirror effect** produces convergent rays. The most commonly used retinoscopes require the sleeve to be raised to achieve the plano mirror effect and lowered to achieve the concave mirror effect. These positions are referred to as "sleeve up" and "sleeve down" respectively. To determine the plano mirror position, shine the streak against the palm of your hand in both the sleeve-up and sleeve-down positions. The streak will appear thickest when in the plano mirror position.

When the plano mirror effect of the retinoscope (usually "sleeve up") is being used, the hyperopic eye usually causes the retinoscopic reflex to move in the same direction as the streak of light. This movement is termed **with motion** (Figure 4.23B). The myopic eye usually causes the reflex to move in the opposite direction from the streak, termed **against motion**

(Figure 4.23C). An astigmatic eye causes different types or degrees of movement in the two principal meridians; astigmatic retinoscopic reflexes vary greatly and can be difficult to interpret, and further discussion of them is beyond the scope of this text.

As might be imagined, with and against motions are reversed if the examiner uses the concave mirror effect. However, for the purposes of this text, the succeeding discussions will assume that the plano mirror effect is in use.

The examiner can affect movement of the retinal reflex by placing corrective lenses between the patient's eye and the retinoscope. The objective is to find the lens power that will "neutralize" the reflex and fill the pupil with light (Figure 4.23D). The lens that achieves this **neutralization point** is the approximate correction for the patient's refractive error. Such a lens will neutralize the reflex regardless of the retinoscope's movement or the mirror effect used. If the eye has an astigmatic error, neutralization will have to be done for both the maximum and the minimum meridians and the axis identified.

During retinoscopy and neutralization, the examiner selects various lenses to introduce before the patient's eye by means of a **trial lens set** and **trial frame** (Figure 4.24) or with a **refractor**, also called a **Phoroptor** (Figure 4.25A), which stores a range of trial lenses that can be dialed into position (Figure 4.25B). When "with" motion is observed (hyperopia), plus lenses are added sequentially until sufficient power is present to achieve the neutralization point. When "against" motion occurs (myopia), minus lenses are added until the neutralization point is reached.

Because the examiner must be much closer to the patient than 20 feet (optical infinity) to perform retinoscopy and neutralization, an additional adjustment to the dioptric power of the neutralizing lens must be made to correct for the distance between the examiner and the patient (the "working distance"). The amount of adjustment needed can be easily calculated using a variation of the formula D = 1/F previously discussed: D = 1/working distance in meters. As an example, if the working distance is 50 cm, then D = 1/0.5 m = 2 D.

Refinement

The second step in refractometry is **refinement**. Also performed on one eye at a time, refinement consists of a group of procedures that provides a very precise measurement of refractive error and appropriate lens correction. It serves to refine (confirm) the information produced by retinoscopy. Refinement is sometimes referred to as **subjective refractometry** because it requires patient participation and reaction ("I can see better with this lens than with that one"). Because of its subjective nature, refinement is not possible with infants, some toddlers, and other patients who are unable to communicate adequately.

In the first step of the process, the patient views letters of various sizes on a special visual acuity chart placed at a distance of 20 feet from the patient. (This is usually the standard eye chart of letters or numbers that is familiar to many people through school or driver's-license screening procedures.) The examiner leads the patient by presenting a choice of lenses in the refractor or trial frame while asking a series of questions about the relative clarity of the images seen on the chart. The patient's responses guide the examiner to selecting the most appropriate lens to correct the refractive error in each of the patient's eyes.

The **cross cylinder** is a common refinement instrument used to confirm first the axis and then the power of a correcting cylindrical lens for astigmatism. The cross cylinder is a special lens consisting of two cylinders of equal power, one minus and one plus, with their axes set at right angles to each other (Figure 4.26). The technique requires choices and responses by the patient, and is extremely accurate.

FIGURE 4.24

A trial frame allows manual insertion of multiple lenses selected from a trial set.

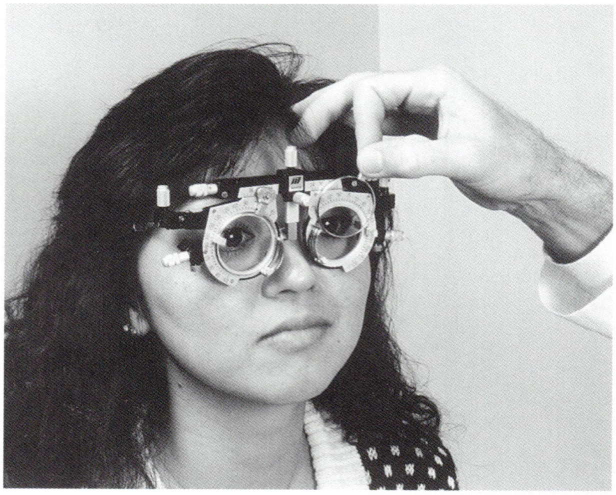

FIGURE 4.25

A Phoroptor (A) stores trial lenses, which (B) may be dialed into position.

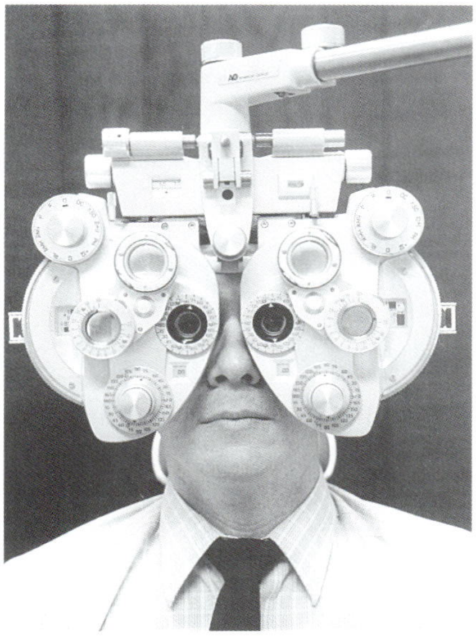

A

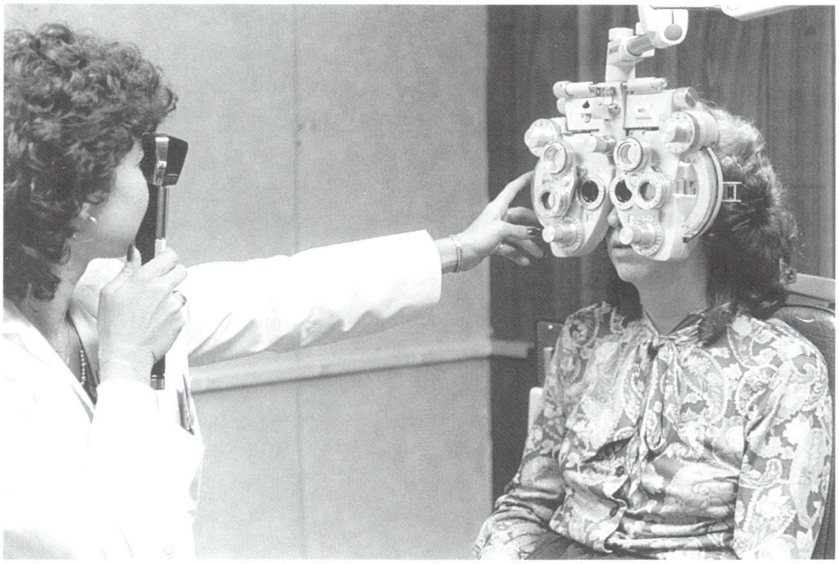

B

FIGURE 4.26

The cross cylinder, used to refine the selection of corrective cylindrical lenses for astigmatism.

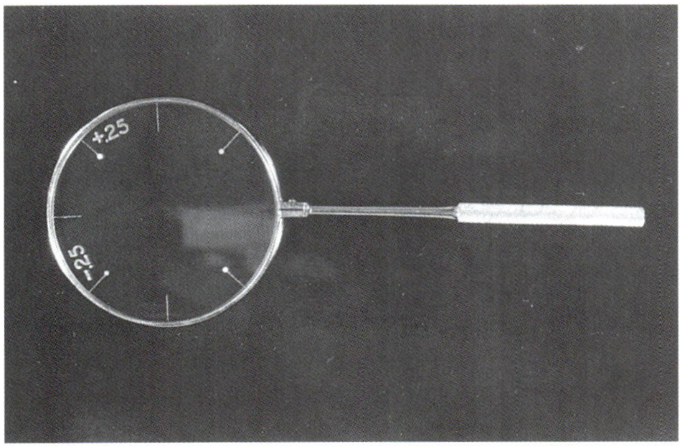

Binocular Balancing

Performed on both eyes at once, **balancing** (sometimes called **binocular balancing**) helps ensure that the optical correction determined by refractometry for distance vision does not include an uneven overcorrection or undercorrection for the two eyes. Such an anomaly can result from errors introduced by the patient's natural accommodation. Obviously, then, this procedure is unnecessary in patients who have undergone cycloplegic refraction or in patients whose accommodation is minimal or absent (patients over 60 years of age or those who have had cataracts removed). It also is not possible in patients with unequal visual acuity.

One technique used for balancing involves "fogging" the end-point refractive correction in both eyes with plus spheres. The rotary prisms on the Phoroptor are used to separate the images seen by the right and left eyes. This allows the patient to compare the clarity of the two images. If the original refraction was correctly balanced, the fogged images will look equally blurred. If one image appears clearer, the refraction may be unbalanced, and the refractometrist must consider making adjustments accordingly. More detailed instruction in balancing techniques can be found in many of the Suggested Resources listed at the end of this chapter.

INTERPRETATION OF PRESCRIPTIONS

The outcome of refraction is an optical prescription—a written description of the optical requirements for correcting the patient's refractive error. The ophthalmologist uses the information gathered during refractometry—power of sphere, and power and axis of cylinder for each eye if cylinder is required—together with other patient considerations only a doctor can evaluate to supply a prescription for corrective lenses. Ophthalmic medical assistants must understand the format used for writing eyeglass lens prescriptions to record accurately the results of refractometry and to interpret refractive data on patient medical charts and forms.

The prescription for spectacle lenses follows a standard format. The power of the sphere (abbreviated *sph*) is recorded first with its sign (+ = plus, or convex, sphere; – = minus, or concave, sphere), followed by the power of the cylinder with its sign and axis if a cylinder is required. The axis is designated by x, followed by a number of degrees. A prescription is recorded for each eye, using the abbreviations **OD** (*oculus dexter*) for the right and **OS** (*oculus sinister*) for the left eye.

A typical prescription for a patient with simple hyperopia might be

OD +2.00 sph
OS +2.25 sph

For simple myopia, the prescription might be

OD –2.50 sph
OS –2.25 sph

No cylinder is required in these cases. A prescription for corrective spherocylindrical lenses might read

OD plano ◌ –0.75 × 90°
OS plano ◌ –0.50 × 90°

In this example, *plano* means "no sphere power"; ◌ is the symbol for "combined with" – 0.75 and –0.50 indicate the sign and power of the cylinders; and 90° indicates their axes. For myopia combined with astigmatism, the prescription might look like the following:

OD –0.75 ◌ +0.50 × 150°
OS –1.00 ◌ +0.50 × 120°

In writing prescriptions, some people omit the ◌ sign and the degree designation. Thus, the previous example might be recorded as

OD –0.75 +0.50 × 150
OS –1.00 +0.50 × 120

For bifocal prescriptions, the word *add*, a plus sign, and the power of the sphere used to correct the presbyopia are appended to the distance correction. A typical bifocal prescription for one eye might read

–2.50 ◌ +1.00 × 90° add +2.00

For a trifocal, a typical prescription for one eye would show first the near add, followed by the intermediate correction:

–2.50 ◌ +1.00 × 90° add +2.50 int +1.25

TRANSPOSITION OF PRESCRIPTIONS

The majority of ophthalmology offices today require refractive measurements and prescriptions involving spherocylindrical lenses to be written in plus-cylinder form, as expressed in the earlier examples, but some prefer to express them in minus-cylinder form. Optometrists and opticians generally use the minus-cylinder form. Conversion from one form of expression to the other, known as **transposition**, may be required to accommodate office preference or to read prescriptions from another office. Ophthalmic medical assistants may encounter the need for transposition in performing lensometry (discussed later in this chapter).

Transposition is nothing more than a simple mathematic manipulation of a lens prescription, as follows:

1. Add algebraically the cylindrical power to the spherical power.
2. Reverse the sign of the cylinder, from plus to minus or vice versa as appropriate.
3. Add or subtract 90° to make the new axis 180° or less.

Examples of plus-cylinder expressions with their minus-cylinder forms appear below:

+3.00 +2.00 × 90 = +5.00 –2.00 × 180
–1.00 –3.00 × 135 = –4.00 +3.00 × 45

AUTOMATED REFRACTORS

Automated refractors exist for both objective and subjective refractometry, eliminating the need to use a phoropter or trial frame and lenses. The automated objective refractors use infrared light to provide information similar to that derived by manual retinoscopy. Automated subjective refractors rely totally on patient responses, the same as manual refractometry performed with phoropters or trial lenses and frames. Combination objective/subjective refractors allow the operator to use patient responses to check visual acuity before and after the measurement as well as to refine sphere, cylinder, and axis after the objective measurement has been made.

In general, automated refractors of all types are expensive, which might be a drawback in some practices. Other general advantages and disadvantages of the differing types are described in the sections that follow.

Objective Refractors

Automated objective refractors are simple to operate. Minimal storage and use space is required—a consideration in small offices. However, refractometric results may be variable and are not accurate enough to allow prescription without refinement. Furthermore, accurate results may not be possible in patients with certain diseases or disorders, such as immature cataracts, or certain physiologic characteristics, such as small pupils.

Subjective Refractors

Some subjective automated refractors allow testing of both distance and near vision and permit over-refraction of a patient's present eyeglasses. Some models feature an automated sequence of refracting steps, and others allow two different refractions to be compared with the push of a button. However, despite many automated features, a subjective refractor still requires a skilled, well-trained operator.

FIGURE 4.27

An automated refractor.

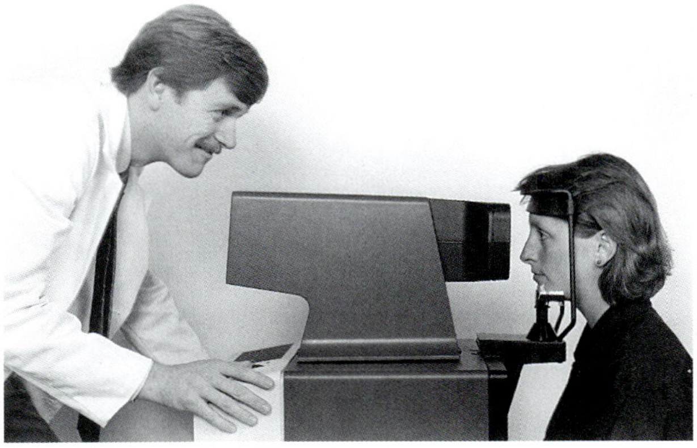

Objective/Subjective Refractors

With both objective and subjective capability in the same instrument, a combination automated refractor may save space in the office, because it eliminates the need for the traditional 20-foot testing distance required by manual refinement. Figure 4.27 shows a typical combination refractor. As with purely subjective refractors though, combination units require operator skill and knowledge for accurate refinement.

LENSOMETRY

Lensometry is a procedure used to measure the prescription of a patient's existing eyeglass lenses or the power of contact lenses. This technique is often called *neutralization*, but should not be confused with neutralization as the word applies to retinoscopy. Lensometry is performed (usually by the ophthalmic medical assistant) with a specialized instrument known as a **lensmeter**.

Lensometry measures four principal properties of lenses:

1. Spherical and cylindrical power in diopters
2. Axes, if the lenses have a cylinder component
3. Presence and direction of a prism incorporated into the lenses
4. Optical centers

Lensometry performed on a patient's eyeglasses before refraction can provide a starting point for the current refraction. This information is also useful in revealing changes in refractive error. Lensometry also serves to confirm that a patient's new glasses have been made in accordance with the doctor's prescription.

Types of Lensmeters

Instruments used to perform lensometry may be either manual or automated. Manual lensmeters are known by several brand names. Figure 4.28A on page 60 shows a manual lensmeter with the significant parts labeled; Figure 4.28B shows a lensmeter in use. To use manual instruments well, the operator needs a thorough understanding of not only lensometry itself, but also the principles of ophthalmic corrective lenses.

PERFORMING BASIC LENSOMETRY

Focusing the Eyepiece

The focus of the lensmeter eyepiece must be verified each time the instrument is used, to avoid erroneous readings.

1. With no lens or a plano lens in place in the lensmeter, look through the eyepiece of the instrument. Turn the power drum until the **mires** (the perpendicular crossed lines), viewed through the eyepiece, are grossly out of focus.
2. Turn the eyepiece in the plus direction, normally counterclockwise. This will fog (blur) the target seen through the eyepiece.
3. Slowly turn the eyepiece in the opposite direction until the target is clear, then stop turning. This procedure focuses the eyepiece.
4. Turn the power drum to focus the mires. The mires should focus at a power-drum reading of zero, which is plano. If the mires do not focus at plano, repeat the procedure from step 1.

Positioning the Eyeglasses

1. Place the eyeglasses on the movable spectacle table with the earpieces facing away from you. You are now prepared to read the back surface of the lenses, normally the appropriate surface from which to measure.
2. While looking through the lensmeter eyepiece, align the eyeglass lens so that the mires cross in the center of the target. It is usually appropriate to measure the right lens first, followed by the left lens.

Measuring Sphere and Cylinder Power

Plus-Cylinder Technique

1. Turn the power drum to read high minus (about –10.00).
2. Bring the closely spaced mires, often called **single lines**, into sharp focus by rotating the power drum counterclockwise while at the same time rotating the cylinder axis wheel to straighten the single lines where they cross the widely spaced perpendicular set of mires, often called **triple lines**.
3. If the single lines and triple lines come into focus at the same time, the lens is a sphere (Figure A). If only the single lines focus, you have identified the sphere portion of a spherocylinder. In either case, record the power-drum reading at this point as the power of the sphere.

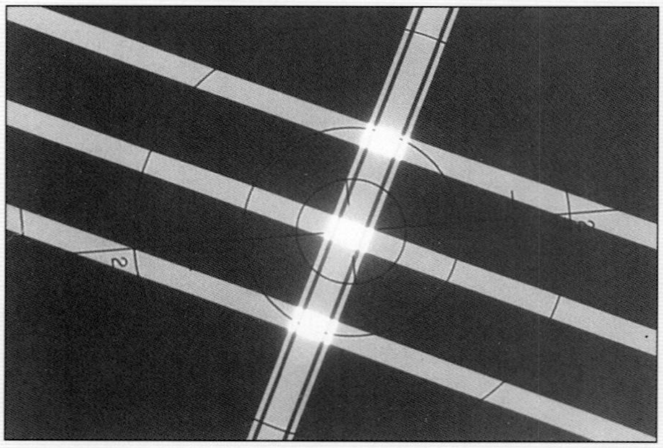

Figure A

Automated lensmeters (Figure 4.29 on page 60) measure an eyeglass lens prescription "at the push of a button." Little understanding of lensometry principles is necessary to operate the instrument. Automated lensometry can be faster than manual methods, but speed depends on the operator. In addition, these instruments are more expensive than manual ones. Because not all ophthalmology offices have automated equipment, ophthalmic medical assistants should develop basic skills in manual lensometry.

Elements of Lensometry

The first three steps in performing lensometry on lenses of all types are

1. Focusing the instrument eyepiece
2. Positioning the eyeglass lens to be measured on the spectacle table (or frame-support platform) of the lensmeter
3. Measuring the sphere power and, if present, cylinder power and axis, either in plus-cylinder or in minus-cylinder form

4. If cylinder power is present, after noting the power-drum reading for the sphere, measure cylinder power by moving the power drum farther counterclockwise or rotating the drum toward you (less minus or more plus), bringing the triple lines into sharp focus (Figure B).

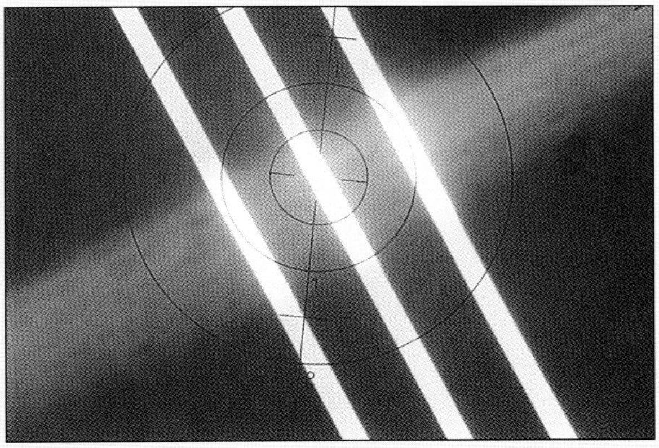

Figure B

5. Calculate the difference between the first power-drum reading for the focused single lines and the second power-drum reading for the focused triple lines, and record this figure as the plus-cylinder power of the lens.
6. Read the axis of the cylinder off the cylinder axis wheel.

Example (plus cylinder):

Single line focused at	–2.50
Triple lines focused at	–1.00
Cylinder power =	+1.50

Minus-Cylinder Technique

1. Turn the power drum to read high plus (about +10.00).
2. Bring the single lines into sharp focus by rotating the power drum clockwise while simultaneously rotating the cylinder axis wheel to straighten the single lines where they cross the perpendicular set of triple lines.
3. If the single lines and the triple lines come into focus at the same time, the lens is a sphere. Record the power-drum reading at this point as the sphere power.
4. If cylinder power is present, move the power drum farther clockwise or rotate the drum away from you (more minus or less plus), bringing the triple lines into sharp focus.
5. Calculate the difference between the single-line reading on the power drum and the triple-line reading on the power drum, and record this figure as the minus-cylinder power.
6. Read the axis of the cylinder off the cylinder axis wheel.

Lensometry always begins with focusing the eyepiece, followed by positioning the lenses. For multifocal lenses, the distance portion is positioned and measured first. Sphere and cylinder power may be measured and expressed in either plus- or minus-cylinder form, but because preference for either method may vary from office to office, ophthalmic medical assistants should be able to obtain these measurements in lensometry in both formats. These steps for performing lensometry on single-vision lenses and the distance portion of multifocal lenses are detailed in the box "Performing Basic Lensometry."

Because incorrect eyepiece focusing can lead to errors in measuring sphere power, proper focus should be verified each time the instrument is used. To avoid errors in measuring the cylinder axis, the lensometrist must ensure that the bottom of the eyeglasses is set firmly on the spectacle table.

FIGURE 4.28

(A) Schematic of a manual lensmeter. (B) A lensmeter in use.

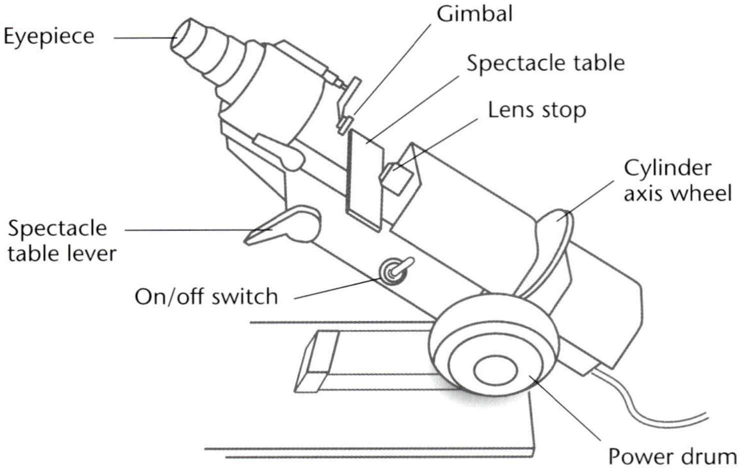

A

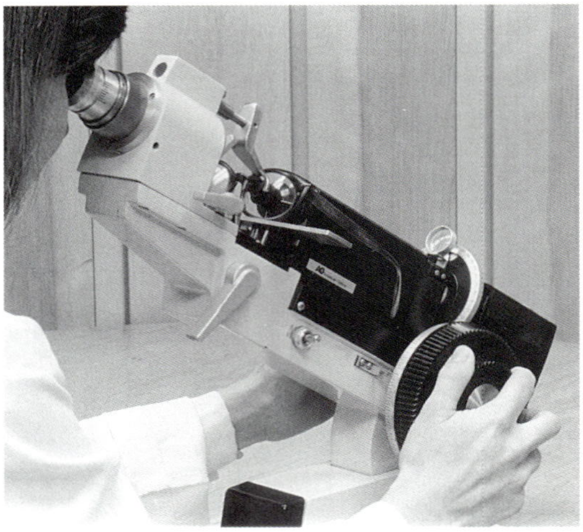

B

FIGURE 4.29

An automated lensmeter.

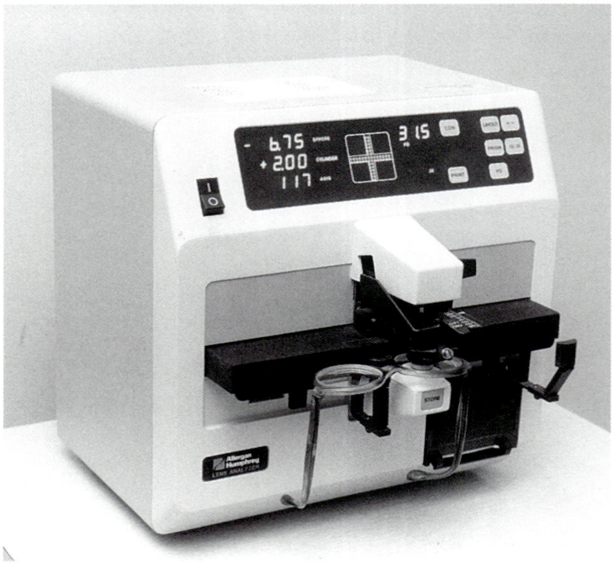

FIGURE 4.30

Progressive-add bifocals. A transition zone (*b*) lies between the distance (*a*) and the near (*c*) portions. That zone, as well as other areas of the lens (*d*), contain optical compromises that may make lensometry readings difficult to obtain.

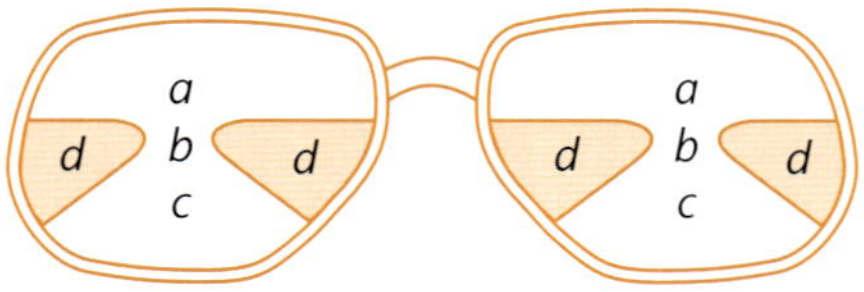

Lensometry Technique for Multifocal Lenses

After measuring the sphere, cylinder, and axis for the distance portion of a multifocal lens, the lensometrist obtains a reading for the bifocal or trifocal add. The procedure for measuring a bifocal and a trifocal segment by lensometry is the same, as described in the box "Measuring Multifocal Power."

Remember that the absolute power of the bifocal segment is always more positive (or less negative) than the sphere power in the upper portion of an eyeglass lens. The add is the total difference in dioptric power between the upper segment and the lower segment. For example, if the distance portion is +1.00 sph and the bifocal measures +3.00 sph, the bifocal add is +2.00. Similarly, if the distance portion is –1.00 sph and the bifocal measures +1.00, the bifocal add is +2.00.

Progressive-Add Multifocal Lenses

Progressive-add multifocal lenses differ from traditional bifocal or trifocal eyeglasses in that no discrete, visible line divides the distance and reading portions of the lenses (Figure 4.30). Optical compromises required by the manufacturing processes used to eliminate the discrete lines on the lens often produce unwanted cylinder power, distortion, or blurred transition zones between the distance and near segments, which poses difficulties in performing lensometry. When looking at progressive-add eyeglasses through the lensmeter, take care to select the area with the

MEASURING MULTIFOCAL POWER

Measuring Bifocal Power

1. After measuring the sphere and cylinder distance portion of bifocal eyeglass lenses, center the bifocal add at the bottom of the lens in the lensmeter **gimbal** (the ring-like frame) and refocus on the triple lines (if working in plus-cylinder technique) or the single lines (if working in minus-cylinder technique).
2. The add, or bifocal reading, is the difference between the distance reading of the triple-line focus (in plus-cylinder technique) or the single-line focus (in minus-cylinder technique) and the new triple- or single-line focus. Always read from the same type of line (single or triple) in the distance part and the bifocal part.
3. If the distance portion of the eyeglass lens is found to be a sphere, measure the sphere power of the bifocal segment. Record as the add the algebraic difference between the distance and bifocal sphere power readings (the distance subtracted from the bifocal). For example, if the sphere power in the distance segment is –1.00 and the sphere power in the near segment is +1.00, the bifocal add is +1.00 – (–1.00) = +2.00. The add is always written as a positive number.

Measuring Trifocal Power

To measure the trifocal segment directly, follow the same procedure as for the bifocal segment, reading the distance segment first, the intermediate segment second, and the near segment last.

least distortion in both the distance and the reading portions of the lenses before taking a reading. Be sure to read the add as close to the bottom of the lens as possible. Once the proper areas are found, the lensometry technique is the same as for conventional multifocals. More specific information about the characteristics and uses of progressive-add multifocal lenses appears in Chapter 8, "Fundamentals of Practical Opticianry."

Lensometry Technique for Prisms

Lensometry measures not only the power of a prism but also the orientation of the prism's base. The prism orientation may be *base in* (toward the nose), *base out* (toward the temple), *base up*, or *base down*. Steps for obtaining these measurements are described in the box "Measuring Prism Power and Orientation" on page 62.

Placement of Optical Centers

For ideal visual correction, the optical center of eyeglass lenses must be placed directly in front of the patient's pupils. The lensmeter may be used to verify the position of the optical center of a lens. Details about the purpose of measuring optical centers of lenses and the lensometry technique for doing so appear in Chapter 8, "Fundamentals of Practical Opticianry."

KERATOMETRY

Performed with a device called a **keratometer** or **ophthalmometer**, keratometry is the measurement of a patient's corneal curvature. As such, it provides an objective, quantitative measurement of corneal astigmatism, measuring the curvature in each meridian as well as the axis. Keratometry is also helpful in determining the appropriate fit of contact lenses. Components of a typical keratometer are illustrated in Figure 4.31. The box "Performing Keratometry" on pages 63–65 describes the procedure for obtaining measurements with this instrument.

MEASURING PRISM POWER AND ORIENTATION

In general, the existence of prescribed prism power in an eyeglass lens is revealed when the lensmeter mires cannot be centered in the central portion of the lensmeter target. Once you have determined the presence of a prism, measure prism power and determine orientation as follows:

1. Count the number of black concentric circles from the central cross of the lensmeter target to the center of the vertical and/or horizontal crossed mires (see the figure). Each circle represents 1 prism diopter.
2. Record the direction of the thick portion (base) of the prism by determining the direction of the displacement of the mires. For example, if the mires are displaced upward, the prism base is base up; downward displacement indicates base down; displacement toward the nose, base in; and displacement toward the temple, base out.

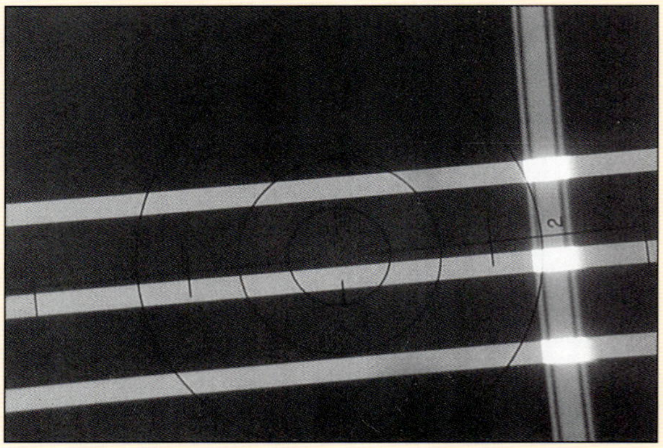

Prism-compensating devices are incorporated into some lensmeters. Such devices permit the measurement of prism without using the concentric circles. To avoid recording prism power that is not actually present when using these devices, be sure that the prism-compensating device is set to zero. Auxiliary prisms are available for use with some lensmeters to assist in measuring glasses with prism power greater than the number of concentric circles.

FIGURE 4.31

A typical keratometer. (A) Side view. (B) Rear view (examiner's perspective).

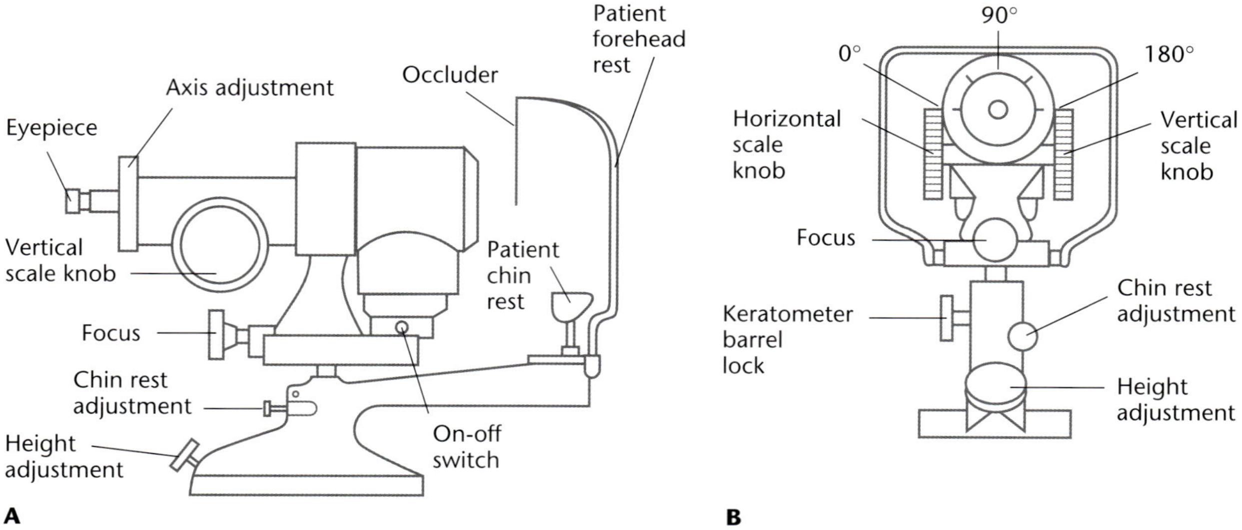

PERFORMING KERATOMETRY

1. Looking through the eyepiece of the keratometer, use the eyepiece to focus the reticle (cross hair) in the same way as for the lensmeter.
2. Adjust the height of the keratometer table or platform so that the patient can comfortably put the chin and forehead on the appropriate rests.
3. Instruct the patient to place the forehead and chin firmly against the rests. Use the occluder attached to the keratometer to cover the eye not being measured.
4. Use the instrument's chin-rest adjustment knob to position the keratometer to the patient's eye roughly in line with the keratometer barrel. Then use the height-adjustment knob of the keratometer to position the light reflections at the level of the cornea. Swivel the instrument horizontally to align with the patient's eye. These actions should both make the patient comfortable at the instrument and bring the light reflections from the keratometer into the patient's cornea.
5. Ask the patient to look into the barrel of the instrument for a reflection of the eye or at a fixation light if one is used.
6. Look through the eyepiece and use the focus knob to focus on the general area of the eye.
7. Lock the keratometer barrel when you see three circles through the eyepiece, which represent reflections from the patient's eye.

Steps 1 through 7 may need to be repeated during the remainder of the procedure to readjust the instrument.

8. Further align the keratometer with the eye by raising or lowering the keratometer by means of the height-adjustment knob and horizontal-swiveling capability until the reticle is in the center of the bottom-right circle (Figure A).
9. To obtain proper focus, rotate the focus knob until the bottom-right circles converge to form a fused image (Figure B).
10. Finding the axis is critical when taking an exact measurement. To locate the proper axis, rotate the keratometer until the pluses between the two bottom circles are in the same plane (Figure C).

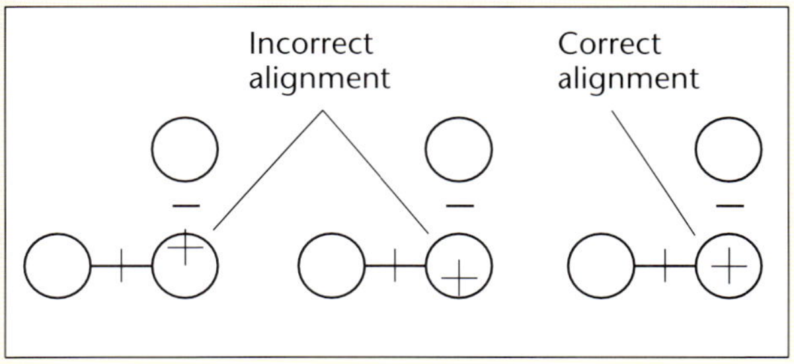

Figure A

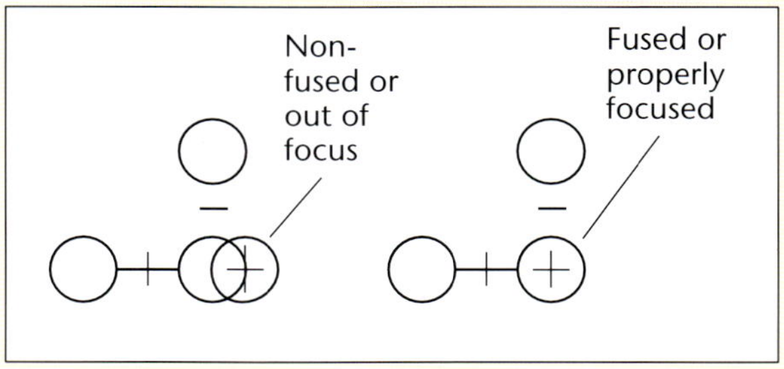

Figure B

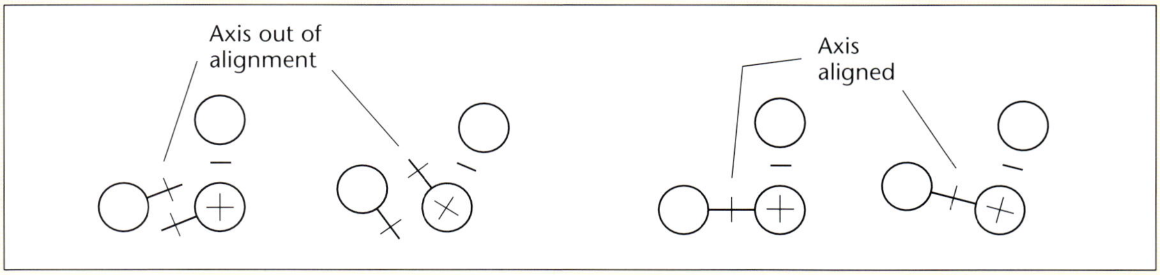

Figure C

(continued)

PERFORMING KERATOMETRY (continued)

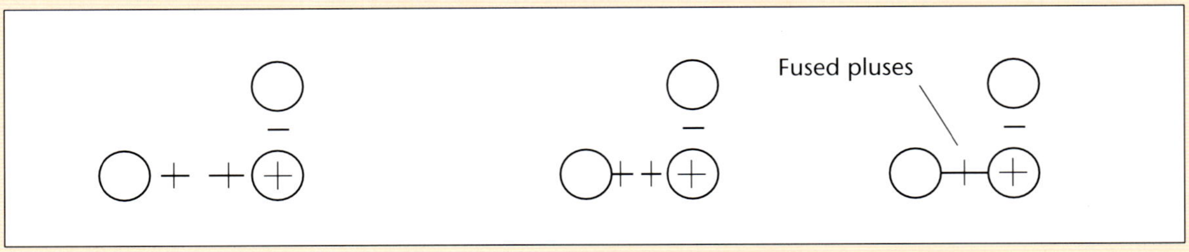

Figure D

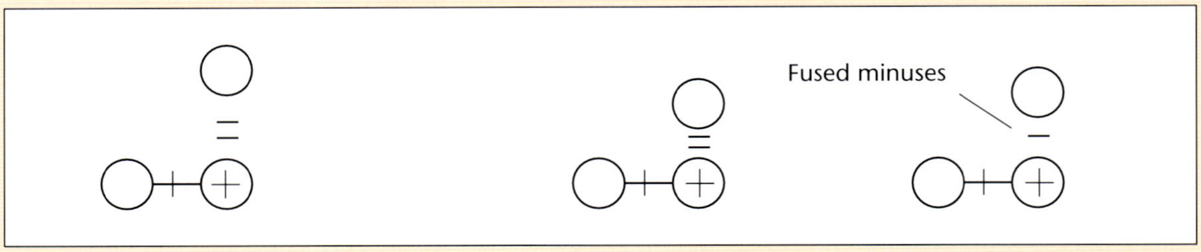

Figure E

11. With the horizontal scale knob on the left, the pluses between the circles can be moved and aligned (Figure D). Some keratometers have different mires. Check with your doctor or read the instruction manual that came with the keratometer.
12. With the vertical scale knob on the right, the minuses between the circles can be moved until they align (Figure E).
13. Often it is not possible to obtain good readings in the vertical meridian using the minuses for alignment. In this case, the keratometer should be rotated 90°, and the pluses aligned using the horizontal scale knob, as described in step 11.

REVIEW QUESTIONS

1. Define the following terms: refractive index, focal point, focal length, diopter.
2. Name the principal refractive property of a convex lens and a concave lens.
3. Distinguish between emmetropia and ametropia.
4. Define and describe the physiologic characteristics of myopia, hyperopia, and astigmatism.
5. Define *presbyopia*.

A proper measurement can be obtained when the following four conditions are met simultaneously:

1. The reticle is in the center of the bottom-right circle.
2. The keratometer is focused with fusion of the bottom-right circles.
3. The pluses between the circles are in the same plane and are fused.
4. The minuses between the circles are in the same plane and are fused.

You may need to readjust one or all of the control knobs until every element of proper measurement is obtained. In addition, it is critical that the eyepiece be properly focused at the start of the procedure.

Recording Keratometry Measurements

Figure F illustrates a possible measurement of an astigmatic cornea. This information can be recorded in one of three ways:

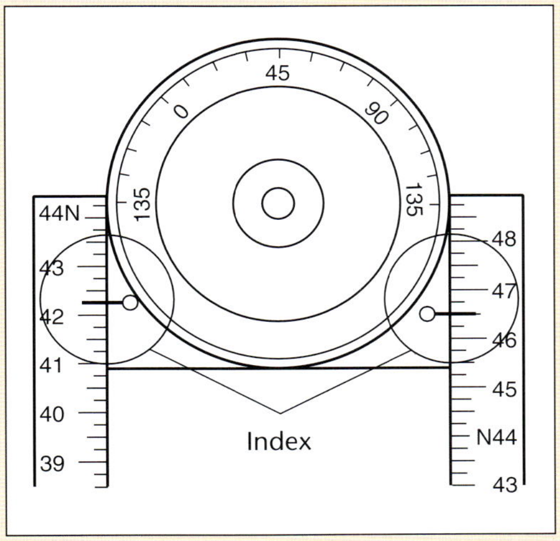

Figure F

1. K $\dfrac{42.25 \times 135}{46.50 \times 45}$

2. K $\dfrac{\text{R } 42.25 / 46.50 \times 45}{\text{L}}$

3. 46.5/A.M. 42.25 × 135 (A.M. = axis meridian)

6. Name at least three methods of correcting refractive errors of the eye.
7. Define and state the purpose of an *add* in multifocal lenses.
8. Define a *spherocylinder*.
9. State the principal refractive characteristic of a prism.
10. State the purpose of incorporating a prism into a corrective lens.
11. The refractive power of a prism is measured in units called __________.
12. A 0.5^{Δ} prism deviates parallel rays of light 1 cm at a distance of __________ m from the prism.

13. Name the kind of ophthalmic lens used to correct the following refractive errors: myopia, hyperopia, astigmatism.
14. Define *refraction* as the term is used in eye care.
15. Name the two main components of refraction.
16. Name the three separate steps of refractometry.
17. Distinguish between cycloplegic refraction and manifest refraction.
18. Define and distinguish between objective refractometry and subjective refractometry.
19. Name four instruments or devices that may be used during refraction.
20. Define *with motion* and *against motion*.
21. Name the three components of the lens prescription shown below:

    +2.75 −1.50 × 135

    a. b. c.

22. Transpose the following lens prescription:

    +4.25 +1.50 × 135

23. Define *lensometry*.
24. List the four properties of lenses that can be measured by a lensmeter.
25. Name the type of lens identified by lensometry when the single and triple perpendicular lines come into focus simultaneously.
26. The lensmeter power-drum reading on the distance portion of a multifocal lens measures −1.50 sph. The power-drum reading for the bifocal is +0.25. What is the bifocal add?
27. Define *keratometry*.
28. List the four conditions that must be met simultaneously to obtain a proper measurement with a keratometer.

SUGGESTED ACTIVITIES

1. Ask a senior technician or an ophthalmologist in your office if you can observe while he or she performs retinoscopy, lensometry, and keratometry. At a convenient time, ask him or her to demonstrate the equipment used in these procedures and allow you to try the procedures.
2. Ask an optician's office staff if you can have damaged or unwanted eyeglass lenses in various styles (single-vision, bifocals, trifocals). With a permanent marker, label each lens in a corner with a different identifying letter or number. Ask your senior technician to read each lens by lensometry and note the identifying letter or number and the lensometry reading for each on a sheet of paper. Then practice your lensometry technique by reading each lens yourself. Compare your readings with those of the technician, and discuss the reasons for any discrepancies.
3. Check the tables of contents and indexes of books included in the Suggested Resources list and read the pertinent chapters or sections for more information on subjects covered in this chapter.
4. Ask the ophthalmologist in your office to consider obtaining the videotapes listed in the Suggested Resources section for your viewing. These tapes demonstrate plus-cylinder retinoscopy, minus-cylinder retinoscopy, and cross-cylinder technique.

SUGGESTED RESOURCES

Azar DT: *Refractive Surgery.* Stamford, CT: Appleton & Lange; 1997; section II: Optics and Topography.

Cassin B: *Fundamentals for Ophthalmic Technical Personnel.* Philadelphia: WB Saunders Co; 1995; section III.

Corboy JM: *The Retinoscopy Book: An Introductory Manual for Eye Care Professionals.* 4th ed. Thorofare, NJ: Slack; 1996.

DiSanto MR: *Technical Options for Professional Service: A Dispensing Manual.* Dayton, OH: Bell Optical Lab; 1994.

Guyton DL: *Retinoscopy: Minus Cylinder Technique* and *Retinoscopy: Plus Cylinder Technique.* Clinical Skills videotape. San Francisco: American Academy of Ophthalmology; 1986. Reviewed for currency: 1999.

Guyton DL: *Subjective Refraction: Cross-Cylinder Technique.* Clinical Skills videotape. San Francisco: American Academy of Ophthalmology; 1987. Reviewed for currency: 1998.

Keeney AH, Hagman RE, Fratello CJ, and The National Academy of Opticianry: *The Dictionary of Ophthalmic Optics*. Boston: Butterworth-Heinemann; 1995.

Milder B, Rubin ML: *The Fine Art of Prescribing Glasses Without Making a Spectacle of Yourself*. 2nd ed. Gainesville, FL: Triad; 1991.

Rhode SJ, Ginsberg SP, eds: *Ophthalmic Technology: A Guide for the Eye Care Assistant*. New York: Raven; 1987.

Rubin ML: *Optics for Clinicians*. 25th anniversary ed. Gainesville, FL: Triad; 1993.

Stein HA, Slatt BJ, Stein RM: *The Ophthalmic Assistant: A Guide for Ophthalmic Medical Personnel*. 7th ed. St Louis: Mosby; 2000.

5 Comprehensive Medical Eye Examination

Patients seek the help of an ophthalmologist for various reasons. They may have injured an eye or developed an infection. They may have noticed a loss of vision or a decline in their ability to see clearly. They may have been referred to the eye specialist by another physician because of a medical problem that might affect their eyesight. They may simply wish to confirm that their eyes are healthy and that their previous refractive correction is still appropriate. Even when no visual complaints are present, periodic ocular evaluation is a wise precaution because some serious abnormalities may produce no symptoms until irreversible damage to sight has occurred.

The purpose of the comprehensive eye examination is to detect and diagnose abnormalities and diseases. This procedure includes an external and intraocular examination by the ophthalmologist with appropriate instruments, together with a series of tests and measurements. The ophthalmic medical assistant may be responsible for initiating the examination by taking the preliminary medical history, which comprises background information on the patient and details of the present condition that will help the doctor make a diagnosis and treat the patient. The assistant also participates in the performance of some of the tests. This chapter discusses the components of the eye examination, with particular attention to those aspects with which the assistant may be involved.

OVERVIEW OF THE EXAMINATION

The comprehensive medical eye examination is designed to reveal both existing and potential eye problems, even in the absence of specific symptoms. The procedure thus helps assure that the patient will receive timely and appropriate treatment to manage or prevent the development or progression of an abnormal condition. The examination may be divided into three major parts:

1. Patient history
2. Examination and testing to assess the functional behavior and anatomic status of the eye and related structures
3. Evaluation of the findings, diagnosis of present or potential abnormalities and disease, if any, and selection of appropriate management or treatment

The ophthalmologist oversees all aspects of the comprehensive eye examination and performs a number of the individual tests. Evaluation of the results and decisions on further studies or treatment are also the responsibility of the ophthalmologist. The ophthalmic medical assistant is often responsible for taking the preliminary medical history and for performing several of the standardized test procedures, particularly those related to eye function. Most of the evaluations of anatomic status require the expertise and training of the ophthalmologist. Even in these procedures, however, the ophthalmic medical assistant helps the ophthalmologist by administering eyedrops, preparing and caring for ophthalmic equipment and instruments, and recording results.

The examination and testing procedures included in the comprehensive examination and the order in which they are performed may vary with the preference of the ophthalmologist and the needs of the patient. However, eight aspects of eye function and anatomy are generally considered in the comprehensive examination. The first five parts involve operation of the visual system; the remaining three are concerned with the physical appearance and condition of the ocular structures. The following is a summary of the components included in the comprehensive eye examination.

Visual Acuity Examination

Visual acuity tests measure the patient's ability to see fine visual detail. A more extensive evaluation of visual acuity includes lensometry to measure the patient's existing optical correction (eyeglasses or contact lenses), refractometry (refraction) to determine the type and amount of refractive error and the proper optical correction, and keratometry or corneal topography to determine corneal curvature as an addition to refraction. Many visual acuity tests and related procedures are performed by the ophthalmic assistant.

Alignment and Motility Examination

Several procedures are used to confirm that the patient's eyes are correctly aligned and can move properly. Misalignment of the eyes or limited movement can interfere with normal vision. Experienced ophthalmic assistants often perform the basic tests.

Pupillary Examination

Reactions of the pupils under various light conditions provide the ophthalmologist with important information about general eye health. Gross pupillary screening procedures may occasionally be delegated to the ophthalmic assistant.

Visual Field Examination

A visual field examination tests the expanse and sensitivity of a patient's noncentral (peripheral) vision, that is, the perception of light and objects surrounding the direct line of sight. Initial rough assessments of visual fields are frequently delegated to the ophthalmic assistant.

Intraocular Pressure Measurement

Measurement of the pressure within the eye, a procedure called *tonometry*, is an important technique for the detection of glaucoma. Most ophthalmic medical assistants are expected to be able to perform this procedure.

External Examination

The ophthalmologist performs the external examination, including a close inspection of the appearance of the patient's lids, lashes, and visible parts of the lacrimal apparatus and external globe. The ophthalmologist may include, or request the ophthalmic assistant to perform, certain additional procedures, such as tests for tear production.

Biomicroscopy

The **biomicroscope**, also called a **slit lamp**, consists of a microscope of low magnifying power (6× to 40×) and a light source that projects a rectangular beam that can be changed in size and focus. This instrument allows close examination of the lids and lashes, cornea, crystalline lens, membranes, and clear fluids within the eye in layer-by-layer detail. The ophthalmologist evaluates the structures to determine whether defects or abnormalities are present. Ophthalmic medical assistants may also use this instrument to perform certain tests and measurements.

Ophthalmoscopy

In this procedure, the doctor uses an ophthalmoscope to examine the interior of the eye, particularly the vitreous and the *fundus* (a collective term for the retina, optic disc, and macula).

FREQUENCY OF EXAMINATION

Office policy and patient need dictate the frequency of a comprehensive eye examination. No matter the precise frequency, however, a regular comprehensive eye examination by an ophthalmologist is of great benefit for three principal reasons:

1. Certain eye diseases may be present but cause no noticeable symptoms until they are far advanced, when treatment may be less effective.
2. Overall eye health can be an important indicator of general health.
3. Some individuals—because of age, race, systemic health, or other factors—may not have existing eye problems but are at risk for developing certain eye diseases. For example, blacks develop glaucoma more frequently and severely than members of other races; many people with diabetes develop retinal disease. These people will benefit from regular ophthalmologic monitoring and, if a condition does develop, early treatment.

Young adults, 20 to 39 years of age, are generally at low risk for ocular problems, unless they are black. Because of the high incidence and more aggressive course of glaucoma in blacks, a comprehensive eye examination every 3 to 5 years is recommended. Other asymptomatic, otherwise normal patients in this age group require a comprehensive evaluation less frequently. Asymptomatic patients between 40 and 64 years of age should be examined every 2 to 4 years, particularly to check for the presence of presbyopia and glaucoma. After age 65, an examination every 1 to 2 years is recommended because of the variety of age-related and other eye abnormalities that may develop. Patients with medical conditions that may affect vision, such as diabetes, should be examined more frequently than healthy individuals of the same age. The frequency of such tests depends on the judgment and recommendations of the patient's ophthalmologist and primary care physician.

Most symptomatic patients and those in whom ocular abnormalities are detected can be diagnosed in the course of the comprehensive ophthalmologic examination and subsequently treated. Thereafter, followup examinations, comprehensive or otherwise, will vary with the abnormalities and the diseases identified. At any time, patients may undergo selected parts of the comprehensive eye examination to diagnose a specific ocular complaint.

OPHTHALMIC AND MEDICAL HISTORY

When the physician requests, the ophthalmic assistant begins the comprehensive eye examination by taking a preliminary ophthalmic and medical history of the patient. This information is entered in the patient's record and is generally reviewed by the physician before beginning the examination.

The purpose of the history is to determine the specific complaint that brought the patient to the office and to obtain information on any present illness or past ocular history that may help the physician in evaluating and diagnosing the patient's condition. Details on nonocular aspects of the patient's medical history and that of the patient's family may also prove useful.

The ophthalmic assistant obtains the history by asking a specific series of questions and recording the information in the patient's file or chart. The type and amount of information to be gathered by the ophthalmic assistant may vary from one practice to another. Some offices have special forms for this purpose. Figure 5.1 shows a sample form that might be used in a general ophthalmology practice. Irrespective of office policy, the history interview usually includes questions in five principal areas:

FIGURE 5.1

One type of form used for taking a preliminary ocular and medical history.

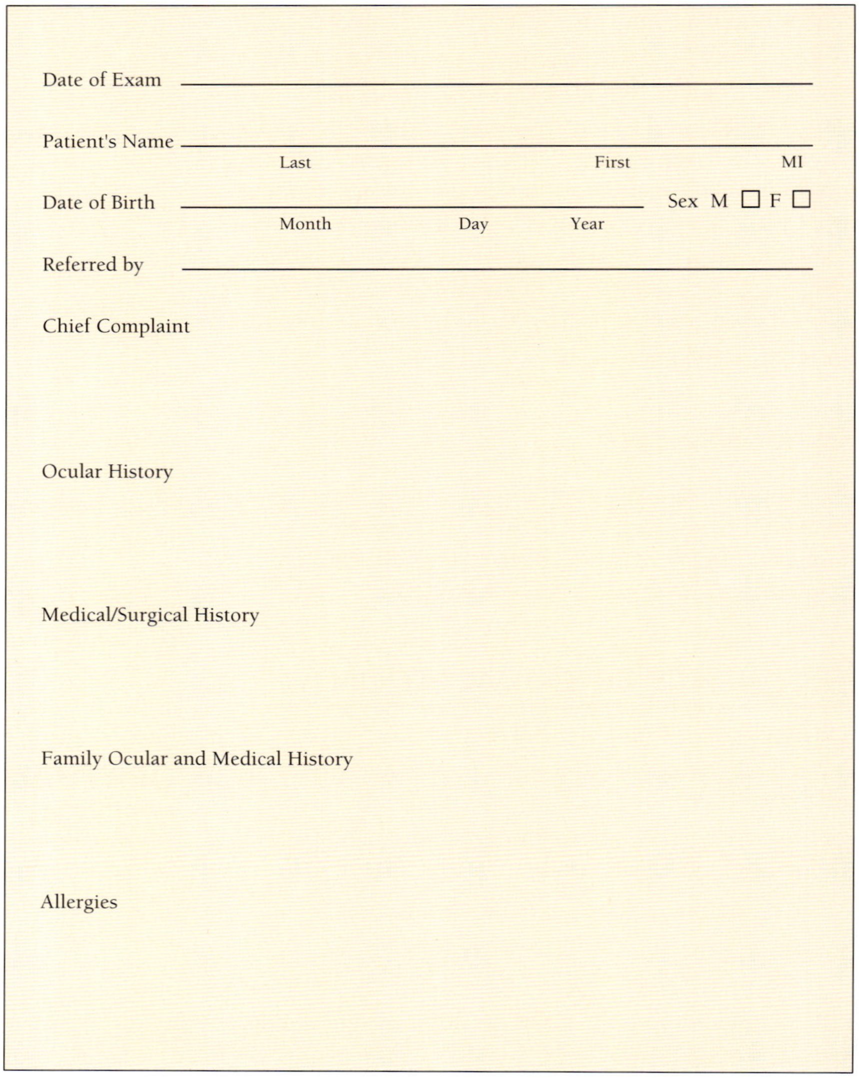

Date of Exam ____________________

Patient's Name ____________________
Last First MI

Date of Birth ____________________ Sex M ☐ F ☐
Month Day Year

Referred by ____________________

Chief Complaint

Ocular History

Medical/Surgical History

Family Ocular and Medical History

Allergies

1. Chief complaint
2. Ocular history
3. Medical history
4. Family ocular and medical history
5. Allergies

Table 5.1 summarizes these principal areas of the history and their related questions, which are described in detail below.

Chief Complaint

The **chief complaint** is the reason for the patient's visit to the doctor, except in those cases where the comprehensive eye examination is a periodic evaluation of an asymptomatic patient. For patients with a specific visual problem, define the chief complaint with the following questions:

- What are your symptoms?
- When did the problem start?
- Does the problem seem to be getting worse?

Depending on the patient's answers, you may have to ask additional questions in the following six areas:

1. *Status of vision*: Have both near and far vision been affected? Has vision been affected in one eye or both?
2. *Onset*: Did the problem start suddenly or gradually?

Table 5.1 Summary of the Five Primary Areas of History-Taking

Medical Area	*Questions to Ask*
Chief complaint	■ What are your symptoms? ■ When did the problem start? ■ Does the problem seem to be getting worse?
Ocular history (Present to past)	■ Do you wear, or have you ever worn, eyeglasses or contact lenses? ■ Have you ever had eye surgery? ■ Have you ever been treated for a serious eye condition? ■ Are you taking any prescription or over-the-counter medications for your eyes, including eyedrops?
Medical history (Present to past)	■ Are you taking any prescription or over-the-counter medications for a health condition? ■ Have you ever required treatment for any serious disease?
Family ocular and medical history	■ Does anyone in your family have any significant eye or other health problems?
Allergies	■ Do you have any allergies to medications, pollen, food, or anything else?

3. *Presence*: Are the symptoms constant or occasional, frequent or infrequent? (Ask the patient to specify the frequency in hours, days, weeks, or months.) Does a specific activity trigger the symptoms or make them worse?
4. *Progression*: Has the problem become better or worse over time?
5. *Severity*: Do the symptoms interfere with your work or other activities?
6. *Treatment*: Have you ever been treated for this complaint? (If yes, ask how, when, and by whom.)

Ocular History

The ocular history describes any eye problems the patient has experienced before this office visit, usually in reverse chronological order, that is, from the present to the past. The following are typical questions used to obtain this information:

- Do you wear, or have you ever worn, eyeglasses or contact lenses? (If yes, ask at what age glasses or contacts were first prescribed and how old the present prescription is.)
- Have you ever had eye surgery? (If yes, ask why, when, and by whom.)
- Have you ever been treated for a serious eye condition? (Ask specifically about glaucoma, cataract, injury, or any other eye condition associated with visual loss.)
- Are you taking any prescription or over-the-counter eye medications, including eyedrops? (If yes, find out the purpose, dosage, and duration of use.)

Medical History

A history of the patient's general medical health can be useful to the ophthalmologist because some health conditions can affect the eye and may influence the physician's choice of treatment (see Appendix B). Ask the following types of questions:

- Are you currently being treated for any disease? (If the answer is yes, ask the name of the physician.)
- Have you ever required treatment for any serious diseases? (Even if the patient answers no, ask specifically about diabetes and hypertension. Encourage the patient to think carefully about the question in order not to overlook a possibly significant disease.)
- Are you taking any prescription or over-the-counter medications for a health condition? (If yes, find out the purpose, dosage, and duration of use. Ask women specifically about contraceptive pills because some patients don't think of them as a medication.)

Family Ocular and Medical History

Many health problems are hereditary, including ocular problems. For this reason, a history of the patient's family ocular and general medical health can be extremely useful. Obviously, only information about family members closely related by blood is required. Ask the following question:

- Does anyone in your family have any significant eye or other health problems now; did anyone in the past? (Again, encourage the patient to think carefully. Ask directly whether any family members have ever had glaucoma, cataract, crossed eyes, poor vision, or blindness. Also ask specifically about diabetes, heart disease, hypertension, cancer, and conditions that run in the family.)

Allergies

Not only can allergies be a source of eye problems, but they also can affect the patient's ability to undergo certain diagnostic tests or use medications or other treatments safely. Ask the following question:

- Do you have any allergies to medications, pollen, food, or anything else? (If the patient answers yes, ask for specifics.)

History-Taking Guidelines

Obtaining a complete and accurate history is a valuable skill that is developed only with experience. The following are some general suggestions to help you develop this skill.

- When you begin the history, introduce yourself to the patient with your full name and explain the purpose of the interview. Address the patient by surname and title, depending on office policy and patient preference (that is, Mr, Miss, Mrs, or Ms). A simple approach is the following: "Mrs ________, my name is ________ ________. I am Dr ________'s assistant. I will be asking you some questions and performing certain tests to help the doctor with your examination." Remember, you are there to serve the patient. Be courteous and caring, but don't lose sight of the primary objective: to take an accurate history.
- Be sure to find out whether the patient has been referred to your office by another person, especially by another doctor. Record the name of the person or doctor as part of the history. Ask if the patient has been seen previously as a patient by the ophthalmologist in your office.
- Ask the name and relationship of anyone accompanying the patient, and determine whether or not the patient wishes these individuals to be present during the taking of the history.
- When documenting the chief complaint, use the patient's words, not your own. Avoid substituting technical terms that the patient has not used. Stick to the facts as they are presented to you.
- Patients may ask questions about their medical problem during the history interview. Handle these questions in a friendly manner but do not provide specific answers. *Always refer the patient to the ophthalmologist for a diagnosis or medical advice*, even if you think you know the answer. If the patient volunteers information you believe could be compromising (for example, drug abuse or sexual practices), write this information on a separate sheet of paper for review by the physician. If the doctor deems the information relevant to the patient's condition, it can be transferred to the permanent chart. Do not include nonmedical information in the history.
- Keep details short and to the point. The interview should take 5 to 10 minutes. Don't rush the process. Do a careful, thorough job, and when you are finished, thank the patient.

VISUAL ACUITY EXAMINATION

Visual acuity refers to the ability to discern fine visual detail. To see fine visual detail, normal central vision is required. The primary acuity test performed as part of the comprehensive examination is the **Snellen acuity test**, which may reveal refractive errors or other optical problems or ocular disease that require additional testing. Ophthalmic medical assistants often perform this basic test and other visual acuity tests.

Distance Acuity Test

This procedure measures a patient's distance vision by testing the ability to read characters at a standard distance from a special target called the **Snellen chart** (Figure 5.2). This is the familiar eye chart most people have seen in school or community vision-screen-

FIGURE 5.2

The Snellen chart used for testing distance visual acuity.

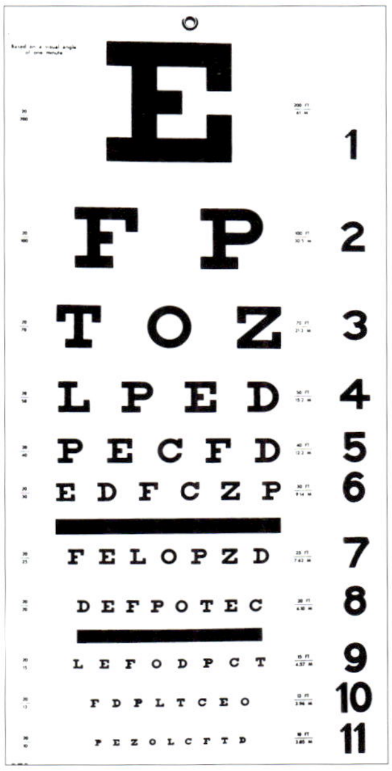

FIGURE 5.3

The tumbling E distance visual acuity chart used with patients unable to read.

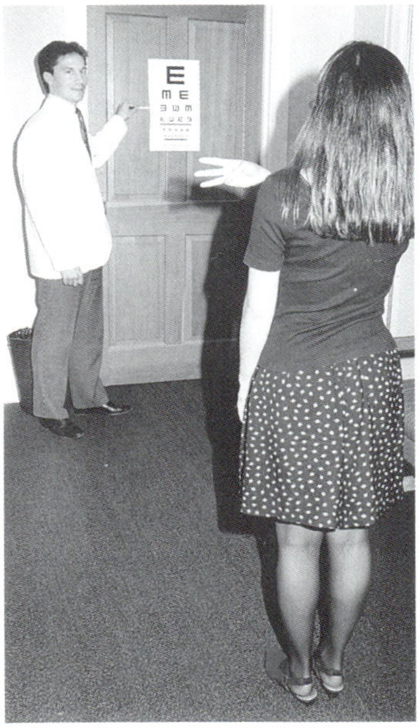

ing programs. The chart consists of **Snellen optotypes**, specially formed letters or numbers arranged in rows of decreasing size. The sizes are standardized so that the letters or numbers in each row should be clearly legible at a designated distance to a person with normal vision. Patients are placed at a specified distance, generally 20 feet, from the chart and asked to read aloud the smallest line they can discern.

Adults who can read are usually tested with the alphabetic or number chart. Illiterate adults and young children may be tested with variations such as the "tumbling E" chart (Figure 5.3) and picture charts. Techniques for testing vision in children and infants are discussed in Chapter 10, "Patients With Special Considerations."

Visual acuity charts may be in printed form for wall display or displayed on a screen from glass slides inserted into a **projector**. Projection with reflection of the image by mirrors permits use of a shorter actual viewing distance in a small office, although the characters appear to the patient as if viewed from the standard distance of 20 feet (Figure 5.4). The distance of 20 feet is used because it approximates optical infinity. Light rays coming from this distance and beyond are considered to be parallel, so that the emmetropic eye need not accommodate to focus them on the retina. If a shorter distance were used, a myopic eye might test at normal acuity.

At the left of each line of Snellen characters appears a numeric notation (for example, 20/50, 20/40, or 20/20). These values are used as measures of visual acuity. The first number (the top number as printed on the Snellen chart) represents the distance in feet at which the test was performed. The second

FIGURE 5.4

The projected visual acuity chart allows an actual testing distance of less than 20 feet.

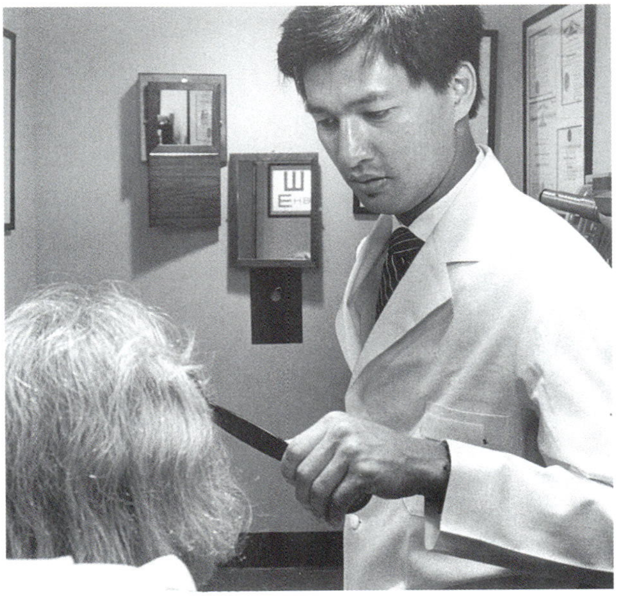

PERFORMING THE DISTANCE ACUITY TEST

Patients who wear eyeglasses or contact lenses should wear them for the test. On a first visit, patients may be tested both with and without optical correction. Test and record the visual acuity in each eye separately, beginning with the right eye. Less confusion results in recording information about the two eyes if the right/left sequence is followed habitually.

1. Position the patient 20 feet from an illuminated Snellen chart. If a projected chart is used, a shorter distance may be used, as specified for the particular projector.
2. Have the patient cover the left eye with an occluder or the palm of the hand. Alternatively, you may hold the occluder over the patient's left eye. With either method, be sure that the eye is completely covered and that the occluder is not touching the eye. Observe the patient during the test to be sure the patient is not peeking around the occluder. This is especially important with child patients.
3. Ask the patient to read the letters from left to right on every other line down the chart until the patient misses more than half the letters on one of the lines. If a tumbling E chart is being used, ask the patient to indicate the symbols visible on the smallest line by stating the direction or pointing the fingers in the direction the three spokes of the E point—left, right, up, or down.
4. Note the smallest line in which the patient read more than half the characters correctly, and record the corresponding acuity fraction (printed at the left or right of each line on the standard Snellen chart) in the patient's record, as well as the number of letters missed (for example, $20/30^{-2}$).
5. Repeat steps 2 through 4 for the left eye, with the right eye covered.
6. Record the acuity value for each eye separately, with and without correction, as shown in the following example:

V OD 20/20 $\overline{cc}$
  OS 20/25

V OD 20/200 $\overline{sc}$
  OS 20/100

The large **V** stands for "visual acuity" (sometimes written as a large **VA**). **OD** and **OS** are abbreviations of the Latin words for right eye *(oculus dexter)* and left eye *(oculus sinister)*. The abbreviations $\overline{cc}$ and $\overline{sc}$ signify "with correction" (eyeglasses or contact lenses) and "without correction," respectively. Because recording methods may differ, check with the doctor or senior assistant for preferred methods of recording visual acuity in the patient's chart.

number (the bottom number on the chart) corresponds to the distance at which the letters could be seen by a person with "normal" visual acuity. If the smallest letters a patient can read correctly are on the 20/60 line, the patient is able to read at 20 feet what the normal eye can read at 60 feet and the visual acuity is recorded as 20/60. If the patient can read the smaller characters in the 20/20 line at 20 feet, the patient's visual acuity is equivalent to that of the normal eye. Actually, some patients are able to read even smaller letters at 20 feet. In this case, their acuity might be recorded as 20/15 or 20/10.

Some offices prefer to express the acuity values in metric terms. Equivalent metric values are listed on the right-hand side of the standard Snellen chart for this purpose. Since 20 feet equals about 6 meters, an acuity value of 20/40 would be expressed as 6/12. Although the Snellen acuity values are written as a fraction, they do not represent a proportion or percentage of normal vision. Rather, they simply compare the distance from which the patient can read a line of characters to the distance from which a person with normal visual acuity can read the same characters.

PERFORMING THE PINHOLE ACUITY TEST

Patients who wear corrective eyeglasses or contact lenses should wear them for the test. Position the patient as for the Snellen distance acuity test, and test each eye separately, starting with the right eye.

1. Have the patient cover the eye not being tested with an occluder or the palm of the hand. Alternatively, you may hold the occluder over the patient's eye.
2. Have the patient hold the pinhole paddle in front of the eye that is to be tested.
3. Instruct the patient to look at the distance chart through the pinhole (or through any of the pinholes on a multihole paddle).
4. Instruct the patient to use very small movements to align the pinhole to produce the sharpest image.
5. Ask the patient to begin reading the line with the smallest letters legible without the pinhole, just as was done with the Snellen distance acuity chart.
6. Repeat steps 1 through 5 for the other eye.
7. Following the Snellen visual acuity data already recorded in the chart, record the pinhole acuity value for each eye. In the example that follows, ph = pinhole.

V	OD 20/80	sc	20/20	ph
	OS 20/100		20/25	

Visual acuity of 20/25 or even 20/30 may be acceptable for some patients but, generally, patients with below-normal visual acuity (20/30 or worse) due to refractive error will require optical correction (eyeglasses or contact lenses) for distance vision or, if that is not possible, some other form of visual assistance. The box "Performing the Distance Acuity Test" presents the basic testing procedure. Because testing standards and procedures vary from office to office, the ophthalmic medical assistant should consult the doctor or senior staff technician regarding the preferred methods of recording visual acuity notations, appropriate room lighting for viewing wall charts, and training in the use of the projector and target slides.

Pinhole Acuity Test

A below-normal visual acuity recording (20/30 or more) may be attributed to a refractive error. The box "Performing the Pinhole Acuity Test" describes the procedure used to confirm whether or not refractive error is the cause of below-normal visual acuity. In this text, the patient views the Snellen chart through a **pinhole occluder** (Figure 5.5). This hand-held device completely covers one eye and allows the other eye to view the chart through a tiny central opening. In some pinhole occluders, the central hole is sur-

FIGURE 5.5

The occluder and pinhole. (A) The occluder covers the right eye so that the left can be tested. (B) The left eye views the chart through the pinhole.

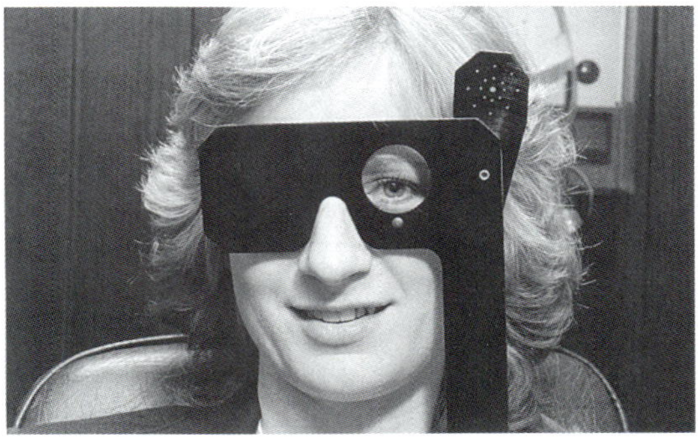

A

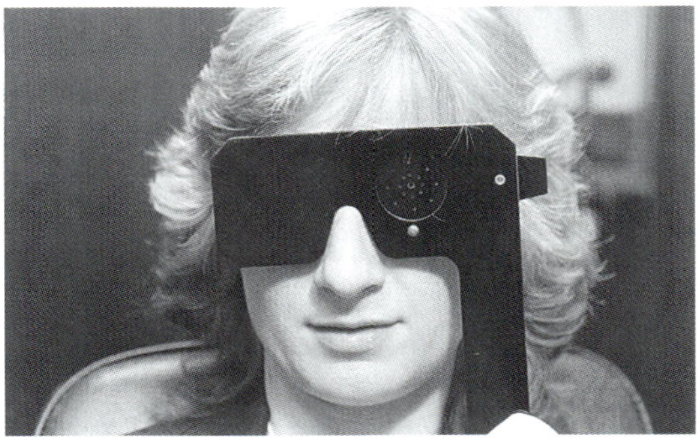

B

rounded by two rings of smaller perforations. Some phoropters also include pinhole devices.

The pinhole admits only central rays of light, which do not require refraction by the cornea and lens. The patient is thus able to resolve fine detail on the visual acuity chart without optical correction. If use of the pinhole improves a patient's poor uncorrected visual acuity to 20/20, or even 20/25 or 20/30, chances are the patient has a significant refractive error. If poor uncorrected visual acuity is not improved with the pinhole and the patient appears to be using it properly, the patient's visual problem is probably due to a cause other than optical or refractive error. In this case, the ophthalmologist may wish to perform additional tests.

Near Acuity Test

The Snellen acuity test measures a patient's ability to see fine detail at a distance with central vision. The procedure is sometimes referred to as a *distance visual acuity test*. However, a similar procedure may be used to test **near visual acuity**, the ability to see clearly at a normal reading distance (Figure 5.6). This test is performed if the patient complains that reading or other close work is difficult or if there is reason to believe the patient's ability to accommodate is insufficient or impaired. On the first visit, some offices record a near vision test regardless of whether or not the patient complains about reading.

As with the Snellen chart, numeric notations are printed next to each line on the near test card as a measure of near visual acuity. However, a near acuity card provides a choice of recording notations based on various units of measurements. One of the two most commonly used is the *distance equivalent*, which assigns an equivalent Snellen acuity fraction to each line on the near vision card (for example, 20/20 for the smallest line). *Jaeger notation*, also commonly used, assigns each line on the card a single arbitrary numeric value corresponding to a Snellen value. For example, Jaeger 2, abbreviated J2 when recording in the patient's chart, is equivalent to the 20/25 Snellen distance-equivalent line on the near vision card. Other notation systems are the *point system* and the *Snellen M unit*. Ophthalmic medical assistants should check their office policy for the preferred testing procedures and proper notation for recording the patient's near visual acuity. The box "Performing the Near Acuity Test" describes the general steps in this procedure.

FIGURE 5.6

The printed card used for testing near vision at a normal reading distance of about 14 inches.

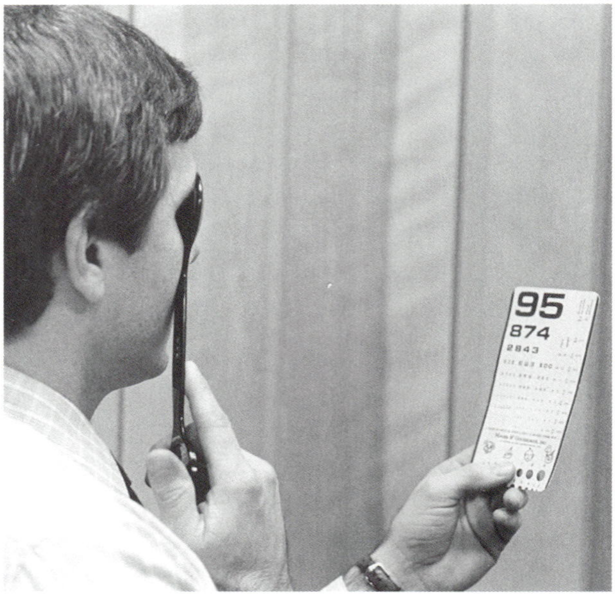

Other Acuity Tests

Patients with severe low vision may not be able to see even the largest Snellen letter (usually, the 20/400 line) clearly at the standard 20-foot or equivalent distance. Repeating the distance visual acuity test at shorter distances is usually the next step in evaluating the patient's visual acuity. If this procedure is unsuccessful, the patient may be asked to count the number of fingers held by the examiner in front of the patient. Alternatively, the patient may be asked to indicate recognition of the examiner's hand motions or to detect light from a small penlight. These specialized acuity tests for visually impaired patients are discussed fully in Chapter 10, "Patients With Special Considerations."

Procedures Following Acuity Tests

If the results of testing indicate below-normal visual acuity, additional procedures may be performed to evaluate the source of the disability in an effort to help the patient achieve visual acuity as close to normal as possible. For patients with eyeglasses or contact lenses, the first step is to determine whether the lenses the patient is wearing are providing appropriate correction of present refractive errors. The optical correction of the existing lenses is measured by

PERFORMING THE NEAR ACUITY TEST

Patients who wear eyeglasses or contact lenses for distance vision should wear them for the test. Some ophthalmologists will also want each eye tested without correction. If the patient has reading glasses, bifocals, or other reading aids, the near vision should be checked with and without the near correction (at least on the first visit); after the first visit, the near vision *with* reading correction is usually enough.

1. Instruct the patient to hold the test card of printed letters at the distance specified on the card, usually 14 inches.
2. Have the patient cover the left eye with an occluder or the palm of the hand. Alternatively, you may hold the occluder over the patient's left eye.
3. Ask the patient to read with the right eye the line of smallest characters legible on the card.
4. Repeat the procedure with the right eye occluded.
5. Record the acuity value for each eye separately in the patient's chart according to the notation method preferred in your office, as shown in the following examples:

near V OD 20/25 / OS 20/25 $\bar{cc}$

near V OD **J2** / OS **J2** $\bar{cc}$

lensometry. The patient's present refractive state is then evaluated by refractometry, a group of optical tests to determine the type and amount of the patient's refractive error and the appropriate lens correction. If the prescription for the patient's existing lenses does not agree with the newly determined correction, the below-normal visual acuity may be due to inadequate correction of the patient's refractive error. In that case, new lenses may be prescribed.

Keratometry and corneal topography are procedures for directly measuring a patient's corneal curvature. This information is useful both as a measure of refractive error and as a guide to fitting contact lenses or intraocular lenses. They may also reveal an irregular surface contour, a sign of past or present corneal disease.

Lensometry, refractometry, and keratometry are discussed in detail in Chapter 4, "Optics and Refractive States of the Eye." Corneal topography is discussed in Chapter 6, "Adjunctive Tests and Procedures." Another test often performed at this stage of the medical eye examination evaluates the patient's color vision. This procedure is discussed later in this chapter.

The ability to overcome glare from objects in the visual field and to discern various degrees of contrast is an important component of overall visual function. Measurement of these two abilities, called *glare testing* and *contrast-sensitivity testing*, may be indicated by the patient's history or the results of the visual acuity examination. The exact purpose and principles of these tests are discussed in Chapter 6, "Adjunctive Tests and Procedures."

ALIGNMENT AND MOTILITY EXAMINATION

Proper alignment of the eyes and unrestricted function of the extraocular muscles are necessary for normal vision. If the eyes are misaligned or if the extraocular muscles are unable to move the eyes in a coordinated manner, the brain may not be able to merge (or fuse) the images from the two eyes. Failure to achieve fusion produces diplopia and possibly amblyopia, with a resultant loss of stereopsis, the ability to perceive depth in three dimensions. While most patients with ocular misalignment readily recognize their diplopia and seek medical help, patients with amblyopia, particularly children, may be totally unaware of their dependency on the vision of one eye and may be ignorant of their loss of stereopsis. For these and other reasons, evaluation of the alignment of the eyes and their motility, that is, the proper function of the extraocular muscles, is an important component of the comprehensive eye examination.

In an ocular alignment and motility examination, patients are observed and tested for three principal properties of their visual system: eye movement (motility), eye alignment, and fusional ability.

FIGURE 5.7

The six cardinal positions of gaze used to evaluate eye movement.

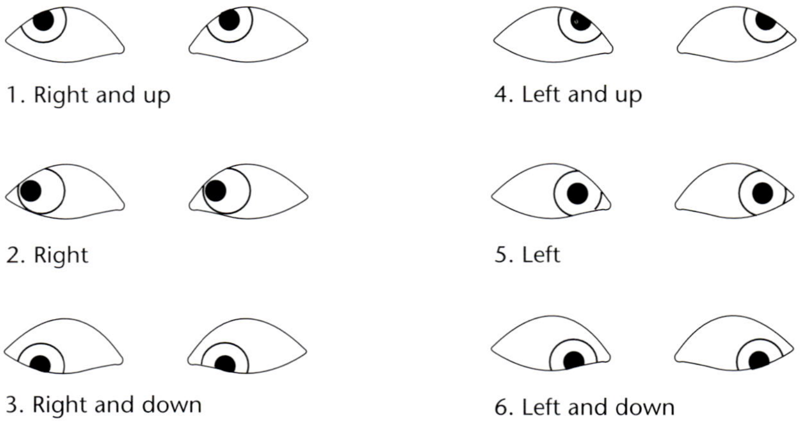

Because these functions are physiologically complex, the methods used to test them are varied and occasionally complicated. Testing usually begins with a gross assessment of ocular motility, followed by additional tests if this screening evaluation indicates the presence of a potential alignment or motility problem.

For the initial, gross evaluation of ocular motility, the examiner holds a small object or displays a finger within the patient's central field of vision and asks the patient to follow its movement with the eyes in the six **cardinal positions of gaze** (Figure 5.7):

1. Right and up
2. Right
3. Right and down
4. Left and up
5. Left
6. Left and down

Movements in these six directions test the function of the six extraocular muscles and reveal possible weakness, paralysis, or restriction. However, detection of functional defects requires skill and considerable experience on the part of the examiner.

Several methods are used to assess alignment of the eyes (also known as *muscle balance*) and to detect the presence and measure the amount of strabismus (misalignment). Most tests are based on an observation of the position and compensatory movements of the eyes. These procedures are considered *objective* because no patient communication is needed. The principal objective test to detect eye misalignments, or strabismus, is the cover–uncover test. The principal method for measuring the extent of the eye's deviation is the prism and alternate cover test. Beginning ophthalmic medical assistants are not usually required to perform these procedures, but they should have an understanding of them.

Cover–Uncover Test

The **cover–uncover** test is performed to determine if a patient's eyes are misaligned. This test requires that the patient fix his or her attention consistently on a target (typically a letter on the Snellen chart several lines above the smallest line that the patient can read). While a cover, or occluder, is introduced in front of one eye, the other eye is observed. This procedure is repeated, introducing the cover over the other eye. If covering either eye causes the uncovered eye to move to fix on the target, then a manifest deviation, or heterotropia, is present. However, if the patient has poor vision in either eye, fixation will not be consistent and this test will not be accurate.

FIGURE 5.8

The prism and alternate cover test.

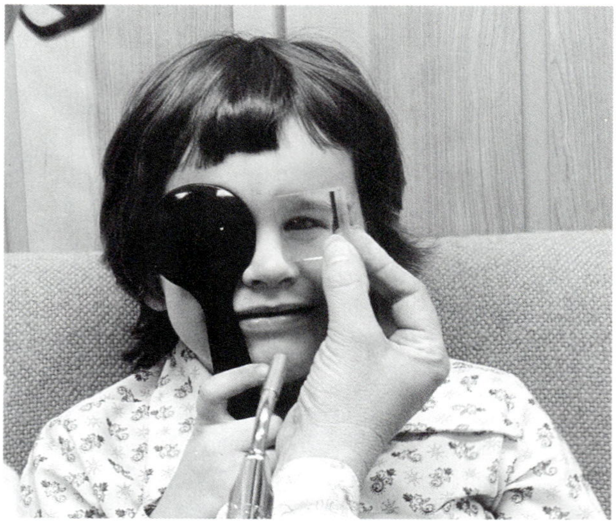

FIGURE 5.9

The Worth four-dot test. (A) The flashlight target, which illuminates four dots: two green, one red, and one white. The eyeglasses are fitted with a red and a green filter. (B) The flashlight is held in front of the patient, who wears the colored eyeglasses.

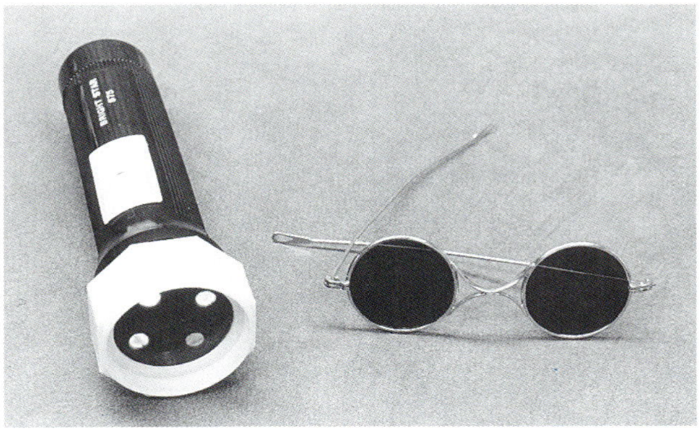

A

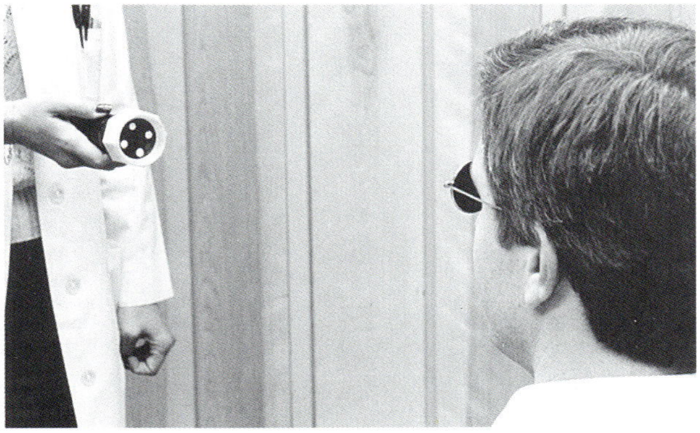

B

Prism and Alternate Cover Test

Consistent patient fixation is also necessary for accurate measurement of ocular misalignments using the **prism and alternate cover test.** As its name suggests, this procedure uses a prism and a cover (Figure 5.8). While the patient fixes his or her attention on a target, one eye is covered. The deviated eye will make a compensatory movement in order to pick up fixation. The occluder is moved back and forth to alternately cover each eye. Corrective prisms are then introduced in front of the deviated eye. The prism alters the apparent position of the fixation target and reduces the extent to which the patient must shift the deviated eye to pick up fixation. The deviation is neutralized by introducing prisms of progressively higher power until the uncovered eye no longer shifts to fixate the test object. Each prism is marked with its power, in prism diopters. The size of the ocular deviation is determined by the power of the prism that neutralizes the compensatory shift on alternate cover test.

Worth Four-Dot Test

The **Worth four-dot test** is designed to determine how a patient uses his or her two eyes together. Three possible states may exist—fusion, diplopia (double vision), or suppression. If the images received by the two eyes are adequately aligned, the brain usually fuses the two images into one visual perception. In the presence of an ocular misalignment or other ocular abnormalities that interfere with fusion, the brain may suppress or ignore the image from one eye. If one image is not suppressed, then two images will be seen, creating diplopia.

For this test, the patient wears a pair of eyeglasses with a red filter over the right eye and a green filter over the left. The patient's gaze is directed at a target displaying four lighted dots: two green, one red, and one white (Figure 5.9). From the patient's responses about the number and color of lights seen, the ophthalmologist can determine whether or not the eyes are normally aligned and whether one eye is being suppressed.

Titmus Stereopsis Test

To perceive depth, both eyes must be able to fixate a visual target accurately and simultaneously. A marked defect in visual acuity, suppression of vision in one eye, or diplopia will interfere with depth perception. The **Titmus stereopsis test** determines whether the patient has fine depth perception, and quantifies it in terms of binocular cooperation.

For the Titmus test, the patient views a series of stereophotographs through a pair of eyeglasses fitted with light-polarizing filters. The patient with normal binocular vision will fuse the images of the stereophotos to perceive a single three-dimensional view. The same principle and method are used for the showing of 3-D movies.

In the first part of the Titmus test, the patient is shown the large photo and asked if the image (a fly) appears to have depth (Figure 5.10). If the answer is yes, the examiner can proceed to quantify the amount of depth perception. For this portion of the test, the

FIGURE 5.10

The Titmus stereopsis test. (A) Light-polarizing eyeglasses and targets. (B) The patient views the target through polarizing filters and reports perception of depth.

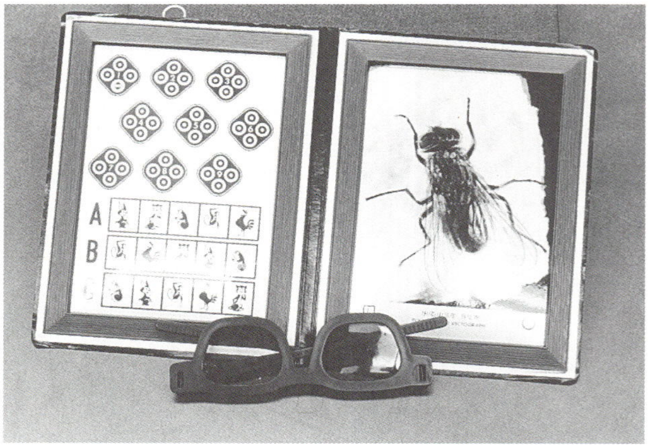

A

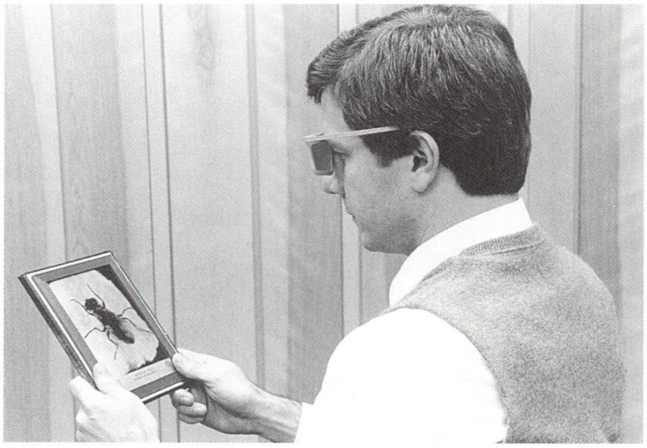

B

patient is shown a group of four circles. Each circle in a group appears the same except one, which appears raised to someone with normal vision.

As the test continues, the patient is shown groups whose "raised" circle requires a higher degree of binocular cooperation to appreciate the sensation of depth. The group of circles requiring the finest binocular cooperation that a patient can distinguish provides a measure of stereopsis. A person with normal binocular vision should be able to appreciate stereopsis in Titmus group No. 9. The highest Titmus circle number reported by the patient as seen with depth is recorded in the patient's record.

PUPILLARY EXAMINATION

Pupillary evaluation can reveal a variety of ophthalmic abnormalities: iris muscle or nerve damage, optic nerve or retina pathology, and diseases affecting the visual pathway and the brain. Pupillary observation and testing may be performed by the ophthalmologist as part of the external examination, but certain elements of pupillary testing are sometimes delegated to the ophthalmic medical assistant.

Pupillary testing is usually scheduled before those portions of the comprehensive test that require pupillary dilation with drugs (cycloplegic refraction, biomicroscopy, and ophthalmoscopy). This test sequence is followed to avoid residual pupillary paralysis induced by the drugs that would affect the accuracy of subsequent tests on the pupil.

Four procedures are used in pupillary evaluation. The first three include measurement of pupil size in dim illumination, speed of pupil constriction when a bright light is directed into the eyes, and pupillary response to a near dim target. The fourth procedure, the swinging-light test, is used to quantify an important normal binocular pupillary response to light, called the **direct and consensual pupillary reaction**.

Normally, when light shines directly into an eye, the pupil of the eye constricts (direct reaction). Even when the light does not reach the other eye, the pupil of that eye normally constricts as well (consensual reaction). In other words, the two pupils react simultaneously to a light stimulus, even if only one eye is directly stimulated. The consensual pupillary reaction occurs even if the nonstimulated eye is blind and cannot itself react to light. Failure of the pupil in the nonstimulated eye to react consensually indicates abnormal function of the iris sphincter muscle or the nerve pathways to or from the brain. In an eye with normal function of the iris sphincter muscle, failure of the pupil to constrict in response to direct light stimulation suggests optic nerve or retinal damage.

As with most other pupillary tests, the swinging-light test for direct and consensual reaction is a complex measurement that requires the judgment of the ophthalmologist. In some offices, however, the ophthalmic medical assistant might be required to perform a less complex screening for the presence or absence of this pupillary response. This procedure is described in the box "Checking Direct and Consensual Pupillary Reaction."

CHECKING DIRECT AND CONSENSUAL PUPILLARY REACTION

1. Seated opposite the patient in ordinary room light, observe the patient's resting pupil size for both the right and the left eyes. Both pupils should be dilated equally (Figure A).
2. In the patient's chart, record the resting pupil size for each eye in millimeters. To gauge size, you may either hold a millimeter rule close to the patient's eye or compare the patient's pupil size with relative pupil sizes printed on most near vision cards.
3. As shown in Figure B, shine a penlight (a small flashlight) into the patient's right eye and observe if the pupil constricts in response to the direct light stimulus. Look immediately at the left pupil to see if it constricts consensually.
4. Remove the penlight from the patient's vision briefly to allow the pupils to return to resting state and then repeat step 3 for the left eye.
5. In the patient's chart, record the results for each eye. If the results are normal, record "Reactive to light, direct and consensual"; if the results are abnormal, record either "No direct response" or "No consensual response," whichever applies.
6. Discuss any abnormal pupillary response, such as dilation, with the ophthalmologist before instilling dilating eyedrops.

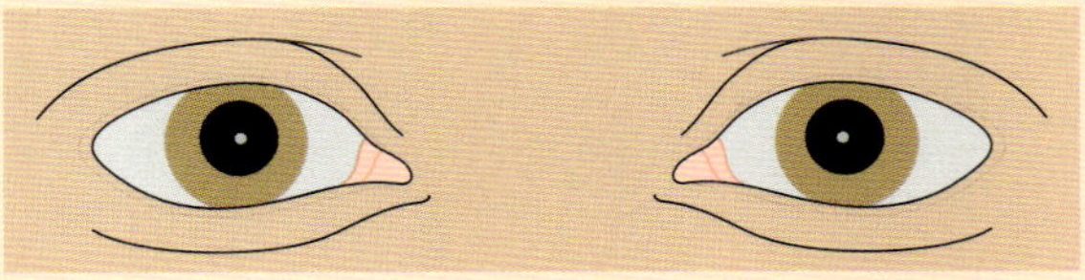

A

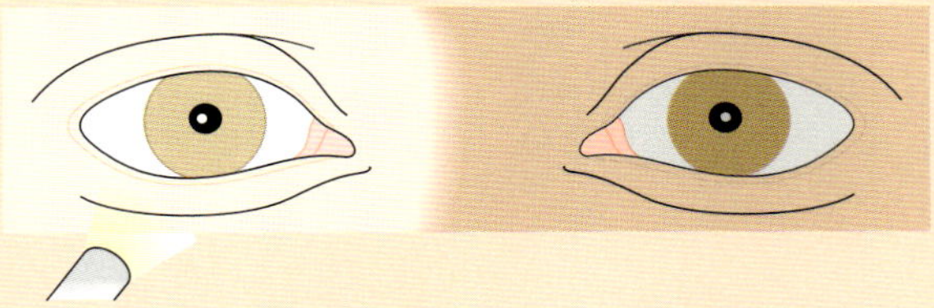

B

VISUAL FIELD EXAMINATION

The visual field examination measures the expanse and sensitivity of vision surrounding the direct line of sight, that is, peripheral vision. Unlike most losses of central vision, defects in peripheral vision can be subtle and are often unnoticed by a patient. Disturbances in peripheral vision are commonly due to diseases of the retina, optic nerve, or structures of the visual pathway in the brain. These last diseases can be life-threatening as well as vision-threatening. Early detection of these abnormalities by a visual field examination permits treatment to be initiated that may halt further progression of the disease and prevent irreversible loss of central, as well as peripheral, vision.

The visual field examination consists of a number of different testing procedures, discussed in Chapter 7, "Principles and Techniques of Perimetry." However, two relatively simple techniques are included in the comprehensive visual examination to obtain a gross evaluation of the patient's peripheral vision, *confrontation visual field testing* and *Amsler grid testing*. Performance of these tests is often the responsibility of the ophthalmic medical assistant. The results of these two tests may indicate the need for the more exact procedures of perimetry.

PERFORMING THE CONFRONTATION TEST

1. Seat the patient at a distance of 2 to 3 feet from you. Confront (face) the patient, cover or close your left eye, and have the patient cover the right eye. You and the patient should fixate on each other's uncovered eye.
2. Extend your arm to the side at shoulder height and slowly bring two fingers from beyond your peripheral vision toward your nose into the field of vision midway between the patient and yourself. Ask the patient to state when the fingers are visible.
3. Repeat the process of moving fingers into the visual field from four different directions. If you picture a clock face in front of the patient's eyes, you perform the hand movement from about 2 o'clock, 4 o'clock, 8 o'clock, and 10 o'clock, each time bringing the fingers toward the center of the clock face.
4. The patient should see the fingers at about the same moment you do in each of the four **quadrants** (upper-left, upper-right, lower-left, and lower-right quarters) of the visual field. (Note: A quadrant of vision is described from the patient's point of view.) If the patient does not see your fingers at the same time you do, the breadth of the patient's visual field in that quadrant is considered to be smaller than normal and additional perimetric studies will probably be required.
5. Record the patient's responses in the patient's chart by indicating simply that the visual field is comparable to yours (normal) or that it is reduced in any of the four quadrants for that eye.
6. Repeat the procedure with the patient's other eye and record the results similarly.

Confrontation Field Test

The **confrontation field test** compares the boundaries of the patient's field of vision with that of the examiner, who is presumed to have a normal field (Figure 5.11). This procedure is described in the box "Performing the Confrontation Test."

Amsler Grid Test

The **Amsler grid test** determines the presence and location of defects in the central portion of the visual field. The Amsler grid is a printed square of evenly spaced horizontal and vertical lines in a grid pattern, with a dot in the center. The chart grid and dot may be either white on a black background or black on a white background (Figure 5.12). See the box "Performing the Amsler Grid Test" for step-by-step instructions in this procedure.

FIGURE 5.11

The confrontation test.

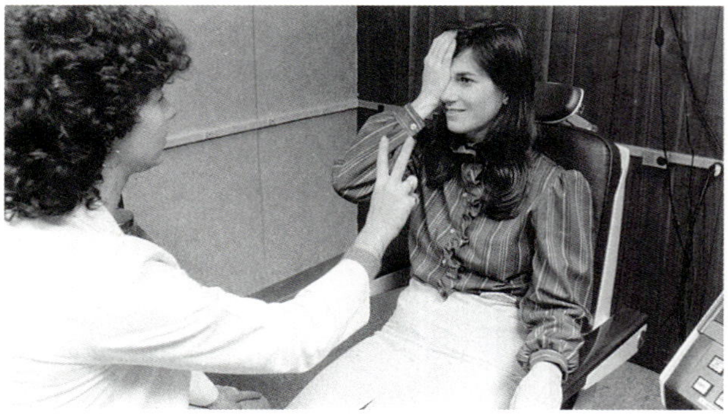

INTRAOCULAR PRESSURE MEASUREMENT

Pressure within the eye is maintained by a delicate balance between the continuous flow through the anterior chamber of aqueous fluid and its steady drainage through the trabecular meshwork. Disturbance or malformation of any of the structures involved may impede aqueous flow, causing intraocular pressure to rise and leading to glaucoma. This condition can permanently damage the optic nerve and produce blindness.

Abnormal intraocular pressure and glaucoma may be present long before a patient notices any symptoms such as visual loss. For this reason, early detection of the disease by measurement of intraocular pressure is a critical part of the comprehensive eye examination. If glaucoma is detected early, intraocular pressure can be reduced to normal or tolerable levels by medication or surgery, and the progression to blindness can be halted or slowed. The examination to determine intraocular pressure is called **tonometry**; instruments used for this purpose are known as **tonometers**.

PERFORMING THE AMSLER GRID TEST

1. Have the patient hold a white-on-black test card about 16 inches away with one hand and cover one eye with the other hand, an occluder, or a patch.
2. Direct the patient to stare at the center dot and to report if any portions of the grid are blurred, distorted, or absent. The patient should not move the gaze from the center dot, so that the presence of any distortion can be assessed.
3. If the answer is yes, you may repeat the test with a black-on-white Amsler recording chart, on which you ask the patient to mark the location of visual difficulties.
4. If test results are normal, state so in the patient's record. If abnormal, state so and include the Amsler recording chart in the patient's record. If visual disturbances are noted, the patient is a likely candidate for further studies (see Chapter 7, "Principles and Techniques of Perimetry").

The patient may also repeat this convenient procedure independently at home and report any changes to the ophthalmologist's office. Instruct the patient to perform the test monocularly (one eye at a time), always at the same 16-inch distance and under the same illumination.

FIGURE 5.12

The Amsler grid test. (A) The typical white-on-black Amsler grid. (B) The patient marks the nature and location of his central field defect on the black-on-white grid.

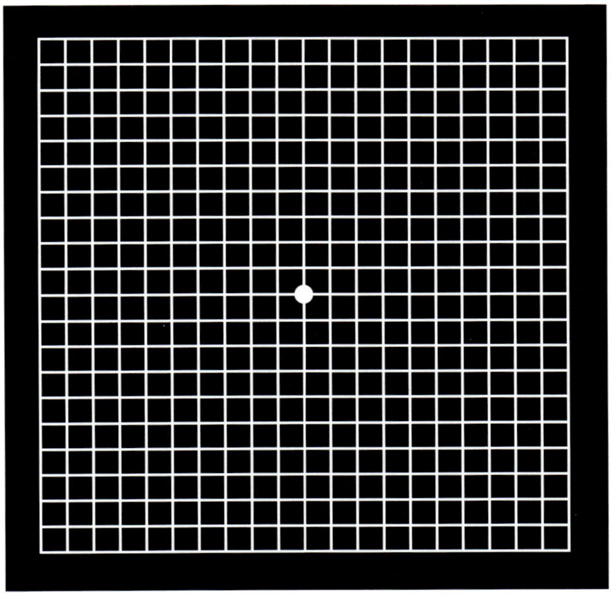

A

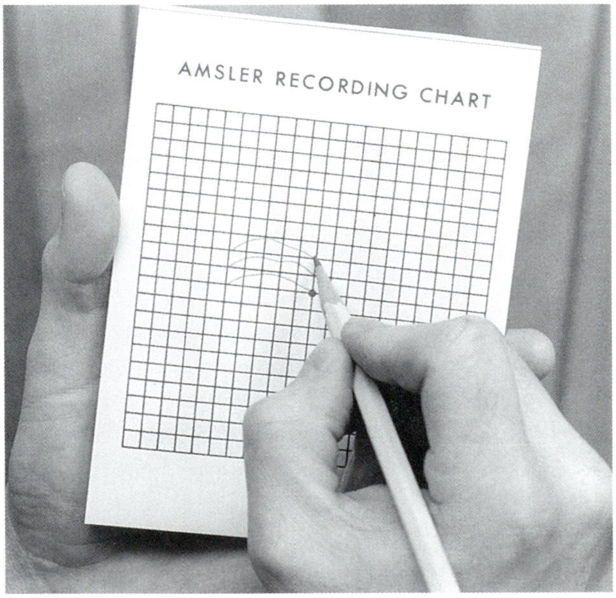

B

Principles of Tonometry

Tonometers measure intraocular pressure by one of two principles: **applanation**, measurement of the force required to flatten a small area of the central cornea; or **indentation**, measurement of the amount of corneal indentation produced by a fixed weight. By convention, intraocular pressure is expressed in millimeters of mercury (mm Hg), the same units used in common mercury weather barometers. Normal intraocular pressure ranges between 10 and 21 mm Hg. The scales or indicators on some tonometers provide direct readings of intraocular pressure in millimeters of mercury. Other tonometers indicate corneal resistance to applanation or indentation in values that are converted to millimeters of mercury by a simple calculation or the use of conversion tables.

PERFORMING GOLDMANN TONOMETRY

1. Ensure that the tonometer tip is clean or, if a disposable cover is used, that a fresh cover is in place.
2. Instill eyedrops of a local anesthetic and fluorescein dye into both of the patient's eyes. (Information on these drugs and instillation techniques appears in Chapter 11, "Basics of Ophthalmic Pharmacology.") Instead of separate solutions, some offices use a single solution containing both the anesthetic and the dye. *Caution: Fluorescein dye can permanently stain soft contact lenses. Be sure a patient's soft contact lenses are removed before instilling fluorescein dye.*
3. Seat the patient comfortably at the slit lamp with the forehead firmly against the headrest. Seat yourself opposite in the examiner's position, and instruct the patient to look straight ahead or to gaze steadily at your ear.
4. On the slit lamp, turn the dial or lever that places the cobalt-blue filter in the instrument's light path. (The resulting cobalt-blue light causes the fluorescein dye on the patient's eye to fluoresce a bright yellow-green.) Using the magnification-adjustment knob on the slit lamp, set the magnification at low power. Adjust the beam from the cobalt-blue light so that it shines on the prism at a wide angle, about 45° to 60°.
5. Looking from the side of the slit lamp, align the prism with the patient's cornea. Adjust the numbered dial on the force-adjustment knob to read between 1 and 2 (10 and 20 mm Hg). Instruct the patient to blink once (to spread the fluorescein dye) and then to try to avoid blinking. If it is necessary to hold the patient's lid open, push up on the skin of the lid with your thumb and secure the lid against the bony orbit; do not apply pressure to the globe.
6. Using the slit-lamp control handle (joystick), gently move the prism forward until it just touches the central cornea. Looking through the slit-lamp oculars, confirm that the prism has touched the cornea: the spot of fluorescein will break into two semicircles, one above and one below a horizontal line. Raise and lower the slit-lamp biomicroscope until the semicircles are equal in size.

While all methods and instruments used for tonometry produce satisfactory measurements of intraocular pressure, each system has advantages and disadvantages. Because almost all tonometers actually touch the highly sensitive cornea, anesthetizing eyedrops are used in patients before testing. Some tonometers also require instillation of **fluorescein**, a dye solution, to aid in positioning the testing device correctly against the cornea.

Applanation Tonometry

The most commonly used instrument for performing applanation tonometry is the Goldmann tonometer. Other devices include the hand-held Perkins tonometer, the electronic MacKay-Marg tonometer, the compact Tono-Pen, and the pneumatonometer. The last-named instrument uses compressed gas to applanate the cornea and measure the intraocular pressure. The air-puff tonometer is a noncontact applanation device that employs a burst of air to applanate the cornea.

All applanation tonometers measure the force required to flatten a small area of the central cornea. The precise area to be flattened is predetermined and varies with the instrument used. The Goldmann tonometer, for example, flattens a circle 3.06 mm in diameter. More force is required to flatten a circle on the cornea when intraocular pressure is high (a "harder" eye), and less force with lower intraocular pressure (a "softer" eye).

The **Goldmann tonometer** is usually attached to a slit lamp (biomicroscope). The tonometer itself consists of a double-prism head (the tonometer tip), attached by a rod to a housing that delivers measured force controlled by an adjustment knob (Figure 5.13). Positioning of the tonometer tip can be observed through the slit-lamp oculars (Figure 5.14). Force is increased by turning the tonometer's force-adjustment knob until a circle of cornea 3.06 mm in diameter is flattened. The

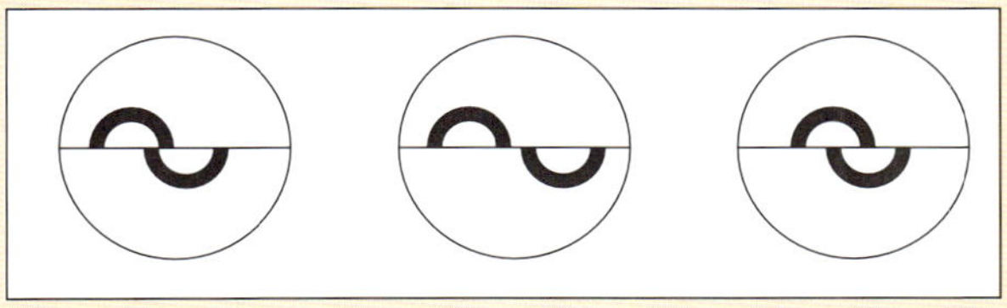

7. Slowly and gently turn the force-adjustment knob of the tonometer in the direction required to move the semicircles until their inner edges just touch, not overlap, as shown at the left in the figure. If the semicircles are separated, as shown in the center figure, the pressure reading will be too low. If the semicircles overlap, as shown in the right figure, the pressure reading will be too high.
8. With the slit-lamp control handle, pull the tonometer head away from the patient's eye. Note the reading on the numbered dial of the tonometer's adjustment knob. Multiply the number by 10 to obtain the intraocular pressure in millimeters of mercury.
9. Record the pressure in the patient's record, followed by the abbreviation for the eye to which it applies, for example,

T 20 OD (A) / 21 OS (A) *or* TA 20 / 21

TA stands for "applanation tension" or "tension by applanation." Also indicate the type of tonometer used, abbreviating the instrument as follows (or with the standard abbreviations used in your office): **A** = applanation (Goldmann) tonometer, **S** = Schiøtz (indentation) tonometer, **P** = pneumatonometer, **AP** = air-puff tonometer, **TP** = Tono-Pen. As always with ophthalmic data, record the measurements for the right eye (**OD**) first, and for the left eye (**OS**) second.

10. Clean and decontaminate the tonometer as required in your office (see Appendix A, "Care of Ophthalmic Lenses and Instruments").

An incorrect pressure reading can occur from too much fluorescein dye (semicircles too fat) or pressure from the examiner's fingers on the patient's eye when holding the eyelids open. Be sure the pressure from your fingers holding the eyelids open is against the orbital rim and not on the eye.

FIGURE 5.13

The Goldmann applanation tonometer.

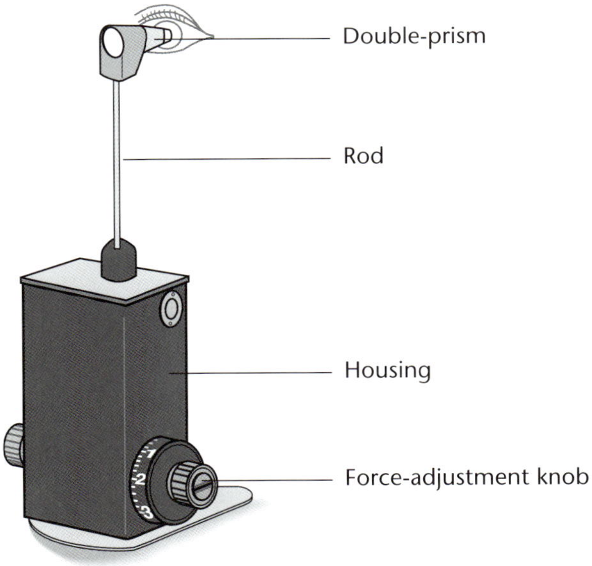

FIGURE 5.14

Applanation tonometry with the Goldmann tonometer.

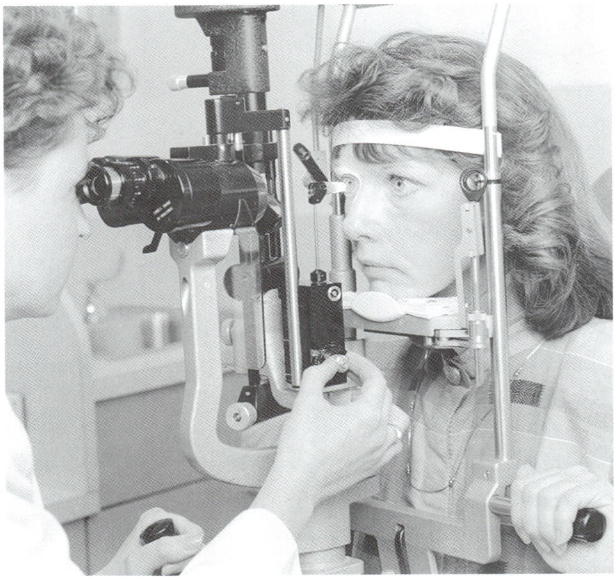

FIGURE 5.15

The Schiøtz indentation tonometer.

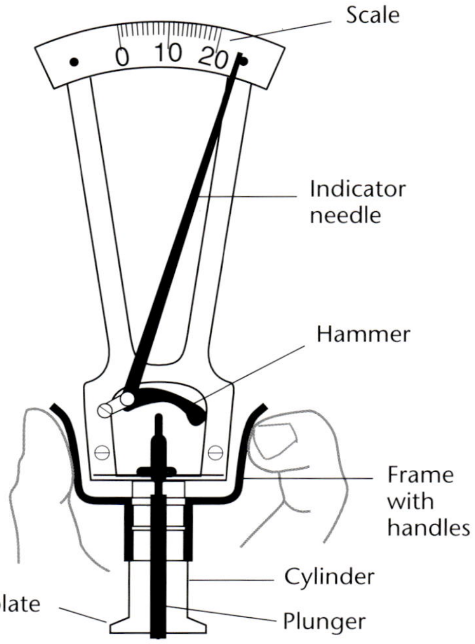

FIGURE 5.16

Indentation tonometry with the Schiotz tonometer.

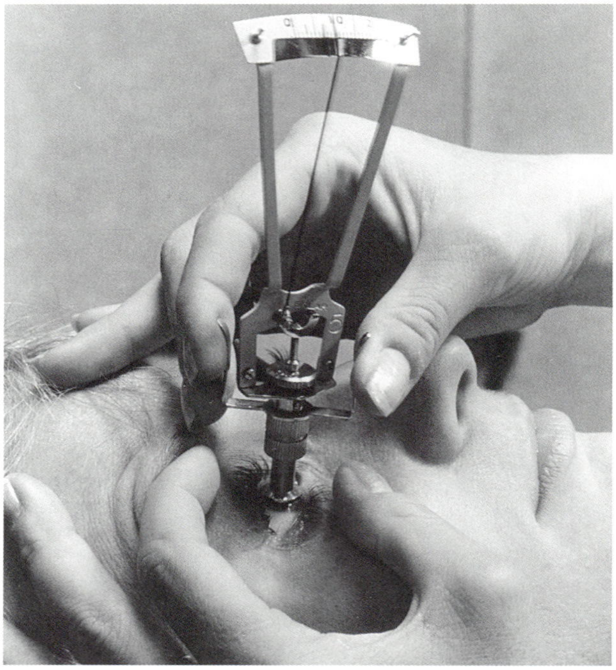

amount of force required is indicated by a number on the calibrated dial on the adjustment knob. This reading is simply multiplied by 10 to express the intraocular pressure in millimeters of mercury.

Goldmann tonometers are popular and common in ophthalmic practice because they make correct alignment with the cornea easy and they are highly accurate. In addition, intraocular pressure is directly related to the readings on the drum. The main disadvantages are their cost and nonportability. These devices also require a relatively normal corneal shape for accurate measurement. The box "Performing Goldmann Tonometry" on pages 86–87 describes the steps of the procedure.

Tono-Pen

As mentioned, the Tono-Pen is a portable electronic device that is used to estimate intraocular pressure. Pen-like in shape, it consists of a stainless steel probe containing a solid-state strain gauge that converts intraocular pressure to an electrical signal. A protective, disposable latex membrane is placed on the tip of the Tono-Pen before use with each patient.

IOP is measured by lightly touching the patient's anesthetized cornea with the tip of the Tono-Pen. Four measurements are recorded for each eye, resulting in an average IOP measurement. Measurements can be taken with the patient either sitting or supine, which adds to the versatility of the instrument. Although the Tono-Pen is not as accurate as the Goldmann applanation tonometer, its size and versatility make it useful for screening purposes and with patients who are unable to cooperate for applanation tonometry.

Indentation Tonometry

Indentation tonometry provides an estimate of intraocular pressure by measuring the indentation of the cornea produced by a weight of given amount. The technique is commonly performed with a relatively simple mechanical device called a **Schiøtz tonometer**. This instrument consists of a cylinder, the bottom of which forms a concave footplate that contacts the cornea (Figure 5.15). Surrounding the cylinder is a frame with a pair of handles by which the examiner holds the device while positioning it. Through the cylinder passes a plunger. The upper end of the plunger moves a hammer, which, in turn, moves a needle across a calibrated scale fixed to the top of the device.

The examiner chooses a weight of a given size (5.5 to 15.0 grams), attaches the weight to the top of the plunger, and gently lowers the device to rest on the patient's anesthetized cornea (Figure 5.16). The amount of corneal indentation by the weight is registered on the scale of the tonometer in increments of 0.05 mm. The units are then converted to intraocular pressure in millimeters of mercury by the use of standard conversion tables supplied with the instrument. The examiner records in the patient's chart the weight used in the test, the indentation units observed, and the conversion to intraocular pressure in millimeters of mercury.

Applanation vs Indentation Tonometry

Schiøtz indentation tonometry is popular for use by nonophthalmologist physicians because it is easy to perform and does not require expensive instrumentation. Like Goldmann tonometry, the Schiøtz procedure requires relatively normal corneal curvature for accuracy. However, the indentation technique assumes that the rigidity of the sclera is normal, which may not be the case with young subjects or patients with high myopia. If resistance of ocular tissues to stretching is higher than normal (ie, scleral rigidity is high), intraocular pressure will be overestimated; conversely, if ocular rigidity is low, the pressure will be underestimated.

Careless techniques can result in inaccurate readings by any tonometric method. For all methods, and particularly Schiøtz, patients must be relaxed, with tight collars loosened. Schiøtz tonometry also requires the examiner to hold the patient's lids apart, but done improperly, this maneuver can apply pressure to the globe and produce a false reading. Most inaccuracies in Schiøtz tonometry result in falsely low, rather than high, readings.

For instructions on cleaning tonometers after each use to avoid the possibility of spreading infection, see Appendix A, "Care of Ophthalmic Lenses and Instruments."

EXTERNAL EXAMINATION

The purpose of the external eye examination is to provide an assessment of the ocular adnexa, external globe, and anterior chamber. During this examination, the ophthalmologist visually inspects the orbital soft tissues around the eyes, the eyelids, the lacrimal apparatus, the visible portions of the external globe, and the anterior chamber angle. **Palpation** (touching) and specialized measurement procedures may be used, as well as visual inspection. Together with the patient's history, the results of this examination provide the ophthalmologist with numerous clues to the patient's general eye health and any specific ocular complaint. Abnormalities revealed in the external examination may be further investigated in other portions of the comprehensive eye examination.

In examining the orbit, the doctor looks for evidence of exophthalmos, inflammation of the orbital tissues, and other visible abnormalities. The extent of proptosis may be measured by a special procedure called *exophthalmometry*, described later in this chapter. The ophthalmologist inspects the lids for general health, function, and normal positioning. If infection or abnormalities are found or the history suggests that they may be present, the lids may be further examined by biomicroscopy or other methods.

If the patient's history and a general examination of the lacrimal system suggest a tear deficiency, biomicroscopy may be employed for a closer inspection. *Schirmer testing*, described later in this chapter, is a specialized test of tear production that the ophthalmic assistant may be required to perform. The pupillary examination, described earlier in this chapter, is sometimes performed as a component of the external examination.

Anterior Chamber Evaluation

The anterior chamber is the dome-shaped space between the back of the cornea and the front of the iris. In a small percentage of individuals, this chamber is more shallow than normal. As these people age, the natural increase in the size of the crystalline lens may block aqueous flow through the pupil, causing the iris to bend forward in a convex shape and creating a narrow angle between the outer edges of the iris and cornea. When this happens, the flow of aqueous fluid out of the anterior chamber through the trabecular meshwork may be slowed and even eventually blocked, producing a sudden rise in intraocular pressure and, possibly, acute glaucoma. In addition, certain ophthalmic drugs commonly used to dilate the pupil during testing and examination can cause a dangerous rise in intraocular pressure if used in a patient with a narrow chamber angle. Determining the patient's chamber depth and angle is an important part of the external examination in that it can reveal patients at risk for acute glaucoma and those in whom certain pupillary dilating drugs should be avoided.

The **flashlight test** is a simple procedure used to estimate the depth of the anterior chamber and the chamber angle. This test, commonly performed by the ophthalmic medical assistant, helps screen for the presence of narrow-angle glaucoma and can alert the physician to avoid using drugs that would dilate the patient's pupil. The test is described in the box "Performing the Flashlight Test" on page 90.

PERFORMING THE FLASHLIGHT TEST

1. Hold a penlight near the limbus of the right eye from the temporal side of the patient.
2. With the penlight parallel to the plane of a normal iris, shine the light across the front of the patient's right eye toward the nose.
3. Observe the appearance of the side of the iris closest to the patient's nose. In an eye with a normally shaped anterior chamber and iris, the nasal half of the iris will be illuminated like the temporal half (Figure A). In an eye with a shallow anterior chamber and narrow chamber angle, about two thirds of the nasal portion of the abnormally curved iris will appear in shadow (Figure B).
4. Record your observations in the patient's record, and repeat the test on the patient's left eye. Consult the physician for the appropriate way to express your observations in the chart.

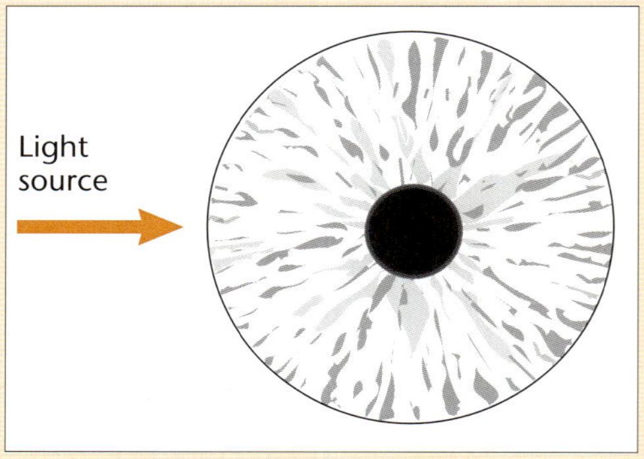

Figure A

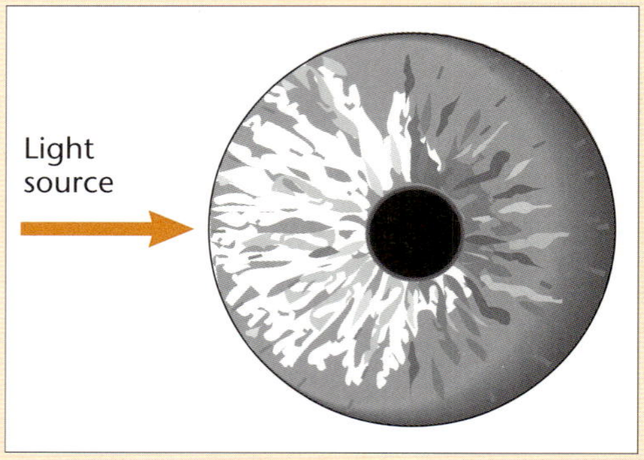

Figure B

FIGURE 5.17

The biomicroscope, or slit lamp.

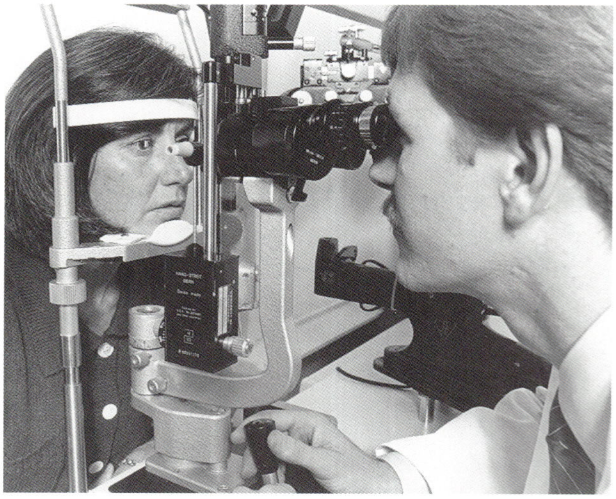

BIOMICROSCOPY

The **biomicroscope**, commonly called a **slit lamp** (Figure 5.17), consists of a magnification viewing system and a source of illumination that delivers an adjustable narrow beam, or slit, of light. The ophthalmologist uses this instrument to obtain a magnified view of the patient's ocular adnexa and anterior segment structures: lid margins and lashes, conjunctiva, sclera, cornea and tear film, anterior chamber, iris, lens, and anterior vitreous. The ophthalmic medical assistant may also use the slit lamp when performing applanation tonometry with the Goldmann tonometer, as already noted.

The ophthalmologist may also use the biomicroscope to examine the fundus: retina, retinal vessels and periphery, macula, and optic nerve head (Figure 5.18). A funduscopic examination is performed to determine the health and physical status of this portion of the eye. A variety of hand-held and attachment lenses used in conjunction with the slit lamp are available; principal among them is the **Hruby lens**, attached to the slit lamp. A noncontact lens attached to the slit lamp, the Hruby lens is useful for examining the optic nerve head and small areas of the posterior retina and vitreous.

Gonioscopy

A careful examination of the structures of the anterior chamber is important for the detection of conditions

FIGURE 5.18

The normal fundus as seen through a slit lamp.

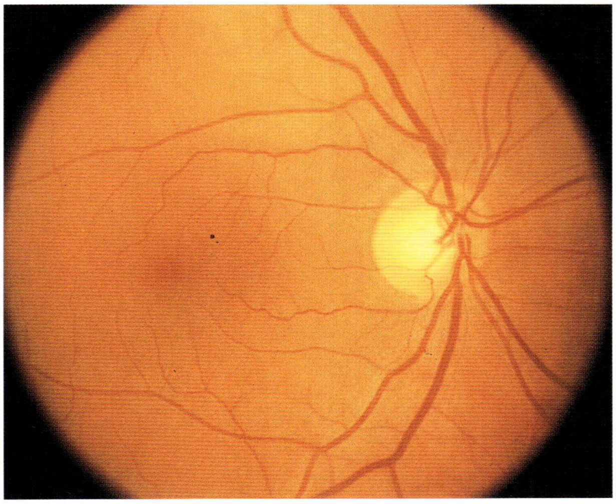

FIGURE 5.19

Preparing for gonioscopy with a slit lamp and a Goldmann goniolens.

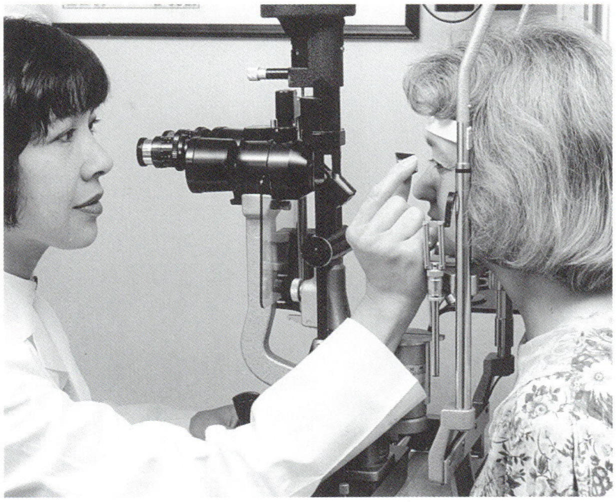

producing, or likely to produce, glaucoma. Because of the curvature of the cornea and its high index of refraction, unaided examination of the chamber angle with a slit lamp is impossible. For these reasons, a specialized viewing method, called **gonioscopy**, is used. In this procedure, the ophthalmologist examines the anterior chamber through a special contact lens placed on the patient's anesthetized eye. One type of gonioscopy, an indirect method, uses the **Goldmann goniolens** (a mirrored contact lens) to reflect the image of the anterior chamber, which is seen through a slit lamp (Figure 5.19). Another, less common type of gonioscopy uses the **Koeppe lens** (a high-plus contact lens) to examine the angle structures as illuminated and observed directly with a hand-held light source and microscope. In both procedures, the contact lenses must be thoroughly cleaned after each use, often by the ophthalmic assistant. Procedures for this purpose are described in Appendix A, "Care of Ophthalmic Lenses and Instruments."

OPHTHALMOSCOPY

Ophthalmoscopy is a method of examining the vitreous and fundus in great detail through the use of an ophthalmoscope. The procedure is sometimes referred to as a *funduscopic examination* or *posterior segment examination*. Ophthalmoscopy is performed exclusively by the ophthalmologist and usually requires the patient's pupils to be dilated with eyedrops to permit the viewing of a greater area of the retina and vitreous. Because pupillary dilation can alter the results of certain visual acuity and pupillary tests, ophthalmoscopy is usually performed after these procedures. The ophthalmic medical assistant is often responsible for instilling the dilating eyedrops. Information about these drugs and their administration is presented in Chapter 11, "Basics of Ophthalmic Pharmacology."

Direct and Indirect Ophthalmoscopy

The two principal types of instruments used for this part of the comprehensive examination are the direct and indirect ophthalmoscopes. The **direct ophthalmoscope** is a hand-held instrument with a light-and-mirror system that affords an upright, monocular survey of a narrow field of the fundus, magnified 15-fold (Figure 5.20). Rechargeable batteries located in the handle of the instrument supply power to the light source. Holding the instrument at close range, the ophthalmologist shines the light at the patient's eye and observes the fundus through the instrument's magnification viewing system.

The **indirect ophthalmoscope** is worn on the physician's head. The headset consists of a binocular viewing device and an adjustable lighting system wired to a transformer power source. The ophthalmologist holds one of a variety of magnifying lenses a few inches from the patient's eye, and the ophthal-

FIGURE 5.20

Ophthalmoscopic examination with the direct ophthalmoscope.

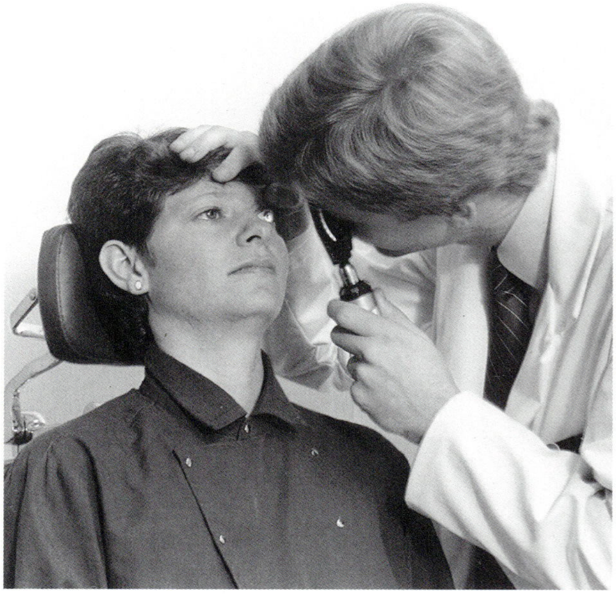

FIGURE 5.21

Ophthalmoscopic examination with the indirect ophthalmoscope.

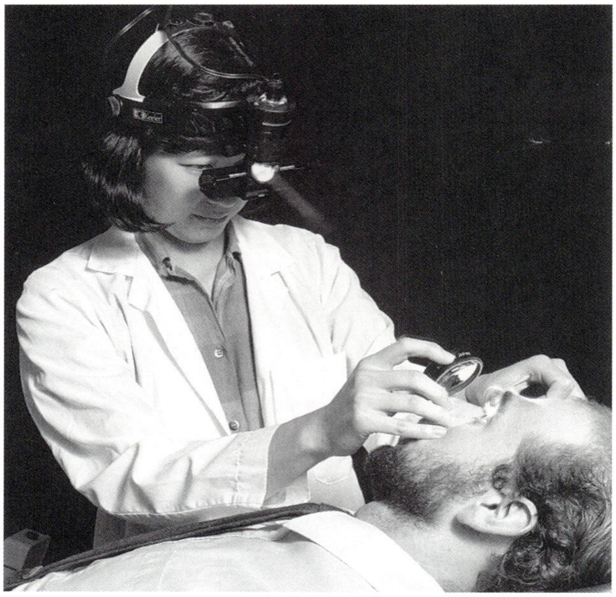

moscope headset provides both the lighting and the stereoscopic vision for the examination. Unlike the upright (direct) view provided by the direct ophthalmoscope, the view of the fundus as seen by the physician is inverted, but provides a wider field of view, in this case magnified 2- to 4-fold (Figure 5.21).

ADDITIONAL TESTS

Information from the patient's history and the results of any portion of the comprehensive eye examination may suggest an abnormality that requires further investigation. Conditions that may require specialized tests include color vision deficit; dry eye; corneal abrasions, lesions, or infections; and proptosis. Dozens of specialized ophthalmic diagnostic and measuring procedures are available. The following are a few of the principal procedures that may require the help of beginning ophthalmic medical assistants or become their responsibility.

Color Vision Tests

The impaired ability to perceive color is most commonly an inherited condition, passed from the mother to a male child usually. Optic nerve or retinal disease may also cause defects in color vision. For the majority of patients with impaired color vision, the color red appears less bright than for normal individuals, preventing accurate perception of color mixtures that include red. While a deficit in color vision is not usually disabling, it can hinder individuals from pursuing certain specialized careers.

Evaluation of color vision is often performed with **pseudoisochromatic color plates** (Figure 5.22). Each eye is tested separately. Patients are instructed to look at a book of these plates, which display patterns of colored and gray dots. Patients with normal color vision can easily detect numbers and figures composed of, and embedded in, the multicolored dots. Patients with color vision deficits cannot distinguish the numbers and figures. Various combinations of colors are used to identify the nature of the color vision deficit.

The **15-hue test**, or **Farnsworth-Munsell D-15 test**, provides a more precise determination of color vision deficits (Figure 5.23). The test consists of 15 pastel-colored chips of similar brightness but subtly different hues, which the patient must arrange in a related color sequence. The sequence is obvious to patients with normal color vision, but patients with color deficiencies make characteristic errors in arranging the chips.

FIGURE 5.22

Pseudoisochromatic color plates used to test color vision. The patient must detect numbers or figures embedded in an array of colored dots.

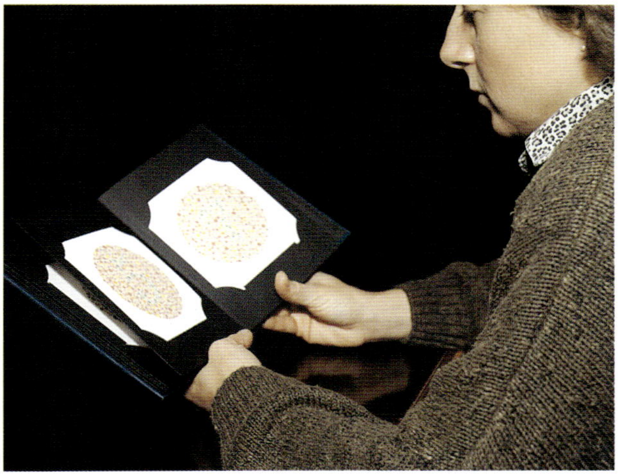

FIGURE 5.23

The 15-hue test of color vision.

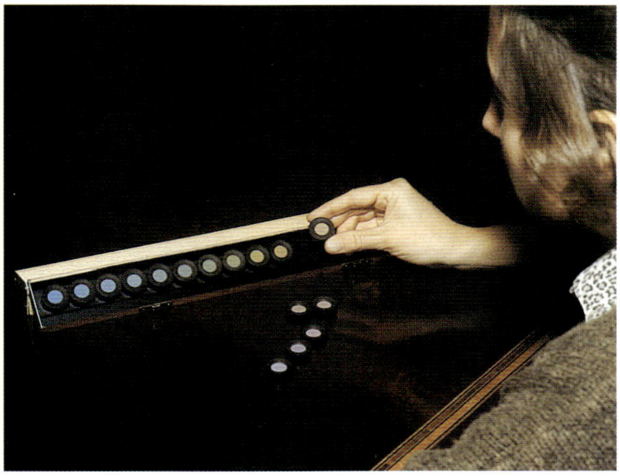

FIGURE 5.24

The Schirmer test, in which the amount of wetting of the paper strips is a measure of tear flow.

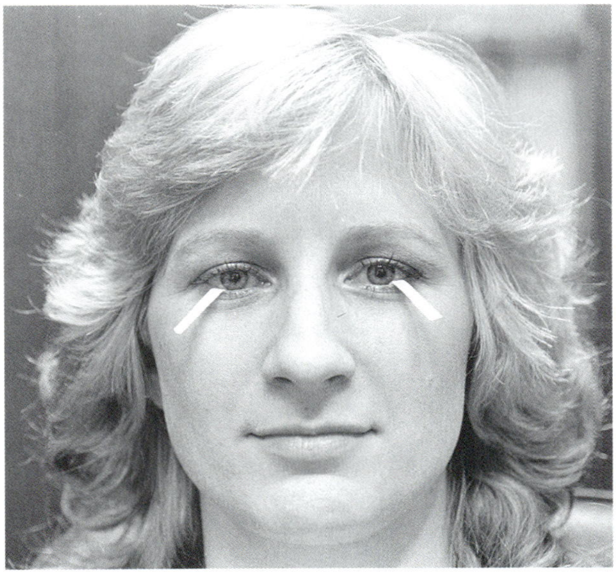

Tear Output Test

The patient's history and external and slit-lamp examinations may suggest the presence of a dry-eye condition. The **Schirmer test** measures the patient's tear output and helps confirm the diagnosis. To perform this test, the examiner places a strip of filter paper in the patient's lower fornix (Figure 5.24). After 5 minutes, the examiner removes the filter paper and measures in millimeters the extent to which the patient's tears have wet the strip. If performed with topical anesthetic, the test measures basic secretion of accessory glands; without anesthetic, the test measures tearing from lacrimal glands (reflex tearing). Less than 10 mm of wetting indicates a dry eye.

Evaluation of the Corneal Epithelium

Fluorescein and rose bengal are dyes used to test the structural and physiologic integrity of the corneal epithelium and to check for conditions such as dry eyes, corneal abrasions, and corneal lesions. When a solution of one of the dyes or an impregnated filter-paper strip is placed in the eye, the dye selectively stains abraded or diseased epithelium (Figure 5.25). The cobalt-blue light of the slit lamp enhances the fluorescence and thereby the visibility of fluorescein. Essential information about these dyes and their use in ophthalmic testing appears in Chapter 11, "Basics of Ophthalmic Pharmacology."

Corneal Sensitivity Test

Certain diseases, such as herpes simplex infections of the cornea and some brain tumors, result in the loss of normal corneal sensitivity. Testing for the existence of corneal sensitivity can help confirm a diagnosis of these conditions. This test may be required by

FIGURE 5.25

A corneal abrasion, stained with fluorescein.

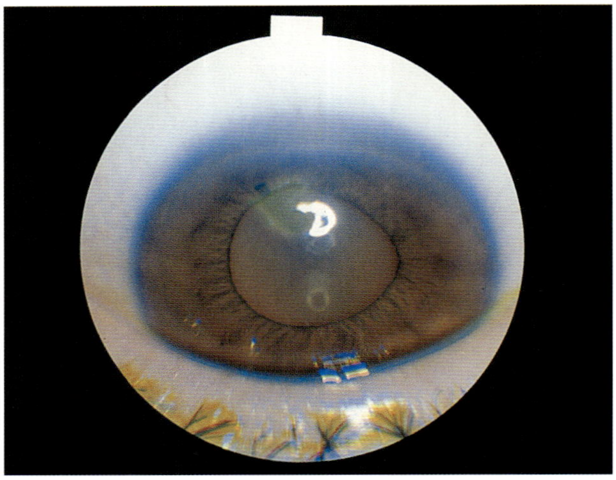

FIGURE 5.26

Measurement of proptosis with an exophthalmometer.

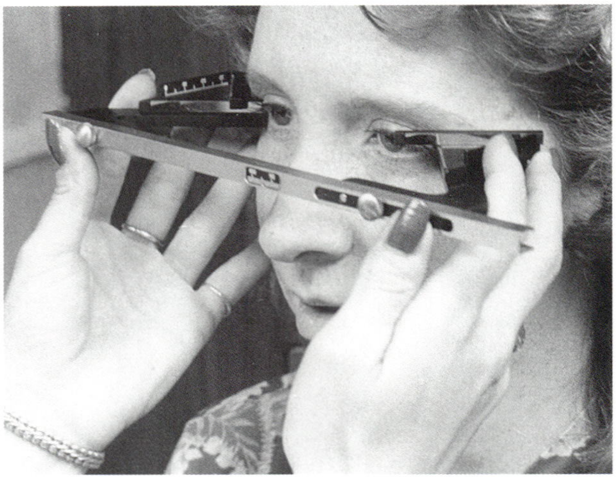

the patient's history or by the results of the external examination or slit-lamp examination. The test is simple but effective. The examiner merely touches the central portion of the cornea with a sterile wisp of cotton to determine whether or not the patient has a normal corneal sensation. A normal response is a blink. With decreased corneal sensitivity, the patient does not blink.

Exophthalmometry

Exophthalmometry measures the prominence of the eyeball in relation to the bony orbital rim surrounding it. The measurement is performed with an instrument called an **exophthalmometer**. The test is useful to record the existence and extent of proptosis caused by such conditions as thyroid disease and orbital tumors (Figure 5.26).

REVIEW QUESTIONS

1. State the purpose of the comprehensive medical eye examination.
2. Name three reasons why a regular comprehensive eye examination may be beneficial.
3. Name the five principal areas covered by the history-taking interview.
4. How should you respond to a patient's request for medical advice or a diagnosis of the patient's condition?
5. Define *visual acuity*.
6. A patient's visual acuity measures 20/40. What does the first number represent? What does the second number represent?
7. You have measured a patient's visual acuity without eyeglasses in place. The measurement was 20/60 in the right eye and 20/40 in the left eye. How would you record this patient's visual acuity in writing?
8. What information is given by the pinhole acuity test?
9. Give two reasons for including the near acuity test in the comprehensive examination.
10. Which three principal properties of the visual system are evaluated by the ocular alignment and motility examination?
11. Name the six cardinal positions of gaze.

12. State the purpose of the prism and alternate cover test.
13. State the purpose of the Worth four-dot test.
14. State the purpose of the Titmus stereopsis test.
15. What important binocular pupillary response to light does the swinging-light test check?
16. State the purpose of the visual field examination.
17. During the confrontation field test, where do the patient and examiner fixate?
18. What does the Amsler grid test determine?
19. Why is the measurement of intraocular pressure a critical part of the comprehensive eye examination?
20. What are the two principles by which tonometers measure intraocular pressure?
21. Which of the four illustrations shows how the semicircles should appear through the slit-lamp oculars when intraocular pressure has been measured correctly with a Goldmann tonometer?

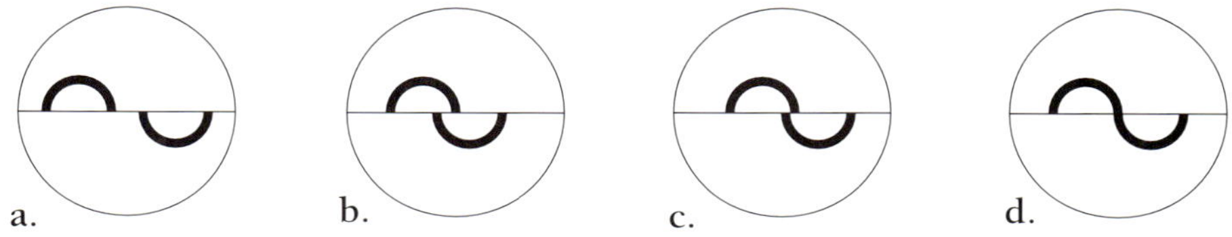

22. State the purpose of the external eye examination.
23. Describe the purpose of the flashlight test and state the two principal reasons it is performed.
24. State four possible uses of the biomicroscope (slit lamp).
25. Describe the Hruby lens and its use.
26. Define *gonioscopy*.
27. Name the two types of ophthalmoscopy.
28. Name two tests used to evaluate color vision.
29. What is the purpose of the Schirmer test?
30. What is the purpose of staining the cornea with fluorescein or rose bengal dye?
31. Describe the corneal sensitivity test and its purpose.
32. Describe the purpose of exophthalmometry.

SUGGESTED ACTIVITIES

1. Discuss with the ophthalmologist or senior staff members in your office which tests will be your responsibility to perform or assist with. Request that you be permitted to observe trained members of the staff perform the tests and that you be allowed to practice the procedures under supervision.
2. Review the elements of the comprehensive medical eye examination with the ophthalmologist in your office. Ask specifically how much and what type of information you should discuss with the patient before the examination.

3. Confirm with the ophthalmologist the specific questions to be included when taking the patient's preliminary history.
4. With a senior staff assistant acting as a patient, role-play the taking of an ophthalmic patient history. Discuss your performance together afterward, and ask for specific tips to improve your technique.
5. Ask permission to observe a senior technician or the ophthalmologist performing the following procedures with patients: visual acuity testing; testing direct and consensual pupillary reaction; confrontation visual fields; applanation tonometry; and the flashlight test. Then, over a period of time, schedule sessions with the technician or doctor to train you in each of these procedures, using other assistants as volunteer "patients" before graduating to testing actual patients.
6. Ask permission to observe a senior technician or the ophthalmologist performing the following procedures with patients: alignment and ocular motility examination; visual inspection of the external eye; biomicroscopy; ophthalmoscopy; and other additional tests selected by the technician or doctor. In a later meeting with the training technician or doctor, go over the names and purposes of the types of instruments used, discuss the purposes of the tests, and determine whether and how you will participate in any of these procedures as a part of your job responsibilities.

SUGGESTED RESOURCES

Bradford CA, ed: *Basic Ophthalmology for Medical Students and Primary Care Residents.* 7th ed. San Francisco: American Academy of Ophthalmology; 1999.

Cassin B: *Fundamentals for Ophthalmic Technical Personnel.* Philadelphia: WB Saunders Co; 1995; chaps 15, 19–22.

DuBois LG: *Fundamentals of Ophthalmic Medical Assisting.* Clinical Skills videotape. San Francisco: American Academy of Ophthalmology; 1999.

Farrell TA, Alward WLM, Verdick RE: *Fundamentals of Slit-Lamp Biomicroscopy.* Clinical Skills videotape. San Francisco: American Academy of Ophthalmology; 1993. Reviewed for currency: 2000.

Movaghar M, Lawrence MG: *Eye Exam: The Essentials.* Clinical Skills videotape. San Francisco: American Academy of Ophthalmology; 2001.

Lewis RA: *Goldmann Applanation Tonometry.* Clinical Skills videotape. San Francisco: American Academy of Ophthalmology; 1988. Reviewed for currency: 1998.

Stein HA, Slatt BJ, Stein RM: *The Ophthalmic Assistant: A Guide for Ophthalmic Medical Personnel.* 7th ed. St Louis: Mosby; 2000.

Wilson Jr ME: *Ocular Motility Evaluation of Strabismus and Myasthenia Gravis.* Clinical Skills videotape. San Francisco: American Academy of Ophthalmology; 1993. Reviewed for currency: 1999.

6 Adjunctive Tests and Procedures

A comprehensive medical eye examination comprises basic assessment and testing of eye function and health in eight principal areas, as detailed in Chapter 5. The results of these basic assessments and tests may reveal an ophthalmic condition that requires further testing to determine the exact diagnosis and treatment. Dozens of adjunctive (additional) tests and procedures are available to complement the comprehensive eye examination. Ophthalmologists generally perform the procedures, but many of these may be delegated to the ophthalmic medical assistant.

This chapter describes several of the most common specialized adjunctive tests and procedures in four principal categories: (1) vision testing in patients with media opacities, (2) tests for corneal disease, (3) photography of the external eye and fundus, (4) ultrasonography. Many of the tests require the use of technical equipment; all of them require some degree of training, skill, and experience to be performed competently. For this reason, the ophthalmologist may delegate them not to a beginning ophthalmic medical assistant but to a more experienced technician. Nevertheless, beginning ophthalmic medical assistants should understand the nature and purpose of these tests not only to increase their effectiveness as members of the office team, but also as the first step toward becoming skilled performers themselves of the adjunctive procedures.

VISION TESTS FOR PATIENTS WITH OPACITIES

The term **ocular media** refers to the eye's three transparent optical structures that transmit light: cornea, lens, and vitreous. **Media opacities** is the general term used to describe a variety of conditions that cloud, obscure, or otherwise affect these structures and may, ultimately, disrupt vision. The principal media opacities are cataracts, which affect the lens, and diseases that cause cloudiness of the cornea, such as corneal edema or corneal scarring from infection or trauma.

Patients with cataracts and cloudy corneas due to certain aging processes or diseases may not have perfectly clear vision, but they are by no means blind as long as the other visual structures of the eye (for example, the macula) are normal. Treatments such as cataract removal surgery, corneal transplantation, intraocular lens implantation, drug therapy, or low-vision optical aids often can restore vision to an adequate functional level.

Visual Potential Tests

A number of testing procedures exist to determine the potential visual status of a patient with a media opacity. The results of these tests help the ophthalmologist determine the extent to which surgery or other types of therapy may potentially improve the patient's vision. With information about a patient's visual potential, the ophthalmologist can recommend the most appropriate treatment. In general, testing for visual acuity potential uses methods that essentially bypass the opacity by measuring the visual abilities of the retina and other optical structures that are unaffected by the opacity. Three commonly used devices are the *potential acuity meter, super pinhole,* and *interferometer.*

Potential Acuity Meter

A principal testing device in the presence of media opacities is the **potential acuity meter** (PAM). This device projects a brightly lighted Snellen acuity chart through the least dense areas of an opacity onto the patient's retina (Figure 6.1). The result of this type of visual acuity testing provides information about the integrity of the visual system and about whether the vision will improve if the opacity is removed.

FIGURE 6.1

Testing with a potential acuity meter (PAM).

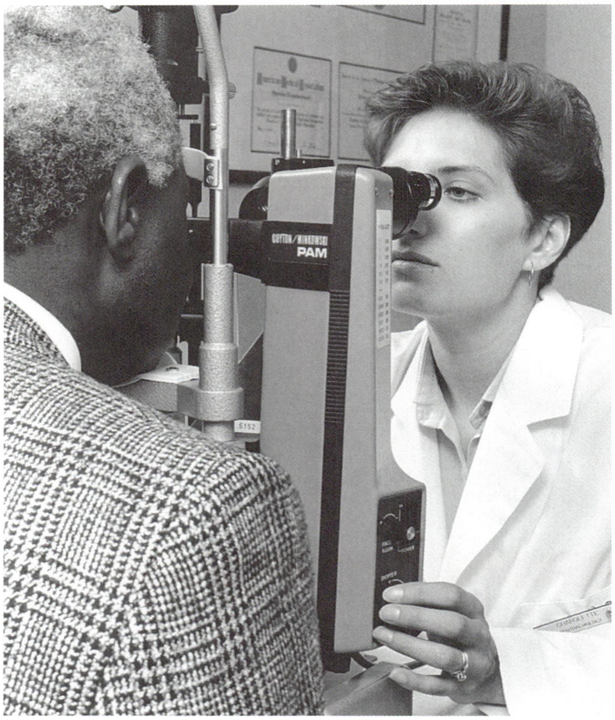

Super Pinhole

The **super pinhole** is a device that helps determine macular function in patients with opacities. In this test, the patient's pupils are dilated with eyedrops and the patient looks at an acuity chart through small pinholes in an opaque disc held before the eye (see Figure 5.5). By moving the disc around, the patient may be able to find tiny openings in the cataract or corneal opacity through which potential vision can be assessed.

Interferometer

The **interferometer** uses the laser or other special light beams to determine visual acuity in the presence of an opacity such as a cataract (Figure 6.2). Sometimes attached to the slit lamp, this instrument measures visual acuity subjectively by projecting a series of parallel lines, separated by varying distances, onto the patient's macula. The patient is then asked to report the orientation of the lines. Visual acuity is measured by the smallest separation of lines whose orientation is reported correctly. The interferometer resembles the pinhole test method in that the inter-

FIGURE 6.2

An interferometer.

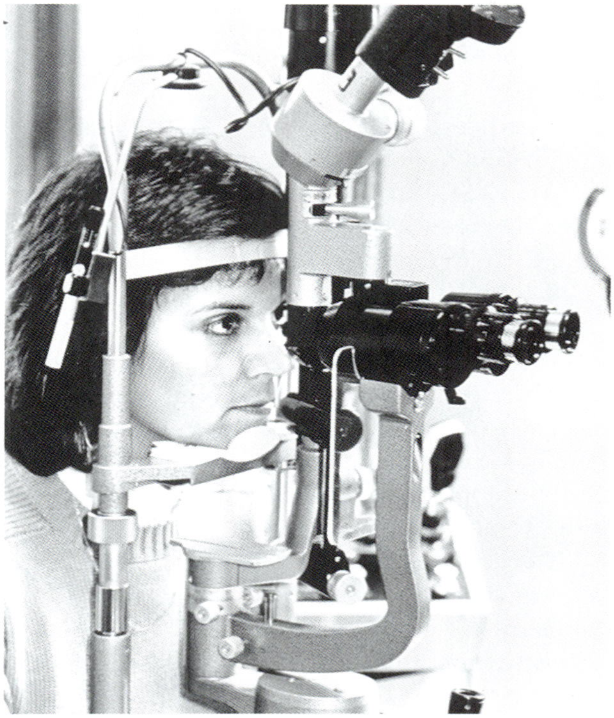

FIGURE 6.3

Contrast-sensitivity testing.

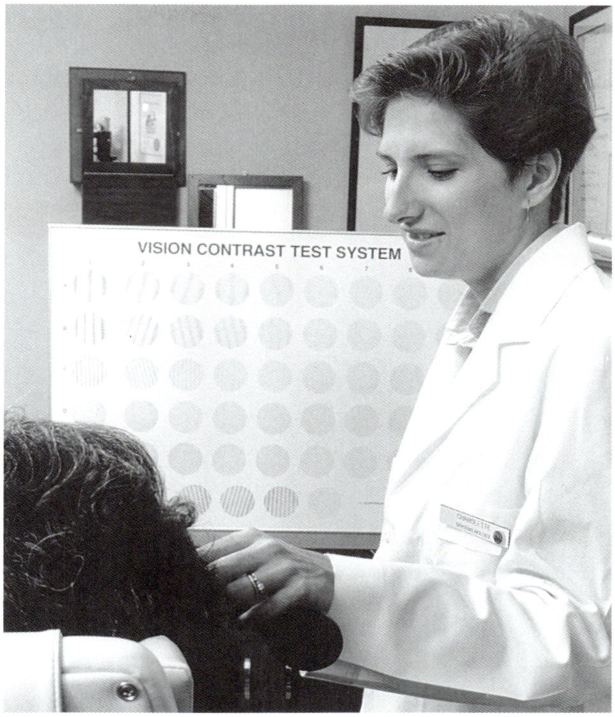

ferometer bypasses refractive errors and the less dense media opacities.

Contrast-Sensitivity and Glare Tests

To perceive objects visually, some contrast of dark and light must be present between the object and its surroundings. Obviously, no one can see any object in absolute darkness. But even in dense fog or deep twilight, shapes at least can be discerned by their relative lightness and darkness. This ability of human vision is called **contrast sensitivity**.

Even if a patient's Snellen visual acuity is sharp, a cataract, corneal opacity, or some other disease can reduce an individual's contrast sensitivity. In these medical conditions, vision can become somewhat like viewing objects in fog or twilight. **Contrast-sensitivity testing** is useful in determining whether a patient's visual complaints are caused by cataract, especially if the patient has shown good Snellen acuity. This testing method also helps the physician determine the need for surgery in patients with cataracts.

The simplest contrast-sensitivity test presents the patient with a printed chart showing letters or symbols in a faint gray print rather than the usual sharp, black-on-white characters of standard charts (Figure 6.3). Other types of charts exist for contrast-sensitivity testing as well as more technical methods involving the presentation of graded patterns or letters on an oscilloscope screen.

Glare occurs when light from a single bright source, such as the sun or an automobile headlight, scatters across the entire visual field. Such scattering of light often dazzles the sight and markedly reduces the quality of image received by the retina. Glare not only can cause the vision to be distorted but also can actually be painful. Patients with cataracts or other ocular opacities often experience this type of optical distortion. **Glare testing** assesses the patient's vision in the presence of a bright light to determine if sensitivity to glare is contributing to a patient's visual symptoms (Figure 6.4).

TESTS FOR CORNEAL DISEASE

Two common procedures used to test for corneal disease are *pachymetry*, which measures corneal thickness, and *specular microscopy/photography*, which allows the cells of the endothelial layer to be counted.

Pachymetry

The normal cornea is about 0.56 to 0.58 mm thick at the center and about 0.80 to 1.00 mm thick at its outer edge. Several diseases, especially some inherited ophthalmic disorders called *corneal dystrophies*, create swelling and cause the cornea to thicken. The cornea then becomes cloudy, leading to visual disturbances.

FIGURE 6.4

Glare testing.

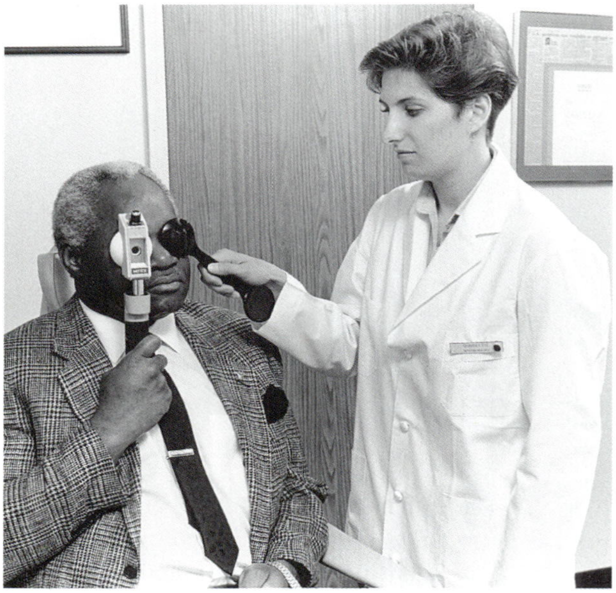

FIGURE 6.5

Pachymetry.

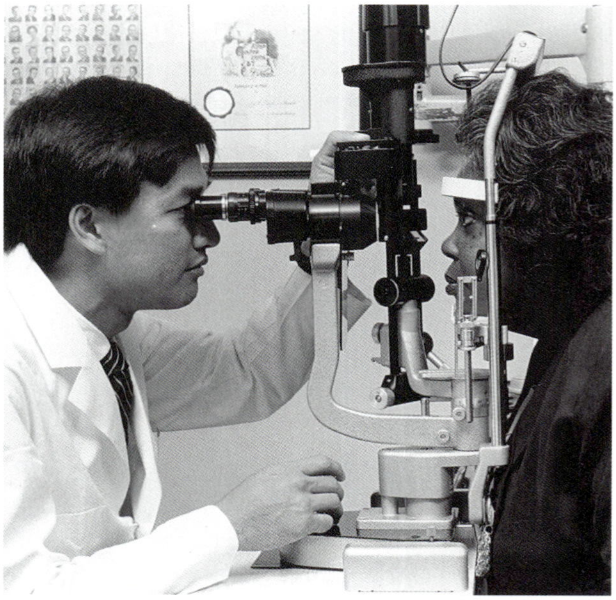

Pachymetry (sometimes spelled *pachometry*), a procedure for measuring corneal thickness, can help diagnose and determine the extent of these conditions, allowing the ophthalmologist to provide timely treatment of the patient's symptoms. Pachymetry is also performed before cataract surgery and other surgical procedures to help estimate the cornea's ability to withstand the stress of an operation.

A device called a **pachymeter** (sometimes spelled *pachometer*) attached to the slit lamp operates on optical principles to measure the distance between the epithelium (front or outer layer of cells) and the endothelium (back or inner layer of cells) of the cornea (Figure 6.5). An ultrasonic pachymeter, which uses reflected sound waves to measure corneal thickness, also is available. Most ultrasonic pachymeters have corneal mapping display programs, which are used to supply information about the potential and actual results of refractive surgery procedures.

The development of many new corneal refractive surgical procedures and the many people wearing contact lenses have promoted the development of **corneal topography,** with concurrent high technology (Figure 6.6). Corneal topography involves the use of a special camera that photographs a projected **Placido disk** pattern on the corneal epithelial surface. This test produces a picture with a detailed map of the corneal curvature (power), elevation, and, with some topography instruments, pachymetry. Corneal topography is routinely performed to help manage patients for corneal refractive surgery, cataract surgery, and contact lens wear.

FIGURE 6.6

Corneal topography map showing a cornea needing further surgical correction after radial keratotomy.

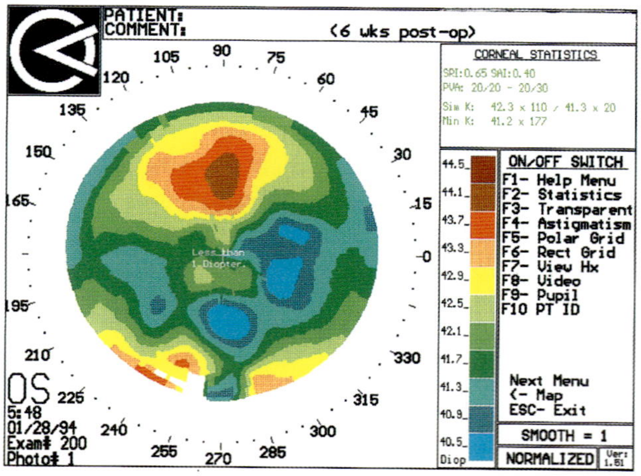

FIGURE 6.7

Specular photograph showing normal endothelial cells.

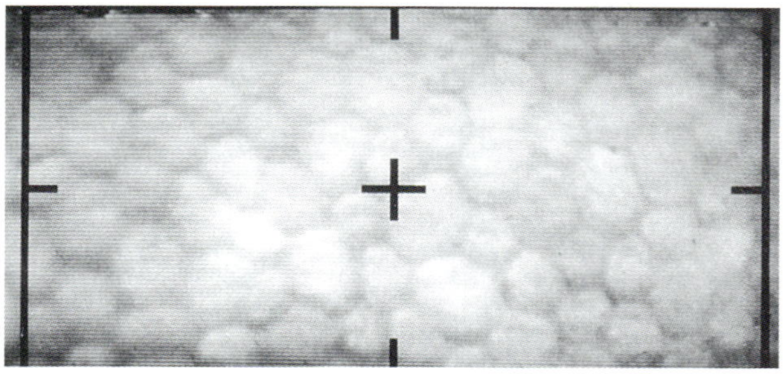

FIGURE 6.8

Slit-lamp photography of the anterior segment of the eye.

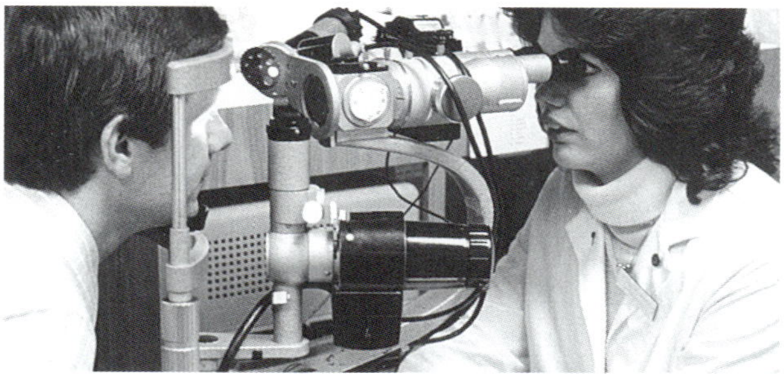

Specular Microscopy/Photography

The cells of the corneal endothelium act as a pump to regulate the amount of fluid in other corneal cell layers, which, in turn, maintain the corneal clarity necessary for proper focusing of light rays. The number of cells in the endothelium serves as an important indicator of the health of the cornea. Too few endothelial cells can indicate the presence of disease and also may affect the ability of the cornea to withstand certain intraocular surgical procedures.

Specular microscopy/photography is a method of microscopically photographing the cornea's endothelial cells at great magnification and producing photographs from which the cells can be counted. Special slit-lamp attachments may be used to produce still photographs, or a video camera may be used to record and display the cells on a video screen. A Polaroid photograph is then taken of the video screen to serve as a permanent part of the patient's medical record (Figure 6.7). Magnification of the photographs is such that cells actually can be counted visually.

OPHTHALMIC PHOTOGRAPHY

Ophthalmic photography serves principally to document ophthalmic conditions for diagnosis and recordkeeping. Some knowledge of photography is required to perform most of these procedures, but a few highly automated photographic devices can be operated effectively, at least in part, by the ophthalmic medical assistant with a minimum of training.

The three general types of ophthalmic photography are

1. External photography
2. Slit-lamp photography
3. Fundus photography

All of these techniques use standard 35-mm still-camera bodies and may produce either color slides or black-and-white negative film for prints.

External Photography

External photography of the eye aids in documenting abnormalities of the eye's outer structures (for example, blepharitis) that do not need high magnification to be seen. This method requires only a 35-mm still camera equipped with a close-up lens and electronic flash attachment.

Slit-Lamp Photography

A 35-mm camera back can be attached to the slit lamp to produce photographs that document abnormalities of the cornea, iris, and lens (Figure 6.8). The optics of the slit lamp replace the camera's normal lens, serving as a viewing and focusing system and providing the necessary magnification of these structures. The slit beam can be used to help determine the depth of a lesion within these structures.

Fundus Photography

Fundus photography encompasses the use of a fundus camera to take color photographs and to produce black-and-white photographs during fluorescein angiography.

Fundus Camera

The modern fundus camera is, in effect, a large ophthalmoscope that can produce color photographs of the retina (Figure 6.9). A fundus camera consists of an optical system for viewing the retina, a light/flash system for illumination, and a 35-mm camera back

FIGURE 6.9

(A) Fundus photography of the retina. (B) Resulting photograph showing normal retina.

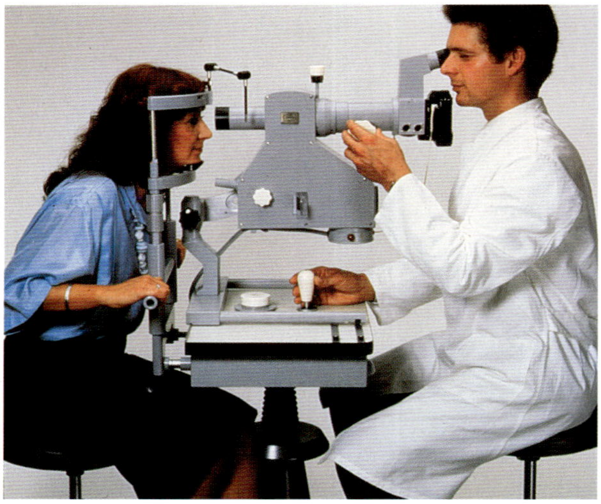

A

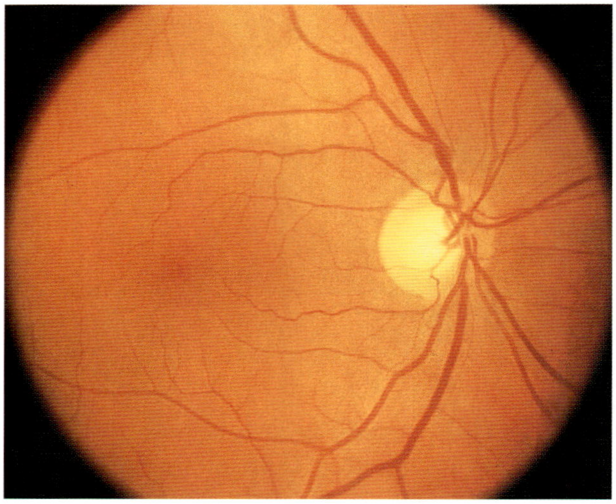

B

FIGURE 6.10

(A) Fluorescein angiogram of a normal retina. (B) Fluorescein angiogram of a diabetic patient. The numerous white dots are tiny outpouchings in abnormal capillaries (microaneurysms) that are filling up with dye.

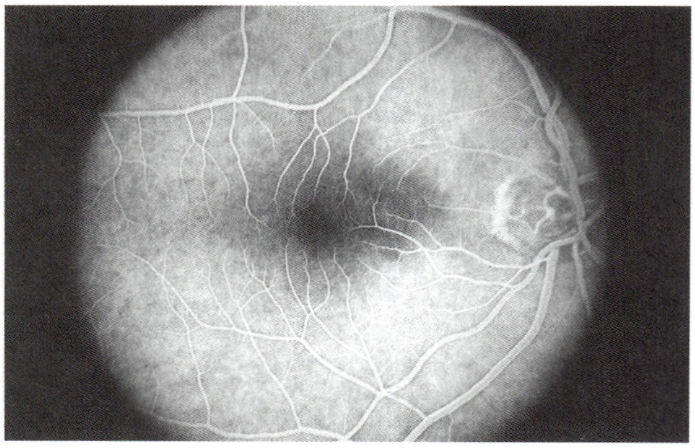

A

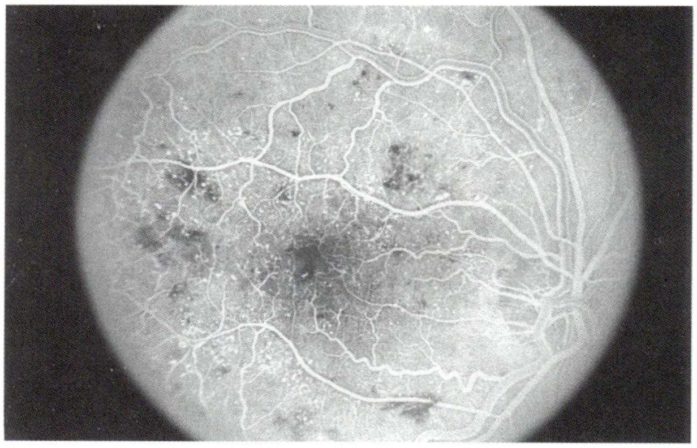

B

containing the film and film-advance mechanism. To allow the photographer the most encompassing view of the fundus, patients usually receive dilating eyedrops to enlarge the pupil before fundus photography.

Fluorescein Angiography

Performed with the fundus camera, **fluorescein angiography** is a specialized technique for viewing detail, such as emboli or other blockages or abnormalities, in blood vessels of the eye (Figure 6.10). In this procedure, a fluorescent dye called *fluorescein* is injected into a vein in the patient's arm. The vascular system quickly delivers the dye to the ocular blood vessels. The fundus camera, equipped with special filters to highlight the dye and a motor drive to take photographs in rapid sequence, captures the appearance of the vessels as the dye courses through the blood vessels. The photographs taken in this manner are called *fluorescein angiograms*.

Fluorescein dye can cause the patient to have momentary nausea or, rarely, a severe allergic reac-

FIGURE 6.11

(A) A-scan ultrasonography. (B) Resulting measurement derived from A-scan ultrasonography.

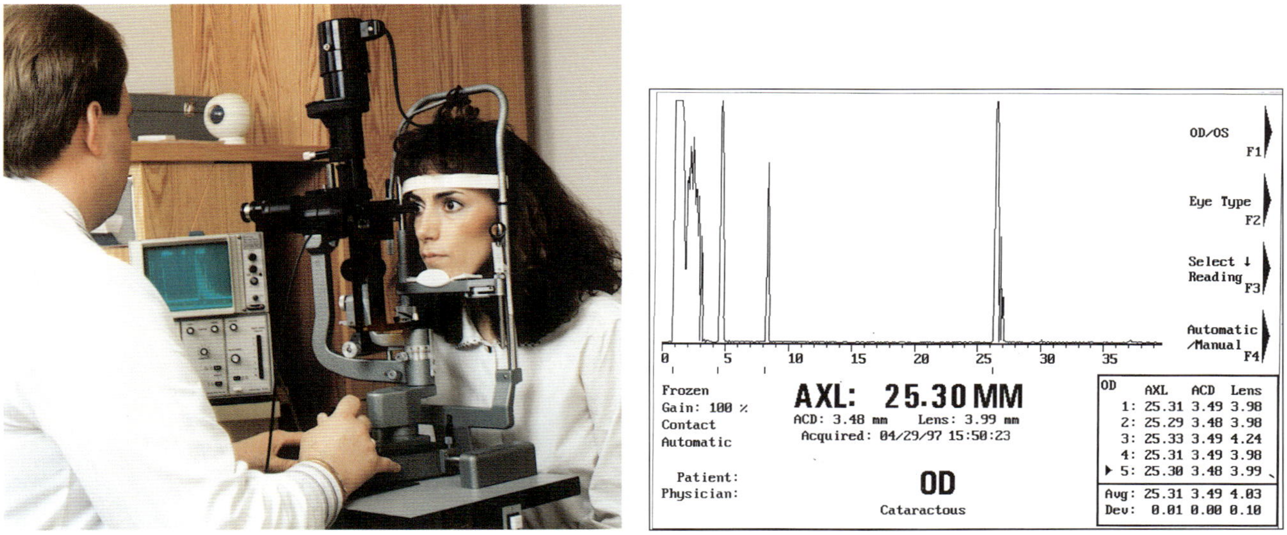

A **B**

tion. Therefore, the doctor and emergency equipment should be on hand during fluorescein angiography. More information about fluorescein and how to deal with an allergic drug reaction appears in Chapter 11, "Basics of Ophthalmic Pharmacology."

ULTRASONOGRAPHY

Ophthalmic **ultrasonography**, or *biometry*, uses the reflection, or echo, of high-frequency sound waves to define the outlines of certain ocular and orbital structures and to measure the distance between structures. Ultrasonography also aids in detecting the presence of abnormalities such as tumors and in determining their size, composition, and position within the eye.

Sometimes ultrasound may be the only nonsurgical method available to observe normal structures or tumors within the eye and to measure their relative or approximate position or their size. Ultrasound procedures are divided into two types: *A-scan ultrasonography* and *B-scan ultrasonography*.

A-Scan

A-scan (or **A-mode**) ultrasonography uses sound waves traveling in a straight line to reveal the position of and distances between structures within the eye and orbit. This method is especially useful for measuring the length of the eyeball, which must be known to properly calculate the power of an artificial intraocular lens (IOL). IOLs may be implanted into the eye either at the time of cataract extraction or later as a secondary surgery. Accurate and consistent measurements are extremely important, because small errors of measurement in axial length will produce large errors in the dioptric power of an IOL implant. The patient will have a large myopic refractive error if the calculation is too large and a large hyperopic error if the calculation is too small; these refractive errors would need to be corrected postoperatively.

To perform A-scan ultrasonography, a probe is placed on the patient's globe. The probe is attached to a device that delivers adjustable sound waves. The measurements are displayed as vertical spikes (peaks) on the screen of an oscilloscope. The appearance of the peaks and the distances between them can be correlated to structures within the eye and the distances between them (Figure 6.11).

B-Scan

B-scan (or **B-mode**) **ultrasonography** delivers radiating sound waves. This technique provides a two-dimensional reconstruction of ocular and orbital tissues. B-scan ultrasonography is especially useful

FIGURE 6.12

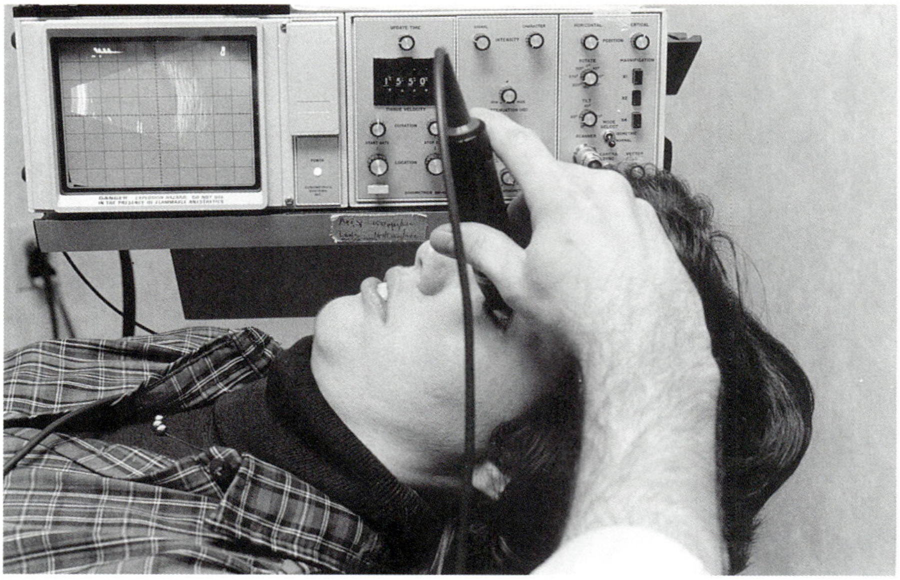

B-scan ultrasonography.

in detecting and measuring the size and position of tumors within the eye.

As with A-scan ultrasonography, the B-scan method employs a probe tip that delivers sound waves when it is touched to the patient's eye. The resulting two-dimensional echo image is displayed on the screen of an oscilloscope (Figure 6.12).

REVIEW QUESTIONS

1. What is the purpose of visual potential testing?
2. Name three principal devices used to measure visual acuity potential.
3. What are the two major reasons for conducting contrast-sensitivity testing?
4. Why is glare testing performed?
5. What does pachymetry measure?
6. State the purposes for performing pachymetry.
7. What is the main use for specular microscopy/photography?
8. The three principal types of ophthalmic photography are
   a. Specular, pachymetry, and contrast-sensitivity testing
   b. External, slit-lamp, and fundus photography
   c. Slit-lamp, pachymetry, and ultrasonography
   d. A-scan, external, and fundus photography
   e. Specular, external, and fundus photography
9. Fluorescein angiography is used to
   a. Count the cells of the cornea
   b. Document abnormalities of the eye's outer structures
   c. Measure the eye's contrast sensitivity
   d. View detail, such as blockages, in ocular blood vessels
   e. Estimate the cornea's ability to withstand the stress of an operation

10. Briefly describe the procedure and process of fluorescein angiography.
11. Name two possible adverse effects a patient can experience during fluorescein angiography.
12. Describe the underlying principle and general diagnostic purposes of ultrasound procedures.
13. The chief purpose for measuring the length of the eye by A-scan ultrasound is to
    a. Calculate the power of the artificial lens to be implanted at the time of cataract removal
    b. View the retinal blood vessels
    c. Determine the size of the cataract for removal
    d. Assess visual acuity
    e. Construct two-dimensional outlines of the retina
14. One of the principal diagnostic reasons for performing B-scan ultrasonography on a patient is to
    a. Determine the size of the cataract for removal
    b. Measure the distances between eye structures
    c. Test for corneal opacity
    d. Measure the distance between the corneal epithelium and endothelium to adjust for cataract surgery
    e. Detect and measure the size and position of tumors in the eye

SUGGESTED ACTIVITIES

1. Determine which of the procedures discussed in this chapter are performed regularly in your office. Ask the ophthalmologist or senior technician which of these procedures you may be expected to learn over time.
2. Ask your ophthalmologist or senior technician for a "guided tour" of the technical instruments discussed in this chapter that are used regularly in your office. Note where these instruments are located in the office, their principal parts, and the purposes for which they are used in your ophthalmologist's practice.
3. Ask your ophthalmologist or senior technician when you may observe either of them performing as many of the procedures described in this chapter as possible. Take notes and meet afterward for questions and discussion.

SUGGESTED RESOURCES

Byrne SF: *A-scan Axial Eye Length Measurements: A Handbook for IOL Calculations.* Mars Hill, NC: Grove Park Publishers; 1995.

Byrne SF: *A-scan Biometry.* Clinical Skills videotape. San Francisco: American Academy of Ophthalmology; 1988. Reviewed for currency: 1998.

Byrne SF, Green RL: *Ultrasound of the Eye and Orbit.* St Louis: Mosby-Year Book; 1992.

Cassin B: *Fundamentals for Ophthalmic Technical Personnel.* Philadelphia: WB Saunders Co; 1995; chap 24.

Cunningham D: *Clinical Ocular Photography.* Thorofare, NJ: Slack; 1998.

DuBois LG: *Fundamentals of Ophthalmic Medical Assisting.* Clinical Skills videotape. San Francisco: American Academy of Ophthalmology; 1999.

Kelly MP: *Basic Principles of Fluorescein Angiography* Clinical Skills videotape. San Francisco: American Academy of Ophthalmology; 1994. Reviewed for currency: 1998.

Kendall CJ: *Ophthalmic Echography.* Ophthalmic Technical Skills Series. Thorofare, NJ: Slack; 1991.

Stein HA, Slatt BJ, Stein RM: *The Ophthalmic Assistant: A Guide for Ophthalmic Medical Personnel.* 7th ed. St Louis: Mosby; 2000.

Wallace P, Evans M: *Fundus Photography.* Clinical Skills videotape. San Francisco: American Academy of Ophthalmology; 1989. Reviewed for currency: 1998.

7 Principles and Techniques of Perimetry

Concerns with vision often emphasize central visual acuity, that portion of eyesight that allows us to see clearly straight ahead in order to read, drive, sew, paint, and perform all the tasks requiring sharp vision. Less attention is paid to **peripheral vision**, the visual perception of objects and space that surround the direct line of sight. Yet this outer field of vision provides the means to move safely within the environment by alerting the brain to potentially dangerous or interesting visual stimuli toward which the gaze can be directed. For example, although central vision plays a large part in driving an automobile, it is the less-sharp but all-important peripheral vision that alerts the driver to cars moving up on either side.

Chapter 4, "Optics and Refractive States of the Eye," discussed the nature, measurement, common defects, and correction of central visual acuity. This chapter discusses the nature of peripheral vision and, most important, the principles of **perimetry**, the testing procedure used to measure the expanse and sensitivity of a patient's peripheral vision and visual field and to pinpoint possible defects in it. Properly performed perimetry is often crucial for the diagnosis and treatment of a variety of ophthalmic conditions, especially those affecting the retina and visual pathway. However, perimetry is a complicated, often highly technical process that requires not only concentration and time on the part of the patient but also skill and knowledge on the part of the person conducting the test. For this reason, this chapter presents only basic principles of perimetry that will introduce you to this complex topic. It includes information about the anatomic basis of the visual field, conventions used in "mapping" the visual field, the purpose and types of perimetry, and the types of visual field defects perimetry can help measure. Also discussed are techniques that can help beginning perimetrists avoid measurement errors as they begin developing their skills.

ANATOMIC BASIS OF THE VISUAL FIELD

The term **visual field** is applied to the entire view or panorama seen by the eye when it is fixated straight ahead. The boundaries of the view and the detail with which its different parts are seen are determined by the composition of the retina (Figure 7.1).

The part of the view focused on the fovea, near the center of the retina, is seen in great detail because of the high concentration of cone cells in this area. The parts of the view focused on the macula, which surrounds the fovea, and on other portions of the retina are seen less clearly; the clarity gradually declines as the distance of the image from the fovea increases. At the outer edges of the retina, where there are no photoreceptor cells, vision disappears altogether.

Close to the fovea on the nasal side of each eye is the optic disc, the point where the arteries enter and the veins and the optic nerve exit the eye. Because there are no rods or cones in the head of the optic nerve, the tiny part of the view focused at this site is not visible. This "hole" in the normal visual field is called the **physiologic blind spot** (Figure 7.2).

FIGURE 7.1

Locations within the retina.

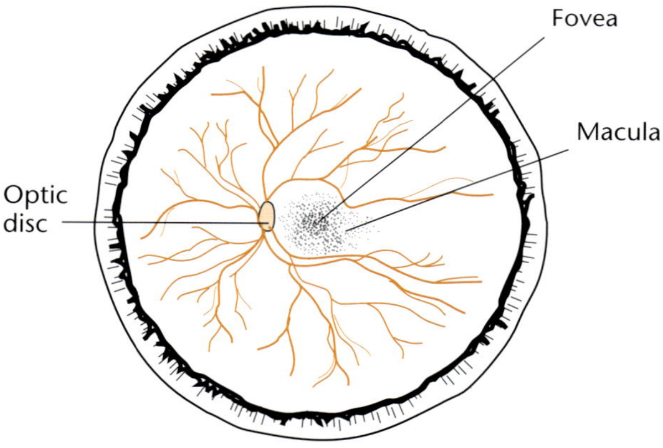

MAP OF THE VISUAL FIELD

The ability to relate the scope of a patient's visual field to physical locations in the eye is important in diagnosing diseases that cause defects in peripheral vision. To provide this ability, a "mapping" system has been devised for use as a tool in measuring the visual field. With this system, locations at any point in both normal and defective visual fields can be expressed in words and numbers.

The visual field may be thought of as an island of vision in a sea not of water but of darkness. Viewed from directly above, the center of this island may be considered to be the patient's point of central visual fixation, which corresponds to the fovea. Placing a series of concentric circles at equally spaced intervals of 10° from this central point provides coordinates that can be used as a reference for mapping the outer boundaries of this island, or, in other words, the extent of peripheral vision. These concentric circles are known as **circles of eccentricity** (Figure 7.3).

Further dividing this circular mapping device into sections that radiate from the point of central fixation provides an additional point of reference for determining locations within the boundaries of the island of vision. These separations, known as **radial meridians**, divide the circular map much as cuts of a knife divide a pie into slices (Figure 7.4). The first cuts divide the pie, or circle, into quarters. These cuts, called the **horizontal and vertical meridians**, are the most significant ones in using the map for diagnostic purposes. The circle can be subdivided by additional radial meridians into almost as many "thin slices," or sections, as needed.

Because a complete swing around a circle represents 360°, a specific meridian can be identified by the

FIGURE 7.2

To demonstrate the physiologic blind spot, close your left eye and fixate on the house at a distance of about 14 inches. The black dot to the right disappears as it falls into the area of your blind spot.

number of degrees, or angle, between the meridian and a baseline—as long as everyone agrees on what point on the circle to start. By convention, the 0° point on the charts for both the right and the left eye is on the extreme right of the horizontal meridian. Moving counterclockwise around the circle, the other meridians are marked in 15° or sometimes 30° steps identified by the angles they form with the horizontal meridian.

The resulting chart for plotting the visual fields of both eyes consists of a pair of adjacent circles with the meridians layered over the circles of eccentricity (Figure 7.5). Plots of the visual field represent the view as seen by the patient. Thus, the circle on the right is used to plot the visual field of the right eye, and the circle on the left, the left eye. The inferior (lower) field is separated from the superior (upper) field by the horizontal meridian, and the nasal (inner) fields are separated from the temporal (outer) fields by the vertical meridian.

Any point in the visual field can be located by noting the number of degrees of eccentricity and the meridian. For example, the physiologic (normal) blind spot is usually located at 15° eccentricity on the 0° or 180° (horizontal) meridian. Can you locate the blind spot of the right and left eyes on Figure 7.5? This spot is always found temporal to fixation (that is, in the temporal field) and serves as a handy reference point to identify which field belongs to which eye.

FIGURE 7.3

Circles of eccentricity in the standard chart form for plotting the visual fields.

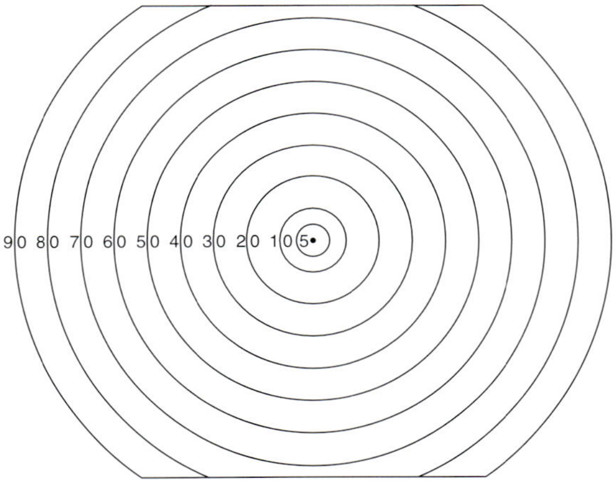

FIGURE 7.4

Radial meridians in the standard chart form for plotting the visual fields.

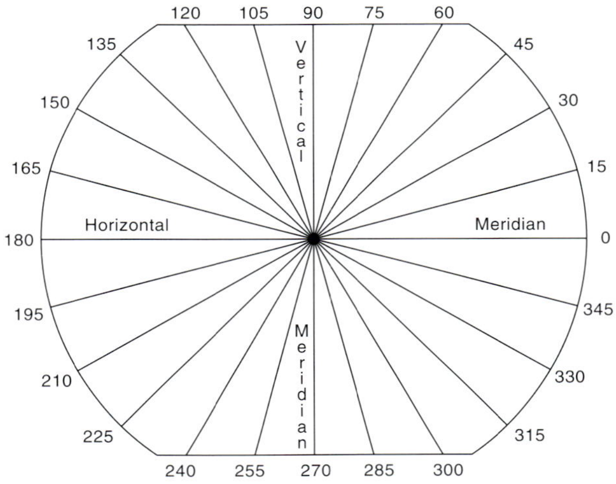

FIGURE 7.5

The standard chart form for plotting the visual fields, with the four quadrants labeled: SN (superior nasal), ST (superior temporal), IN (inferior nasal), and IT (inferior temporal).

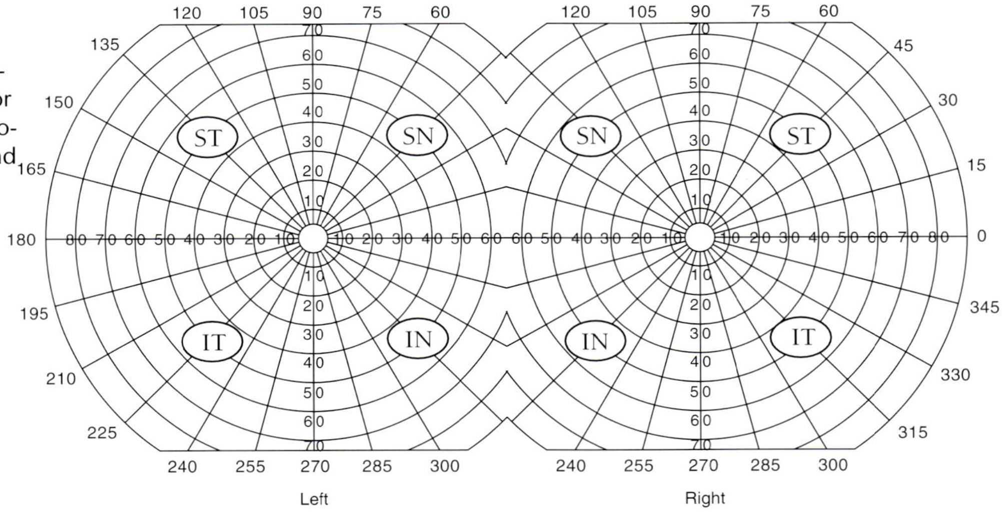

FIGURE 7.6

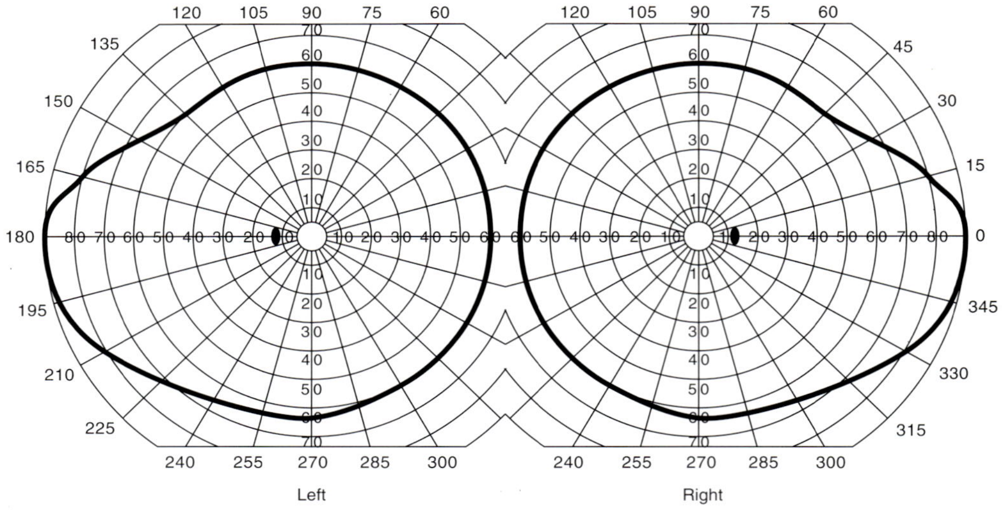

Boundaries of a normal visual field. The black spot in the temporal field of each eye represents the physiologic blind spot.

Figure 7.6 depicts the concept of mapping the boundaries of the patient's visual field by showing the extent of a normal visual field on a standardized visual field "map." The boundary of the normal patient's island of vision—or, in other words, the visual field—extends on the circles of eccentricity to about 90° temporally and about 60° nasally, superiorly, and inferiorly. Objects appearing 110° temporally from the point of central fixation would obviously not be visible, for objects outside of the boundary of the island of vision fall into the "sea" of darkness and cannot be perceived. The result of perimetry is an outline of the shape of the visual field and a map of defects within it.

Another way of perceiving the island of vision is to imagine it as a three-dimensional island might appear, with a peak at its center (corresponding to foveal vision) that slopes gradually to sea level (the outer, nonseeing retina) at the boundaries of the island (Figure 7.7). The slope is steeper on the nasal side of the field and more gradual on the temporal side. The physiologic blind spot may be thought of as a deep vertical well temporal to the peak that extends to sea level. This model of the visual field as an island illustrates how perimetry measures the extent and type of defect in the visual field.

Orientation of the Visual Field Map

Plotting of visual fields traditionally represents the view as seen by the patient. For example, parts of the field that appear to the patient on the temporal side are shown on the temporal side of the chart. When the fields from both eyes are drawn, the field from the patient's right eye is shown on the right. However, it is important to understand that a particular part of the visual field and the corresponding section of the retina do not share the same relative positions. The difference is due to the fact that images of objects focused on the retina are inverted and reversed by the optical system of the eye. In other words, the images appear upside down and backward. Thus, an object that the patient sees in the *temporal* visual field is actually focused on the patient's *nasal* retina. An object appearing in the superior visual field is detected by the inferior retina (Figure 7.8).

The reverse situation also applies. A defect in the patient's superior temporal retina, for example, will affect the patient's inferior nasal field of vision. An illustration of these relationships is the physiologic blind spot. Recall that the absence of photoreceptor cells at the head of the optic nerve is responsible for the absence of vision at this point. Although the optic nerve head is located on the *nasal* side of the eye, the blind spot appears in the patient's *temporal* visual field (see Figure 7.6).

The relationship between locations, sizes, and shapes of defects in the visual field and corresponding parts of the retina and other structures of the visual pathway is discussed later in this chapter. For the moment, the important point to remember is that the map or chart obtained by perimetry represents the visual field as seen by the patient.

FIGURE 7.7

The three-dimensional island of vision.

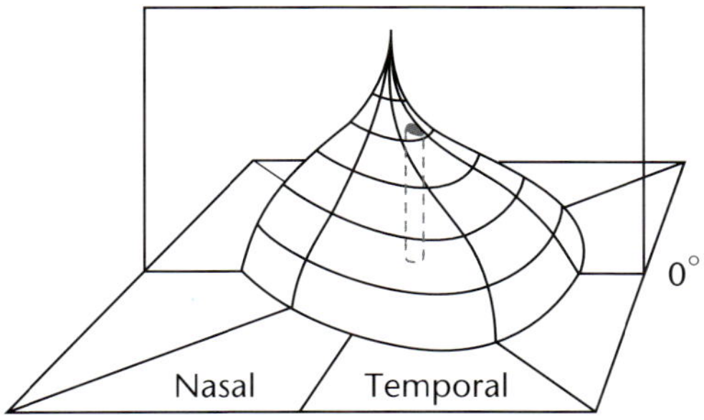

PURPOSES AND TYPES OF PERIMETRY

Perimetry has two important functions. One is to *detect* abnormalities in the peripheral visual field, defects that usually are not apparent with visual acuity measurements. The other function is to *monitor* changes in the normal or defective visual field that may indicate the development, progression, or improvement of diseases affecting the retina and visual pathway. Many diseases of the retina, optic nerve, and brain interfere with peripheral vision before they affect central vision. An accurate mapping of the visual field can help identify the nature and location of these diseases.

Many procedures have been devised to measure the visual field, each with certain advantages and drawbacks. However, all types of perimetry use a test object or target seen by the patient against some specific type of background. The contrast between the test object and the background directly affects the measurements obtained by perimetry; if the target and background were the same color and brightness, no one could distinguish between the two. To illustrate this concept, consider how a small dark bird can be easily seen against a white cloud in daylight, while a large dark tree might be almost invisible when viewed against a dark mountain at dusk. Perimetric measurements are evaluated by taking into account the brightness of the background, as well as the size and brightness of the test object. In most types of perimetry, these qualities can be controlled by the examiner who conducts the test.

The two basic methods employed to survey the field of vision are kinetic perimetry and static perimetry. **Kinetic perimetry** uses a *moving* test object of a predetermined size and brightness, while **static perimetry** employs a *stationary* target that can be changed in size, brightness, and position within the visual field but is not displayed until it has stopped moving.

FIGURE 7.8

The image of an object in the visual field as focused on the retina.

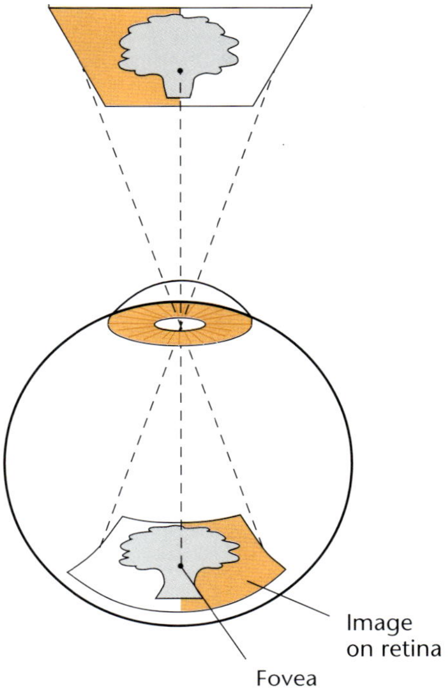

Kinetic Perimetry

A simple demonstration of kinetic perimetry would be to move a hand or finger into the visual field of a patient who is fixating straight ahead, noting when the patient first sees the target. If the action were repeated from several directions around the visual field (that is, at several meridians), the examiner could obtain a rough idea of the boundaries of the patient's vision. This is the basis of the *confrontation field test*, in which the examiner compares the range of the patient's visual field with that of his or her own, which is presumed to be normal. Chapter 5, "Comprehensive Medical Eye Examination," discusses the general principles of this test and describes how to perform it.

Although the confrontation field test is less sensitive than the perimetric methods described in this chapter, its simplicity makes it useful for screening patients for major defects. The test is particularly use-

FIGURE 7.9

The tangent screen test.

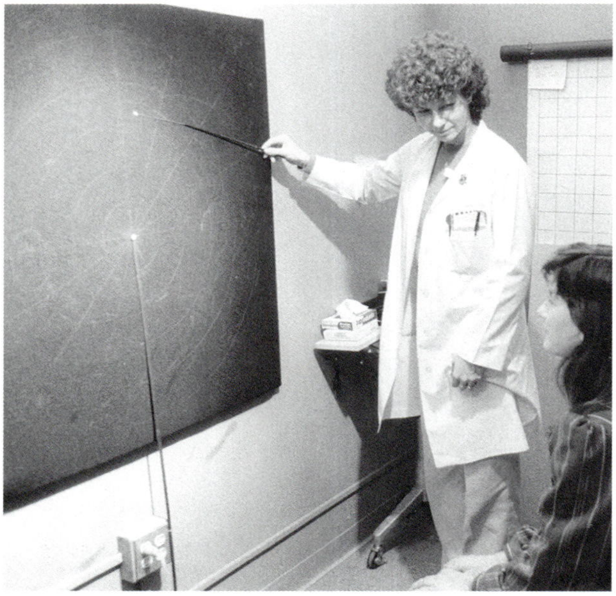

FIGURE 7.10

A series of isopters obtained by kinetic perimetry, and the contours of the island of vision that they represent.

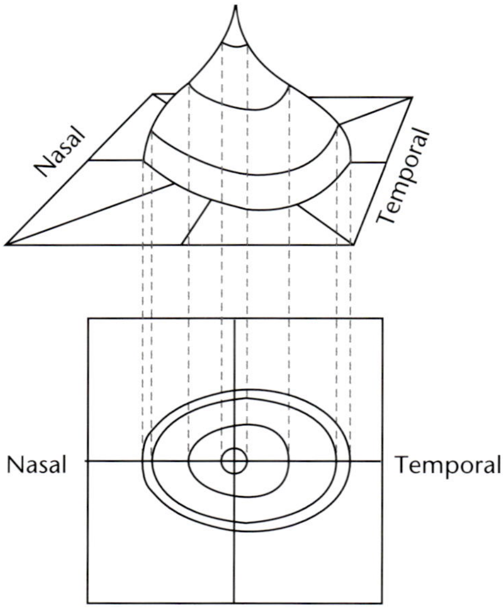

ful with children, the very old, and the mentally impaired—indeed, for any patients unable physically or mentally to undertake the more complex tests.

Tangent Screen Test

A more sensitive type of kinetic perimetry is the **tangent screen test** (Figure 7.9). In this procedure, the patient sits about 3 feet in front of a black felt or metallic gray screen. With one eye occluded by a patch, the patient fixates with the uncovered eye on a center dot on the screen while the examiner slowly moves a black wand with a small white or colored disc at its end into the field of vision. The patient indicates the moment the disc, or target, is seen, and the examiner marks the point on the screen. The process is repeated, moving the target into the field from various directions, each time at the same speed, until a number of points are marked. After the examination, the points are transferred from the tangent screen to a smaller paper chart and joined together by a continuous line. The result is a drawing of the boundaries of the visual field for the particular target used.

The boundaries of the visual field tend to be larger with brighter or larger targets and smaller with dimmer ones, because the less bright or smaller targets require more sensitive vision to be observed. A contour obtained with a single target of a particular size and brightness, such as with the tangent screen test described above, represents a line of equal sensitivity, called an **isopter**. A series of isopters of increasing sensitivity can be obtained through kinetic perimetry by using progressively smaller or dimmer targets. When these isopters are plotted on paper, they look like a stack of irregular ovals seen from the top (Figure 7.10). The shape of the ovals and their exact positions in relation to one another provide a surface contour map of the hilly island of vision, that is, a two-dimensional representation of the sensitivity levels of the visual field.

Surveying the boundaries and contours of the island of vision is only one objective of kinetic perimetry. Another is to discover whether defects are present in the surface of the island and to determine their location and size. Perimetry searches for localized areas within the contours of the visual field where the eye does not see as well as it should. Such an area of reduced sensitivity is called a *scotoma*.

If the island of vision were observed from above, a **shallow scotoma** (mild defect) would appear as a depression in the island surface. A **deep scotoma** (more serious defect) would look like a pit or well. If the defect were so severe that the largest and brightest stimulus could not been seen, it would appear as a well that descends to the sea level of blindness. Such a defect is called an **absolute scotoma** (Figure 7.11). Although it is normal and natural and not pathologic, the physiologic blind spot may be considered an abso-

FIGURE 7.11

Defects in the island of vision. A deep scotoma (left) and an absolute scotoma.

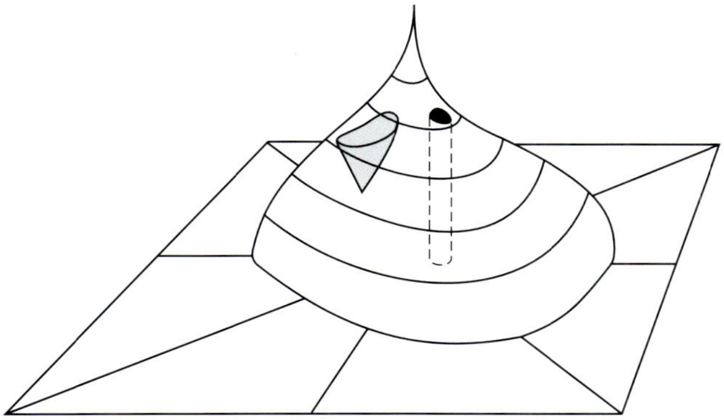

lute scotoma. Detailed information about the causes of scotomas and the manner in which they are charted appears later in this chapter.

The tangent screen procedure is relatively simple to perform and, like the confrontation test, is often used to screen patients for visual field defects. However, results obtained with the tangent screen are difficult to reproduce from one test to another, partly because neither the lighting of the screen nor the brightness of the test objects can be easily standardized. In addition, the tangent screen test measures only the central 30° of the visual field. (The flat screen would have to be excessively large to test the entire visual field.) For these reasons, the tangent screen has been replaced for most purposes by a device called the *Goldmann perimeter*.

Goldmann Perimeter

Instead of a flat screen background, the **Goldmann perimeter** uses a large bowl that can be lighted accurately and reproducibly through a range of desired levels. The target is a projected light that can be preselected for size and brightness and moved over the entire visual field and beyond. Contours of the patient's visual field are measured in much the same way as described with the tangent screen. However, the Goldmann perimeter plots the isopters more easily and covers the entire visual field. Because the test conditions can be standardized and reproduced accurately, results obtained with the same patient at different sessions with a Goldmann perimeter are fairly comparable, even if the tests are run by different technicians on different instruments. However, some differences exist from technician to technician and from instrument to instrument that prevent tests with different technicians and instruments from being exactly comparable.

FIGURE 7.12

The Goldmann perimeter. (A) From the patient's side. (B) From the examiner's side.

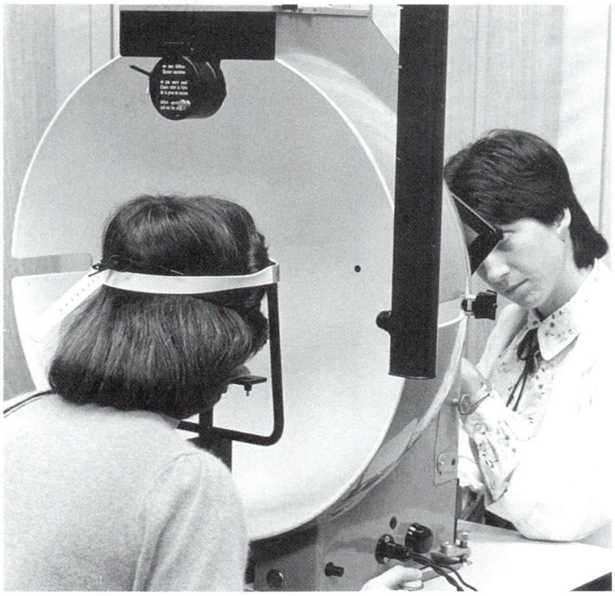

A

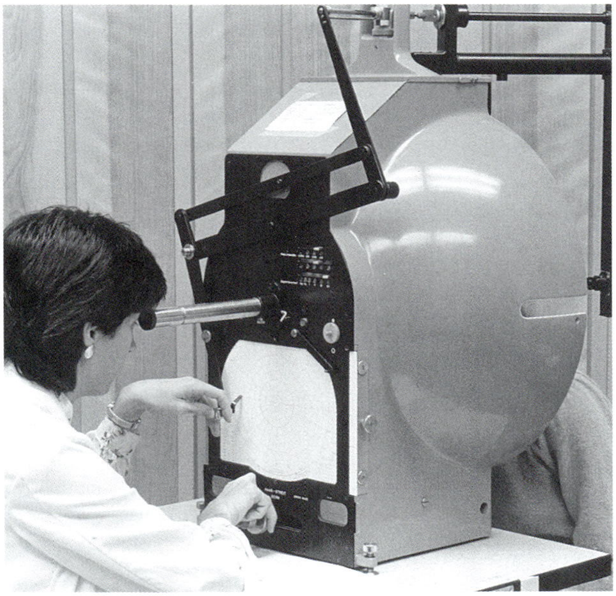

B

In Goldmann perimetry, the patient is seated in front of a lighted bowl set at a specific light level. The technician is seated behind the device (Figure 7.12). One of the patient's eyes is covered. A lens is placed in front of the tested eye to correct for the testing distance and the patient's near correction, if any. The technician moves a small handle attached to a projector from outside the patient's vision toward the center until the patient just sees the projected light. The patient indicates by knocking a key or coin on the table or by pressing a button connected to a buzzer when the light is seen. The handle is connected by a series of levers to the projector in such a way that a paper form representing the patient's visual field on the technician's side of the device and the actual visual field inside the bowl correspond. Thus, the technician can plot the visual field directly on the paper form.

The target can be varied by size and brightness. The targets come in five sizes and are indicated by roman numerals I through V, representing a round light of sizes 0.25 mm^2 to 64 mm^2. The brightness is adjusted by a series of filters placed in the path of the projected light. The gross adjustment for brightness is the 1 through 4 scale. Each unit is 0.5 log unit more intense than the next, with 4 being the brightest. The fine adjustment for brightness is the *a* through *e* scale, with *e* being the brightest and difference between each being 0.1 log unit. Commonly used targets, in ascending order of size and brightness, are I2e, I4e, and III4e.

Other Devices

Devices other than the tangent screen and the Goldmann perimeter are also available for kinetic perimetry. The **Autoplot**, a refined version of the tangent screen, similarly measures only the central 30° of vision. Another device is the **arc perimeter**, which can test the entire field of peripheral vision. Autoplots and arc perimeters are seldom used now and are mostly of historical interest.

Advantages and Disadvantages

Kinetic perimetry has the advantage of being simple to understand for both the patient and the examiner. The procedure also produces a pictorial result that is easy to interpret. The disadvantage of kinetic perimetry is that accurate results depend on the capabilities of the patient and the examiner—human variables that can be difficult to control. For example, if the patient is slow to respond, because of either a long reaction time or a poor understanding of the test, the field will be recorded as smaller than it actually is.

The examiner has the difficult responsibility of moving the target at the same speed in each direction for accurate results. If the examiner moves the target too rapidly, by the time the patient signals that it has been seen, the test object will have moved far beyond the true point of visibility, producing faulty results. If the examiner moves the target too slowly, the patient may become fatigued and unable to respond appropriately. Clearly, for accurate results, kinetic perimetry requires patience and cooperation on the part of the patient, skill and experience on the part of the examiner.

Static Perimetry

Some of the errors associated with kinetic perimetry can be avoided by an alternate approach to surveying the visual field, namely, static perimetry. This procedure tests the ability of the retina to detect a stationary target or light at selected points in the visual field. As with kinetic perimetry, the background can be varied but is usually left at the same levels as with kinetic perimetry. The two static methods used to estimate the light sensitivity of the retina are suprathreshold perimetry and threshold perimetry.

In **suprathreshold static perimetry**, a light or target of a specific size is chosen so that the patient should be able to see it when it is placed at a particular site in the visual field. If the patient does not see it, a defect probably exists at that point. If the brightness of the light or target is considerably above the normal minimal level of brightness for visibility, the defect is probably deep.

Suspicion of the presence and location of a visual field defect determines the placement of targets for exploration. The doctor may direct the examiner in choosing and placing the targets on the basis of a suspected defect or, in the case of computer-driven devices, may direct the computer to certain locations. Automated static perimeters have programs with predetermined locations that are aimed at the kinds of defects seen in certain diseases. Although a shallow defect may be easily missed by suprathreshold static perimetry, the technique is useful as a screening procedure to find gross defects.

Static perimeters use the same test-object sizes as Goldmann kinetic perimetry and the same roman numeral convention (I-V) to indicate that size. On the other hand, brightness of the test objects is indicated by a unit called a **decibel** (one tenth of a log). Whereas in kinetic perimetry the higher numbers indicate brighter test objects, in static perimetry the higher numbers indicate dimmer test objects. Thus, if a patient can see a size III test object at 38 decibels, the patient's eye is more sensitive at that location than an eye that can see the same test object only at 24 decibels.

FIGURE 7.13

Cross-section of the island of vision obtained by static threshold perimetry.

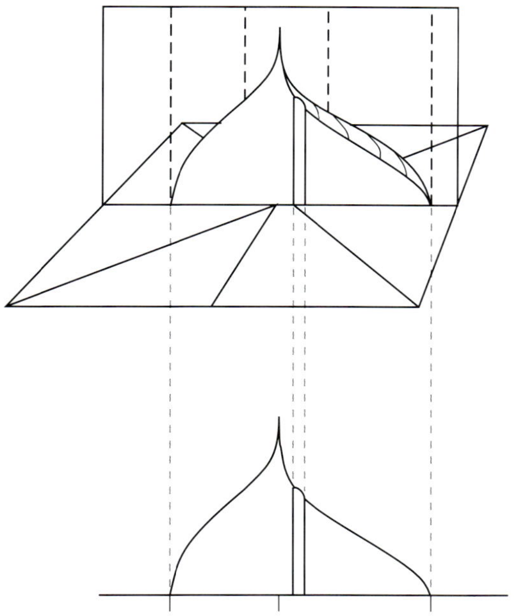

FIGURE 7.14

An automated perimeter.

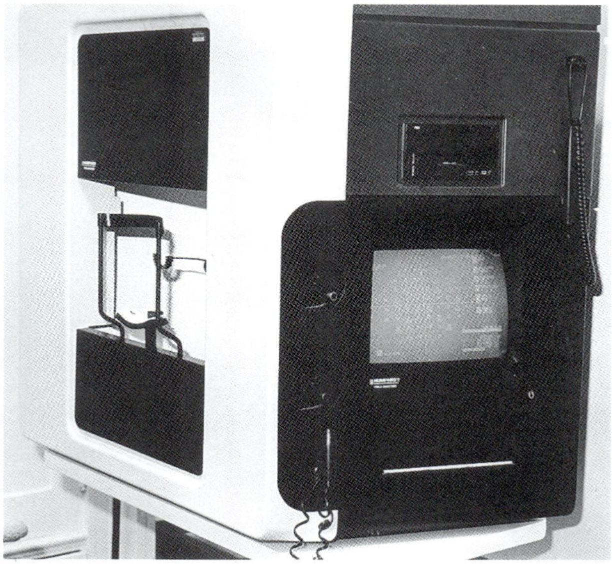

Another, more specific way of performing static perimetry is to place a target of a given size in the visual field and gradually increase its brightness until the patient just sees it. This procedure is called **threshold static perimetry**. The threshold is that level of brightness at which a patient can just detect a given test object about half the time. If the threshold test is repeated at a series of points along one meridian, a cross-section of the island's contours, including the depth of scotomas and other depressions, can be obtained (Figure 7.13). This kind of cross-sectional mapping can be done with manual static perimetry. However, to map multiple meridians, a computerized perimeter is necessary (see the next section).

Several devices are available specifically for performing static perimetry, and new instruments and improved versions of existing units are being added to their number continually. Devices designed for kinetic perimetry can also be used for measurements by static perimetry. Indeed, kinetic perimetry generally includes several suprathreshold measurements. However, such manual performance of the more comprehensive threshold static perimetry is very tedious for both the technician and the patient. For this reason, most static perimetry devices are automated with computer control and recording. These devices usually have the same lighted bowl as the Goldmann perimeter. The patient indicates with a push-button switch when a light (test target) is seen (Figure 7.14).

Computerized Static Perimetry

Computerized threshold perimetry reports the sensitivity to light at a given retinal location in numeric units, which the computer can convert into patterns in shades of gray (Figure 7.15A), resembling the isopter mapping of the visual field with kinetic perimetry (Figure 7.15B). Areas of "normal" sensitivity appear white, and the shades become increasingly gray as sensitivity is reduced. Black indicates total loss of sensitivity for that particular size target.

The values generated by computerized threshold perimetry can be manipulated statistically to determine whether changes seen in a visual field are significantly different from those that might be expected in normal subjects of the same age. The figures can also be compared with the results of previous tests on the same patient. Analysis of multiple serial visual fields with these statistical methods is helpful in detecting trends of deterioration or improvement due to eye disease (Figure 7.16).

Only a limited number of points can be tested by static threshold perimetry at one session before the patient begins to fatigue. For this reason, various computer strategies have been developed, each with the purpose of testing a selected group of points at differ-

FIGURE 7.15

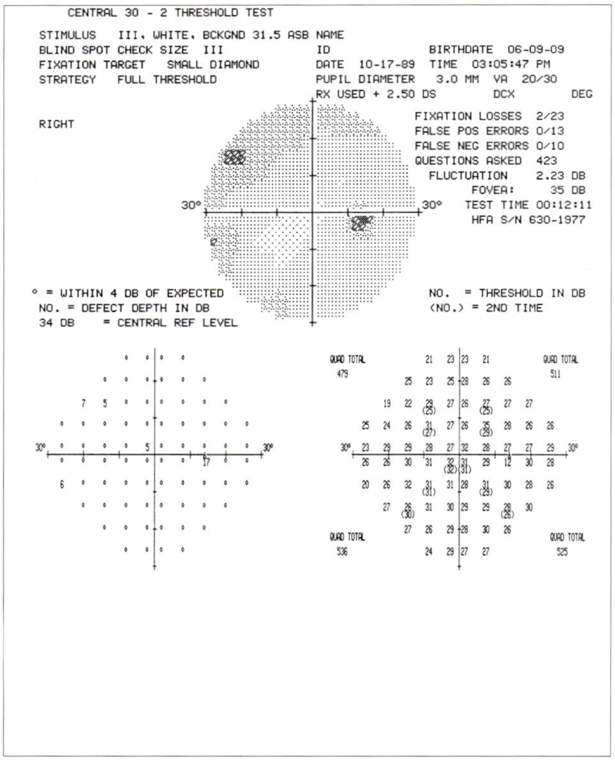

A

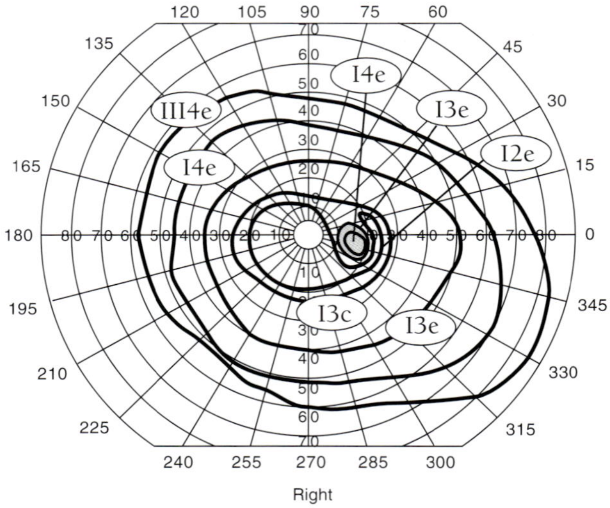

B

(A) A computer-generated grayscale rendering of a visual field as measured by static threshold perimetry. Compare with (B), a kinetic Goldmann plot.

FIGURE 7.16

A series of static visual fields showing progression of glaucoma. Notice the increasingly darker areas at left, denoting progressive visual field loss.

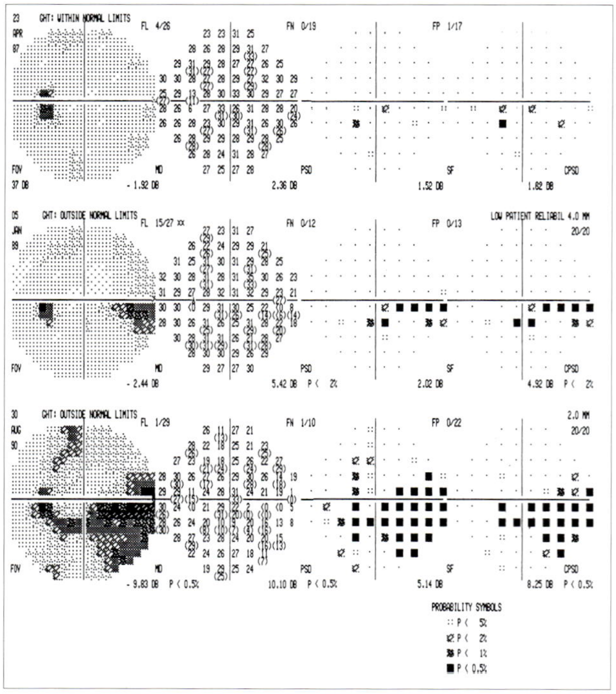

ent sites in the visual field. The most commonly used computer programs, for example, scan the visual field with test points that are 6° apart. With such a program, scotomas 6° in size and smaller could be missed. Generally, these scotomas are not clinically significant, unless they are close to the macula. If a scotoma is suspected near the macula, another computer program can be selected to concentrate on test points in this area.

Some computer programs are designed strictly for screening purposes, others are intended to monitor visual field defects caused by glaucoma, some are directed to macular problems, and still others monitor visual defects resulting from pathology in the brain. Obviously, it is important to know what the doctor is looking for in a particular patient in order to select the program most likely to provide the needed information. As beginning ophthalmic medical assistants work with the perimeter and their ophthalmologist or technical supervisor, they will become familiar with available and newly developed computer programs and their applications.

Advantages and Disadvantages

Computerized static threshold perimetry is more sensitive than kinetic perimetry at detecting small or

FIGURE 7.17

Normal "island" and visual field (A,B) compared with an island and visual field that evidence a general contraction (C,D).

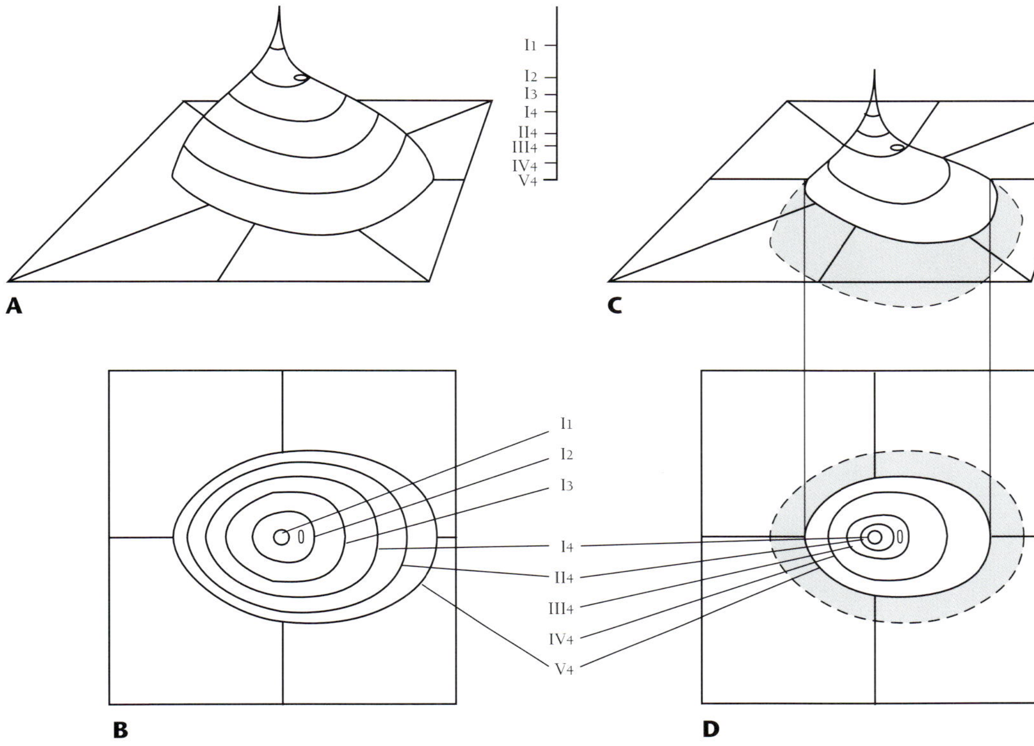

shallow defects in the visual field. The automated procedure also has the advantage of eliminating certain technician- and environment-induced errors, such as moving the test object too rapidly or forgetting to standardize the illumination of the background and test object. However, patient or examiner errors can still occur and may be even more frequent than with kinetic perimetry because, despite automation, computerized threshold perimetry takes longer to perform and is more tedious. In addition, the procedure is more difficult for patients to understand. For patients with limited mobility or attention span and for those with limited understanding of the language spoken by the examiner, Goldmann perimetry may yield more reliable results.

DEFECTS SHOWN BY PERIMETRY

Pathologic changes in the visual field can be divided into two main types: general defects and focal defects. In addition, hemianopic defects involve the right, left, or both halves of the visual field. Other field defects are largely the result of glaucoma.

General Defects

When the field of vision shrinks symmetrically (to the same extent from all directions) or is depressed evenly across the entire retina, a **general defect** is present and the visual field is said to be *contracted* or *constricted*. General defects can be pictured as the whole island of vision sinking into the sea of darkness (Figure 7.17). In Goldmann perimetry, a general defect appears as a symmetric contraction of each isopter; that is, the isopters shrink toward the fixation point. In threshold perimetry, the values at each tested point are reduced.

General contraction of the visual field can result from several disease conditions, including glaucoma, retinal ischemia, optic nerve atrophy, and media opacity, such as a cataract or corneal scar. A gradual, but usually not significant contraction of the visual field can also occur with age, due to the natural loss of retinal sensitivity.

Apparent visual field contraction can also result from poor testing technique. Examples in kinetic perimetry include too rapid movement of the test

FIGURE 7.18

Depression, a focal defect that appears as (A) an indentation of the island of vision or (B) an inward deviation of a portion of several isopters, as measured by kinetic perimetry. The closeness of the isopters at the border of the defect characterizes it as steep rather than gradual.

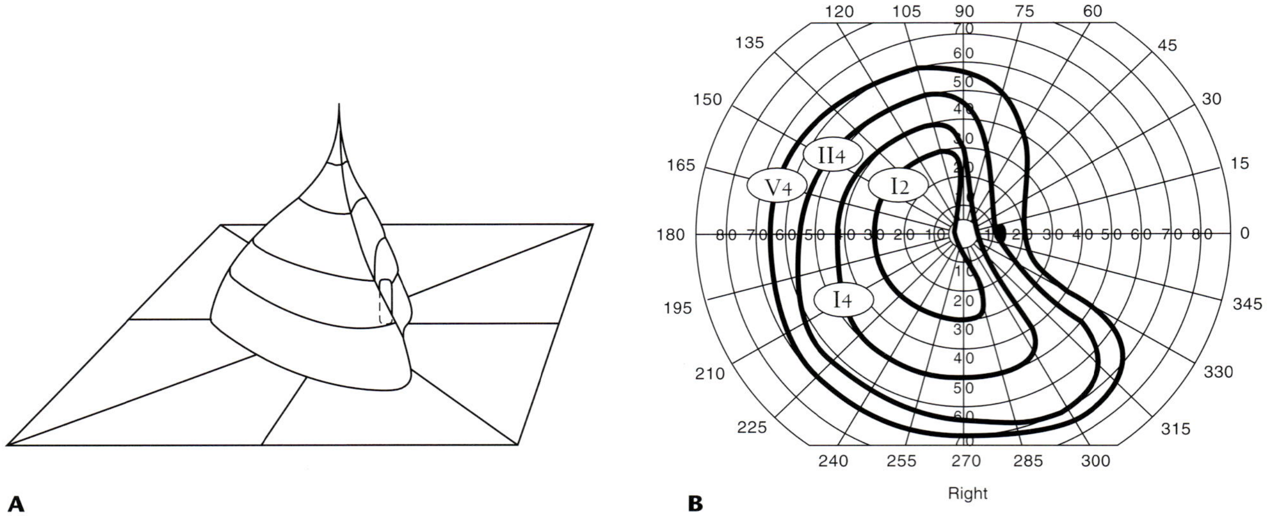

A B

object, poor understanding of the test by the patient, and patient slowness in signaling that the target has been seen. Small pupils, interference with vision by prominent eyeglass rims, aphakia, or a target that seems to be out of focus due to refractive error will also produce a smaller visual field as measured by perimetry.

Focal Defects

Localized changes in the contours of the visual island are called **focal defects.** They may be thought of as a pit or a hole or as a loss of chunks of the island. Small, shallow focal defects can be caused by refractive error, but most are due to an abnormality in the retina, optic nerve, or brain. The size, shape, location, and depth of these visual defects can be helpful in identifying the nature and location of the abnormality.

Two types of focal defects can be distinguished: depression and scotoma. A **depression** is an indentation in the surface of the visual island (Figure 7.18A). On a kinetic field, a depression appears as an inward shift of a portion of several isopters (Figure 7.18B). On a static field, the retinal sensitivity will be reduced at one test site relative to other sensitivities at the same circle of eccentricity. A **scotoma** is a pit or well in the island (Figure 7.19A), represented on the kinetic visual field chart as a circumscribed area in which one or more targets are not perceived (Figure 7.19B). On the static field, a scotoma appears as an area of decreased sensitivity within the outer boundaries of the field (Figure 7.20).

When a visual field defect is mapped, five main features are noted:

1. Location
2. Size
3. Shape
4. Depth
5. Slope of margins

The general concepts of location and size were discussed earlier in this chapter. The shape of a visual field defect depends a great deal on the target size and brightness used to map the defect. One important consideration related to shape and location is whether a defect is aligned with the vertical or horizontal meridian. Due to the anatomy of the visual pathways, defects oriented in line with the vertical meridian suggest a neurologic cause; horizontal defects relate to glaucoma. The distinction can be helpful in assisting the ophthalmologist in locating the source of a visual field defect.

The depth of a defect is the extent to which it "excavates" the island of vision. If the largest and brightest target of the testing device used cannot be seen in a portion of the defect, that part of the defect is said to be *absolute*; less severe defects are considered *relative* (see Figure 7.19).

FIGURE 7.19

Scotoma, a focal defect that appears as (A) a pit or well in the island of vision or (B) a circumscribed area in which one or more targets are not perceived, as measured by kinetic perimetry. The pit represents a relative defect; the well, an absolute defect. The well in this illustration is actually the normal physiologic blind spot.

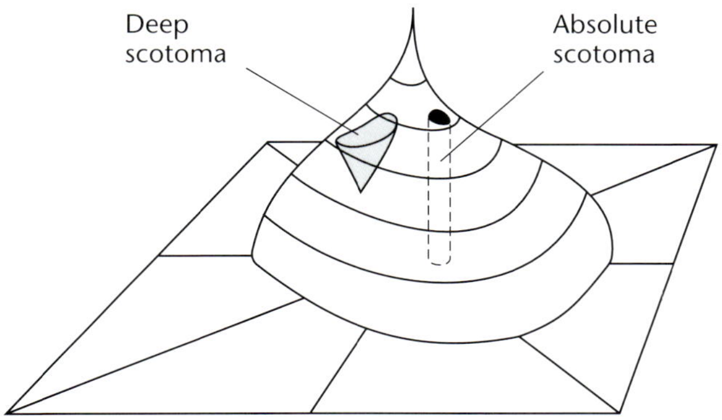

A

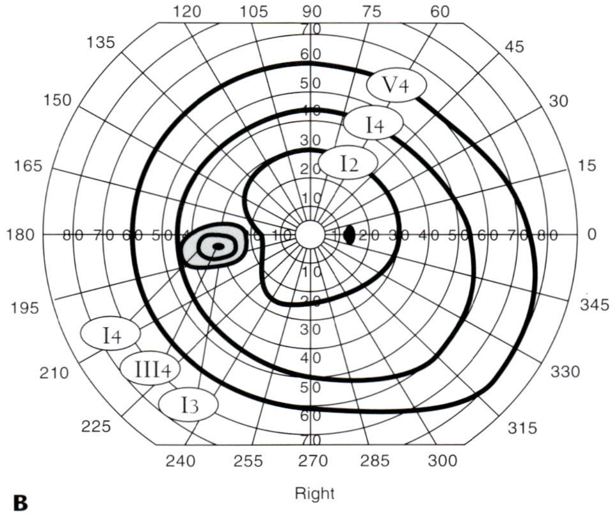

B

The slope of the margins of a defect is determined by how close the defect's borders of different isopters are to one another. For example, if all of the isopters crowd together at the border of the defect, the margins of the defect are said to be *steep* (see Figure 7.18). Steep defects tend to be associated with conditions caused by blood vessel closure, such as strokes. On the other hand, if the isopters showing the defect are widely spaced, the slope of the margin is said to be *gradual*. Gradual slopes tend to be associated more with slowly progressive conditions such as brain tumors and glaucoma. In automated perimetry, slope is determined by differences in sensitivity values of adjacent points.

Hemianopic Defects

Another example of abnormal visual fields is a condition in which the right or left half of the field is missing, a defect called a **hemianopia**. If the right or left half of the visual field is defective or missing in *both* eyes, the defect is called a **homonymous hemianopia**. This visual defect results from damage to the optic tract or optic radiations in the visual cortex due to a stroke or brain tumor (Figure 7.21). A **bitemporal hemianopia**, missing or defective temporal field vision in both eyes, is often due to a tumor or other lesion of the optic chiasm (Figure 7.22 on page 121).

FIGURE 7.20

A scotoma as measured by static perimetry (dark areas except for blind spot at left).

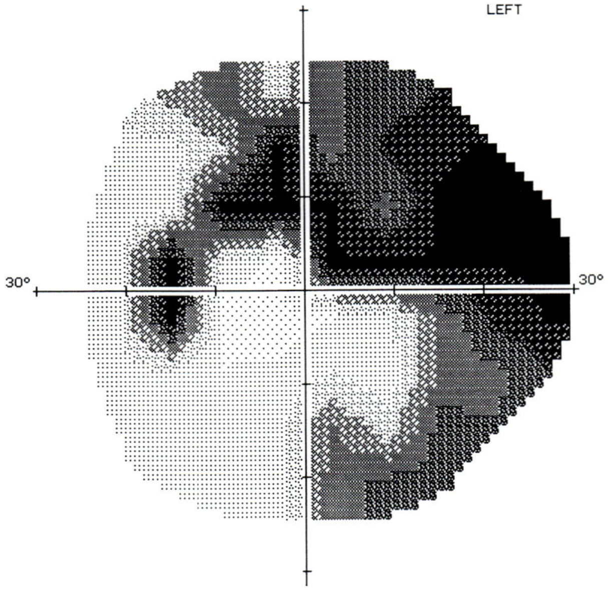

Detection of hemianopic defects is of critical importance because they suggest the presence of a lesion within the brain that may be life-threatening as well as vision-threatening. Early detection increases the chances of recovery because many lesions are treatable, if not curable.

FIGURE 7.21

A right homonymous hemianopic defect resulting from a lesion in the optic tract or in the optic radiation of the visual cortex. (A) The lesion (black rectangles) has destroyed fibers of the optic tract or optic radiation from the temporal retina of the left eye and the nasal retina of the right eye (dotted lines). As a result, objects in the right half of the visual space (gray part of the tree) are not seen. (B) A Goldmann visual field chart of a right homonymous hemianopia. (C) A static chart of a left homonymous hemianopia.

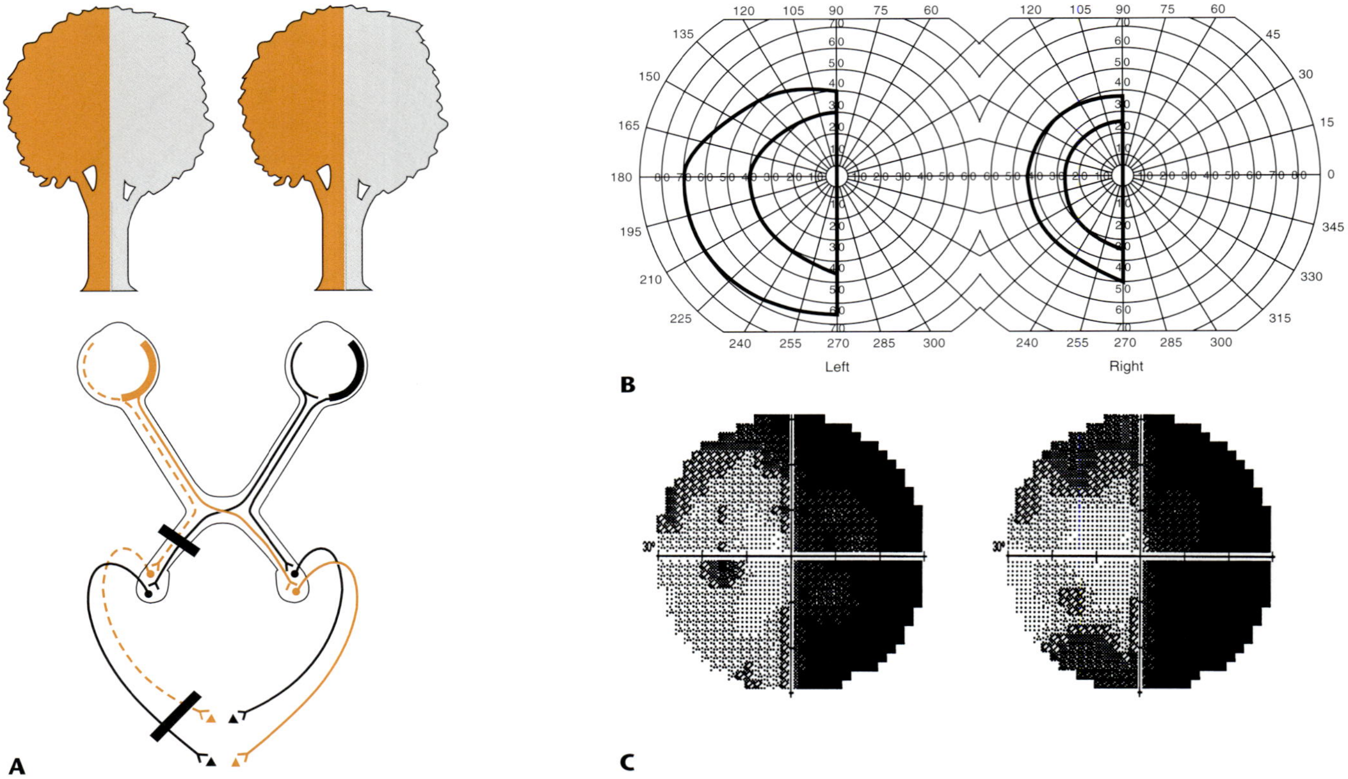

Other Defects

Glaucoma may produce various kinds of defects in the visual field, depending in part on the stage of the disease. Three common types are the Bjerrum scotoma, paracentral scotoma, and nasal step (Figure 7.23 on page 122). The **Bjerrum scotoma** is a small, relatively blind area that appears at about 15° of eccentricity in the upper or lower field. As glaucoma progresses, the Bjerrum scotoma may become enlarged to form an arc-shaped area of reduced sensitivity called an **arcuate scotoma**. A **paracentral scotoma** is a relatively blind area even smaller than a Bjerrum scotoma. This type of scotoma may be seen very near the fixation point above or below the horizontal. The **nasal step** is so called because, when plotted, it appears as a step-like loss of vision at the outer limit of the nasal field. A nasal step and an arcuate scotoma may join and enlarge to cause loss of the entire upper or lower visual field; this type of defect is called an **altitudinal scotoma** (Figure 7.24 on page 122).

In addition to scotomas, advanced glaucoma also may result in large visual field losses that limit vision to small islands, especially on the temporal side of the eye (Figure 7.25 on page 123).

Damage to the optic nerve or lesions involving the macula can produce a **central scotoma**, a defect in the very center of the visual field (Figure 7.26 on page 123). In contrast to most of the visual field losses already discussed, these defects are usually associated with decreased visual acuity.

CONDITIONS FOR ACCURATE PERIMETRY

A visual field test is a complicated procedure regardless of the method or device used. Many conditions must be controlled to secure an accurate result and

FIGURE 7.22

A bitemporal hemianopia due to a lesion of the optic chiasm. (A) The lesion has destroyed chiasmal crossing fibers from the nasal retinas (dotted lines). As a result, objects in the temporal half of the visual space (gray part of the tree) are not seen. (B) A Goldmann visual field chart of a bitemporal hemianopia. (C) A static chart of a similar defect.

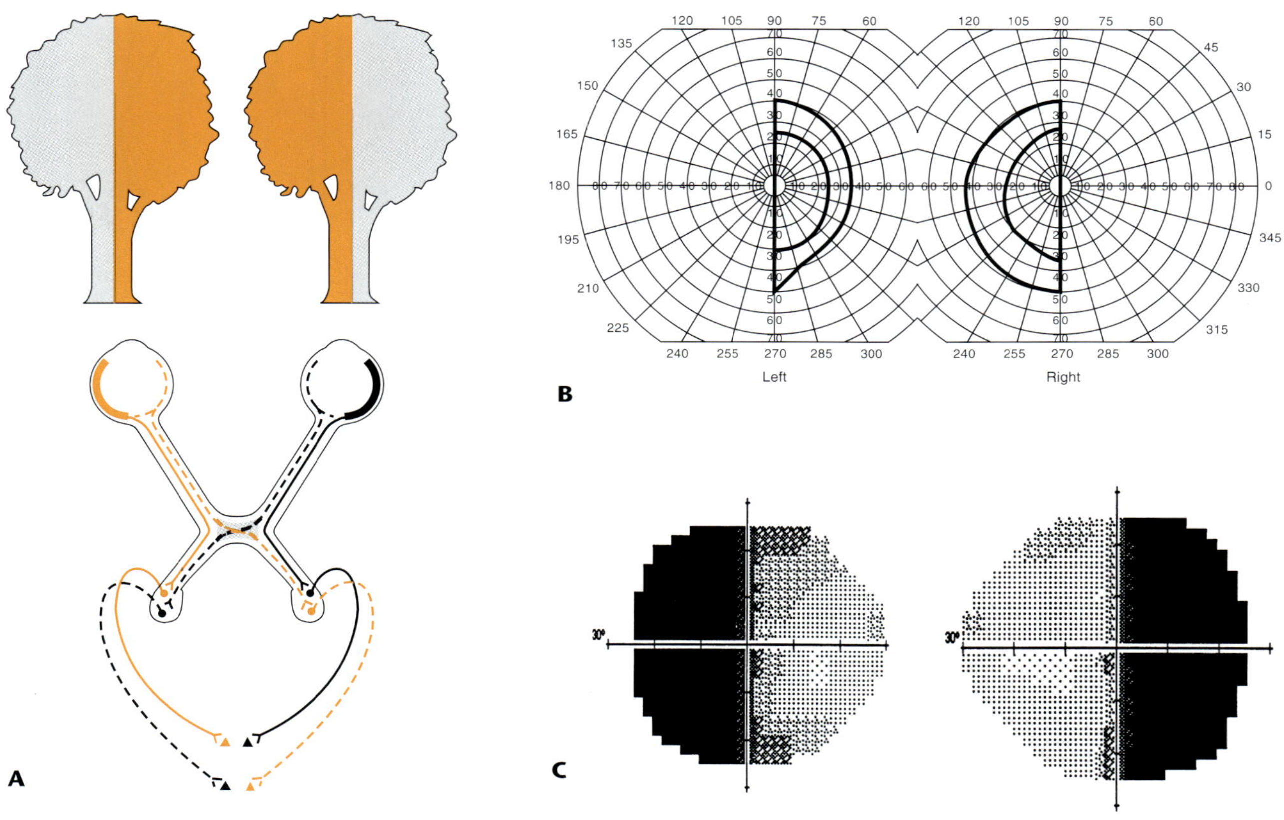

avoid error. Conditions that can lead to errors are usually related to one or more of four factors: the environment, the device, the patient, and the examiner.

Environment-Related Factors

It is the examiner's responsibility to ensure that the testing environment facilitates the test procedure. The room temperature must be neither too warm, which may make the patient drowsy, nor too cold, which can make the patient uncomfortable. The room lighting should be adjusted to the level best suited for the particular test device or method to be used. Room lights that are too bright or that change during the test will affect illumination of the background and that of the test object and, consequently, the results of the test.

Intrusion, movement, and noise should be minimized, so that the patient can concentrate on the test. A crying child in a nearby room can distract both the patient and the examiner. The test should not be interrupted. Even with automated equipment, the examiner should remain in the room in case the patient has questions, grows restless, or needs encouragement. A useful visual field test cannot be expected from a patient who has been seated at an automated perimeter, instructed on its use, and left alone during the test.

The patient should be made physically comfortable during visual field testing. The chair should be comfortable but not too soft. The chair should not permit the patient to sink in as the test progresses or to squirm around. The height of the chair, the table on which the perimeter sits, and the chin rest must be coordinated so that the patient is in a comfortable position and the head is straight, without an up or down tilt or a right or left swivel.

FIGURE 7.23

Glaucoma field defects. (A) In early glaucoma, defects may include (1) a Bjerrum scotoma (shown in the right field), (2) a paracentral scotoma, or (3) a nasal step (both shown in the left field). (B) A static chart of a nasal step. (C) A static chart of a Bjerrum scotoma.

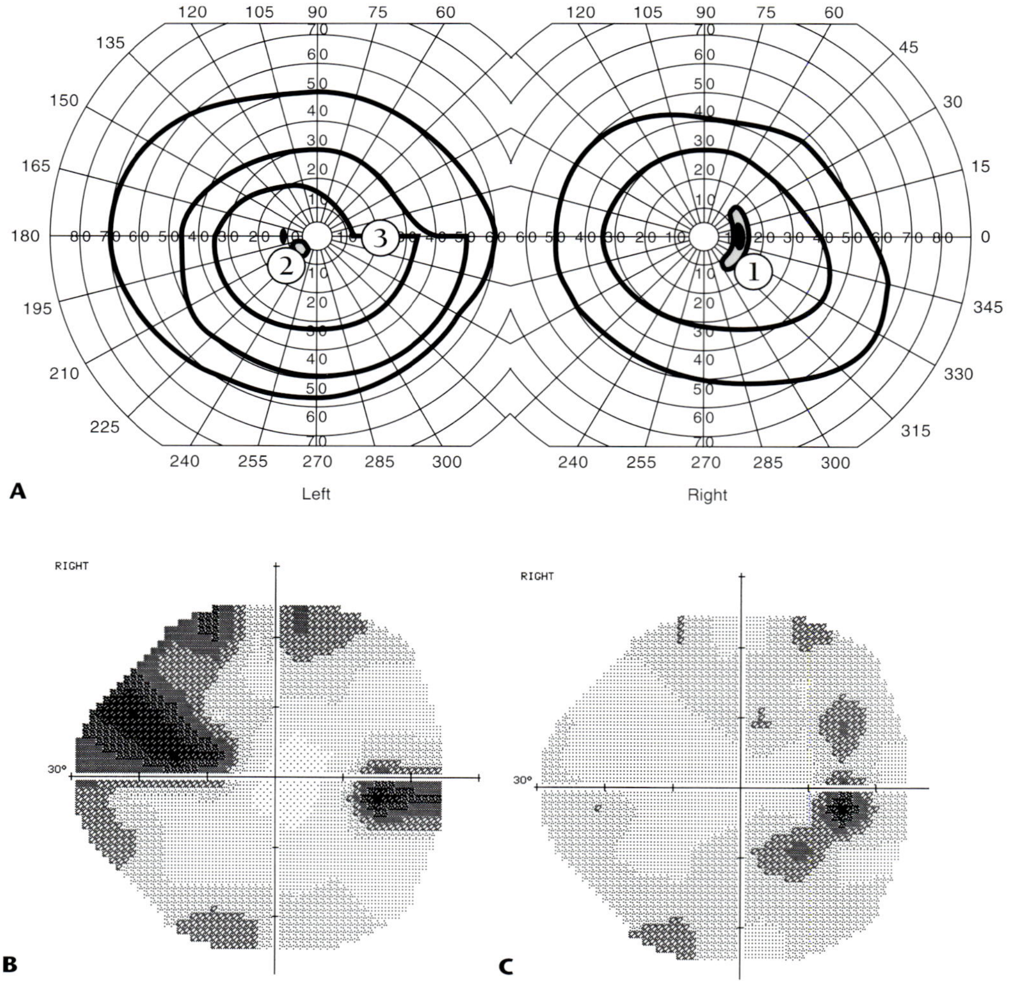

FIGURE 7.24

An altitudinal defect. (A) A Goldmann visual field chart of an altitudinal defect. (B) A static chart of a defect in the same patient.

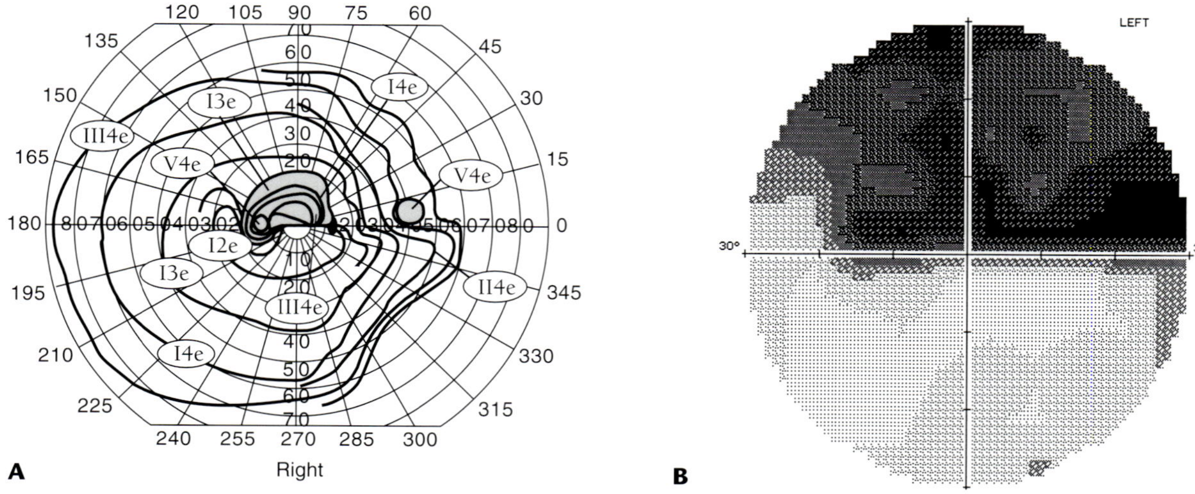

FIGURE 7.25

In advanced glaucoma, the visual field may be limited to small islands, especially on the temporal side.

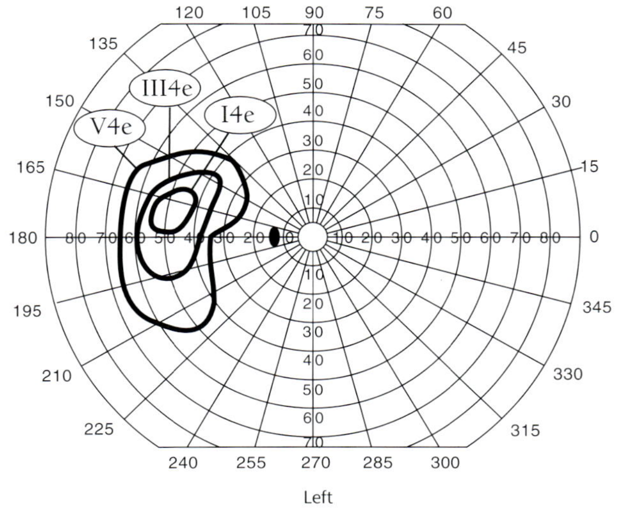

FIGURE 7.26

A central scotoma on a Goldmann visual field chart.

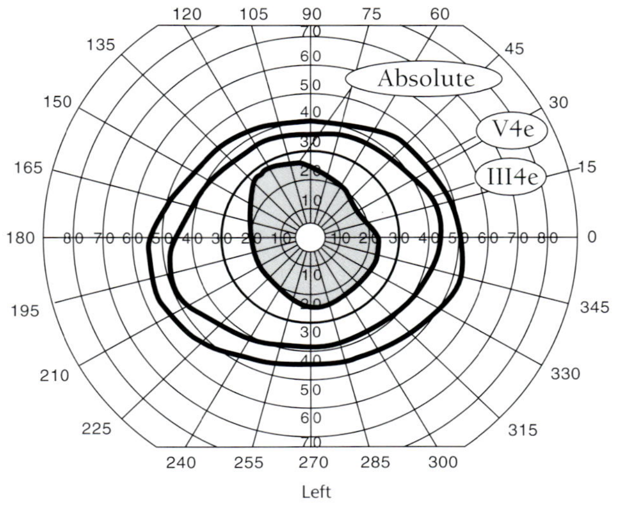

Device-Related Factors

A perimetric instrument must be calibrated before use every day to obtain the desired amount of illumination for both the background and the test object. Often performed by the examiner, **calibration** consists of testing the illumination against a known standard to ensure that the level indicated on the device is in fact the actual level desired. Some automated devices also have automatic calibration. The Goldmann perimeter has a specific calibration protocol, which should be followed at least daily. Calibration may need to be rechecked if a particular patient's clothing is very dark or very light, because these qualities can affect the relative brightness of the background illumination.

Each device has its own checklist of items to monitor and procedures to follow before beginning the test. Some of these items are common to most devices:

- Are the room lights at the right level of brightness?
- Is the room door closed to avoid noise, which may distract the patient, and light, which might affect background levels?
- Is paper in the right place or in the printer?
- Are pencils or other markers present?
- If the perimeter is computer-controlled, is the correct disk for the program in the disk drive?
- Is the door of the disk drive closed?

Patient-Related Factors

Several factors concerning the patient can affect the success of visual field testing. These include the patient's comprehending the test, reaction time, physical condition, distractibility, boredom, anxiety, comfort, pupil size, visual acuity, and refractive error. Some of these factors have been discussed.

With any kind of perimetry, the results will be most accurate if the patient fully understands the test procedure. The technician should not assume that the patient knows what to do simply because the patient has done the test before. Both very young and very old patients may have forgotten how to do the test or may not have understood fully on the previous occasion. The safest course of action is to underestimate what the patient knows or remembers and to explain the purpose and methods of the test, at least briefly, each time. To overcome any awkwardness associated with repeating the information, the examiner might introduce the topic in the following manner: "I know that you have done a visual field test before, but I'm going to repeat the instruments just to be sure we both understand what is going to happen."

Patient anxiety can lead to error and faulty test results. The examiner can help set the patient's mind at ease by a sympathetic, understanding, and gentle manner. Showing impatience and irritation when a patient seems slow to learn or gives inappropriate responses is counterproductive and unacceptable. Some patients approach a visual field test as if taking a final exam and are anxious not to "make a mistake." The examiner must explain that there is no right or wrong and that the patient is expected *not* to see the test object all the time. Reviewing the purpose of the test and making a brief trial run can do much to relieve patient anxiety before beginning the actual test.

Patient fatigue can also lead to errors in testing the visual field. Patients younger than 20 and older than 60 years tend to tire more quickly than others, but anyone can tire in a dark room with a tedious test. The examiner should be alert for signs of fatigue, such as frequent loss of fixation, distractibility, unresponsiveness, and intermittent drooping of the eyelids. Rest periods may help the patient overcome fatigue. If several lengthy tests are required, it may be possible to schedule some of them for another session.

Some patients have severely drooping eyelids (ptosis) that can cut off the upper visual field. In patients with ptosis, the eyelids may need to be held up with tape to get an accurate picture of the upper visual field. Droopy lids should be noted on the test results, together with any other patient problems during the test.

The size of a patient's pupil should always be recorded at the time of perimetry because a pupil 2 mm or smaller will produce a contraction of the visual field independent of any other condition that might be present. The person interpreting the field chart must take into account the pupil size at the time of the test. Recording pupil size is particularly important in patients with glaucoma because these patients often use medications that cause the pupil to constrict. Some ophthalmologists will dilate pupils that are less than 3 mm to avoid this problem.

When the central 30° field of a presbyopic or aphakic patient is tested, the patient's near add or correction must be in place. Because the rims of a patient's eyeglasses can interfere with accurate test results, most perimeters include a special lens holder for this purpose, into which the examiner inserts the appropriate corrective lens or lenses from the trial lens set. The near correction helps the patient properly focus on the target in the perimeter bowl, which is about 33 cm from the eye. In addition, if the image is blurred, the patient may not see the test object, thereby falsely suggesting the presence of a scotoma. The amount of correction needed for different refractive conditions can be determined by the use of printed tables that suggest the amount of add for a given age.

To avoid errors when testing with a correction in place, the lens should be as close to the eye as possible without touching the eyelashes when the patient blinks. This precaution avoids the possibility that the patient may be distracted or that the lens may become smeared when the lashes touch the lens. On the other hand, if the lens is too far from the eye, the lens edge may interfere with the patient's vision. Because it is easy to select the wrong lens in the darkened testing room, the examiner should ask the patient to confirm that the test object can be seen clearly once the chosen lens is in place.

Examiner-Related Factors

As suggested by the foregoing discussions, the examiner contributes to accurate test results by ensuring that the patient is comfortably seated, understands the procedure, and is not worried or anxious about the test. The examiner calibrates the testing device and ensures that the environment is free of distractions, adequately heated, and properly lighted. The examiner also makes sure the eye not being tested is covered with a specially made disinfected patch or other occluder.

The patient should be instructed to maintain fixation on the fixation point and not search for the test object. In automated static perimetry, the computer randomizes the location of the test target. In kinetic perimetry, the examiner can vary the order of presentation so that the patient cannot anticipate where the target will appear.

In kinetic perimetry, the examiner must pay careful attention to the speed of movement of the test object. The usual suggested speed is 2° per second, but this rate should be reduced if the patient's reaction time is slow, as may be the case with elderly patients. On the other hand, moving the test object too slowly will lengthen the test and tire both the patient and the examiner. Presenting test objects too rapidly or too slowly in automated static perimetry can have similar negative effects.

REVIEW QUESTIONS

1. Define *perimetry*.
2. What anatomic structure of the eye determines the boundaries of the visual field and the detail with which its different parts are seen?
3. Why is the part of the visual field focused on the fovea seen in such great detail?
4. Describe the anatomic location of the physiologic blind spot and state why no sight is possible there.
5. Describe briefly the purpose of a mapping system for measuring the visual field.
6. What structure of the eye corresponds to the center of the island of vision?
7. Name the two types of reference coordinates used for mapping the visual field.
8. Where is the physiologic blind spot located in a map of the right and left visual fields?
9. State in degrees of eccentricity the approximate boundaries of the four quadrants of the normal visual field.
10. A person sees an object in the superior temporal quadrant of the visual field. In what quadrant of the retina is the view focused?
11. Name the two principal functions of perimetry.
12. Name the two basic methods used to survey the field of vision, and describe how the targets used differ between the two.
13. Define the term *isopter*.
14. Define the term *scotoma* and explain the difference between a shallow, deep, and absolute scotoma.
15. Name the three main tests used for kinetic perimetry, and describe the advantages of each.
16. Describe the two advantages of kinetic perimetry.
17. Describe two sources of human error in kinetic perimetry.
18. Name two methods of static perimetry.
19. Describe two advantages of computerized static threshold perimetry over kinetic perimetry.
20. Describe at least two disadvantages of computerized static threshold perimetry in comparison with kinetic perimetry.
21. Name the two main types of pathologic changes in the visual field.
22. Name four disease conditions that may produce general contraction of the visual field.
23. Give at least three examples of factors that may cause an apparent contraction of the visual field.
24. Name the five main features of a focal defect that may be noted in mapping a visual field.
25. Define *hemianopia* and *homonymous hemianopia*.

26. Name three common types of visual field defects produced by glaucoma.
27. Describe the visual field defect known as an *altitudinal scotoma*.
28. Name the four types of factors that can lead to errors in visual field testing.
29. List at least two examples of each of the four factors.

SUGGESTED ACTIVITIES

1. To gain a better understanding of perimetry from both the examiner's and the patient's standpoint, ask your ophthalmologist or the perimetrist in your office to perform, over time, several different perimetric measuring procedures on you: confrontation field test, tangent screen test, static threshold (automated if possible), and static suprathreshold. Ask questions as the procedures are being performed.
2. Ask your ophthalmologist or technical staff manager to tell you which perimetric measurements you may be required to perform. Request that regular sessions be scheduled for training in the use of specific techniques and equipment.
3. Read the instruction manuals that accompany the various perimetric devices in your office. Pay close attention to calibration techniques and any information or tips offered for avoiding measurement errors with each device.
4. Request that you be allowed to observe while an examiner in your office conducts a variety of perimetric measurements with different patients. Take notes and schedule a meeting with the examiner to review the test results (the visual field plots) and discuss your questions.
5. Practice administering the test under the supervision of an experienced examiner, first on a volunteer such as someone who works in the office, then on patients.

SUGGESTED RESOURCES

Cassin B: *Fundamentals for Ophthalmic Technical Personnel.* Philadelphia: WB Saunders Co; 1995; chaps 16–18.

Choplin NT, Edwards RP: *Visual Fields.* Thorofare, NJ; Slack; 1998.

Haley MJ, ed: *The Field Analyzer Primer.* 2nd ed. San Leandro, CA: Allergan Humphrey Systems; 1987.

Harrington DO, Drake MV: *The Visual Fields: Text and Atlas of Clinical Perimetry*. 6th ed. St Louis: Mosby; 1990.

Movaghar M, Lawrence MG: *Eye Exam: The Essentials.* Clinical Skills videotape. San Francisco: American Academy of Ophthalmology; 2001.

Stein HA, Slatt BJ, Stein RM: *The Ophthalmic Assistant: A Guide for Ophthalmic Medical Personnel.* 7th ed. St Louis: Mosby; 2000.

Trobe JD, Glaser JS: *The Visual Fields Manual: A Practical Guide to Testing and Interpretation.* Gainesville, FL: Triad; 1983.

8 Fundamentals of Practical Opticianry

Opticianry is a specialized area of eye care that includes the making of corrective lenses from refractive prescriptions and the fitting of both the lenses and the eyeglass frames for proper visual correction. An ophthalmology office may have an optician on staff to support the doctor's patients; however, opticianry services frequently are located elsewhere. Whatever the case, ophthalmic medical assistants often are required to perform certain tasks related to opticianry.

Ophthalmic medical assistants may be called upon to answer patients' questions or solve problems concerning the proper fit or correction of their eyeglasses, serving as an intermediary between the ophthalmologist's office and the optician who filled the prescription. This chapter provides information about types of corrective lenses and materials used in lens manufacture. It introduces you to special optical measurements and techniques used to determine the proper fit and correction of eyeglasses. Frame design, eyeglass care, and adjustments are also discussed. Although opticianry frequently concerns contact lens manufacture and fitting, these subjects are covered in depth in Chapter 14, "Principles and Problems of Contact Lenses."

TYPES OF CORRECTIVE LENSES

Two principal types of eyeglass lenses may be manufactured to correct vision: single-vision lenses, which provide correction for only one distance (that is, far or near); and multifocal lenses (bifocals, trifocals, and progressive-addition multifocals), which combine two or more corrections in a single lens to provide sharp vision at more than one distance. As part of the process of refraction, the doctor decides which type of lens would most benefit a particular patient.

Single-Vision Lenses

Generally speaking, a single-vision lens can focus at only one distance. Single-vision lenses are used to correct a refractive error, such as myopia, hyperopia, or astigmatism, for one working distance, usually either far or near. Patients receiving a prescription for single-vision lenses to correct a vision problem have many lens materials, styles of eyeglasses, and frame designs to choose from.

Multifocal Lenses

Many people, especially those over 40 years of age, need lenses that will focus not only at far distances but at near or intermediate distances as well. One solution is to have two or three single-vision eyeglasses for each working distance. This solution works for some patients, but is inconvenient for many. A more practical solution for most people is a multifocal lens.

Multifocal lenses are used to correct vision for two or more distances. A **bifocal lens** has two powers, usually one for correcting distance vision and one for correcting near vision. A **trifocal lens** has three power zones: one for correction of distance vision, one for intermediate range of sight, and one for near vision. The terms *segment*, *add*, and *near add* are used interchangeably to describe the portion of the multifocal lens (usually the lower part) that provides near vision.

To meet a range of patient needs, segments of various shapes can be placed at different locations within a lens. An **executive** bifocal lens consists merely of a top distance band and a bottom near band, which divide the entire width of a lens into two parts (Figure 8.1A). This same principle may be applied to manufacture a trifocal lens as well (Figure 8.1B). This type of lens provides a large field of vision for reading and intermediate work.

FIGURE 8.1

Executive multifocal lenses. (A) Bifocal. (B) Trifocal.

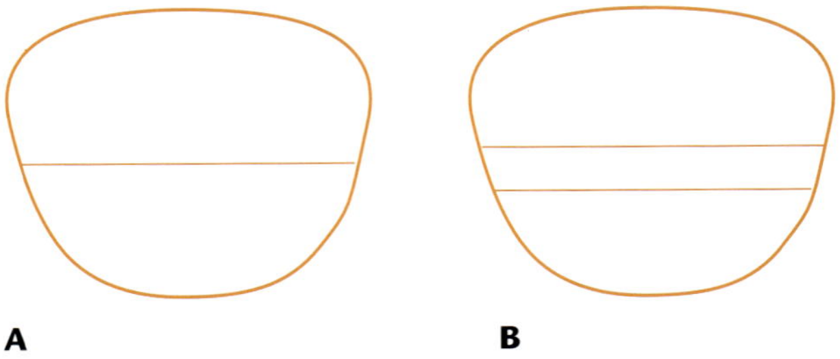

FIGURE 8.2

Round-top segments. (A) Bifocal. (B) Trifocal.

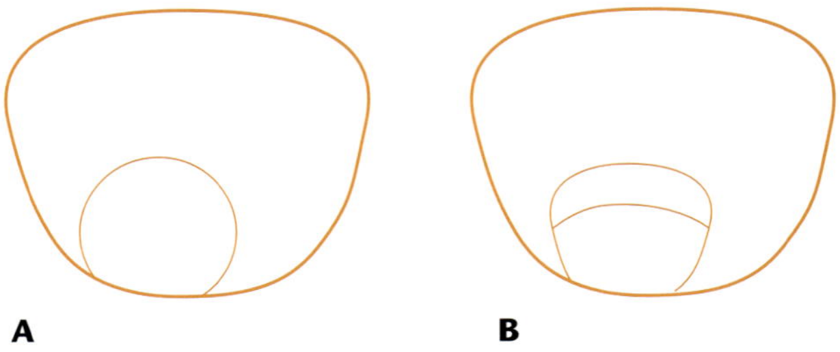

Round-top segments are portions of circles fused or ground into the distance lens. They may be used in bifocals (Figure 8.2A) or trifocals (Figure 8.2B). The straight-top, or flat-top, **D segment** is so called because it is shaped like the capital letter D lying on its side. The D segment may be used in bifocals (Figure 8.3A) and trifocals (Figure 8.3B). The D segments and round segments are the multifocal lenses used most often, some by patient choice but many by the optician's personal preference. They can be manufactured in a variety of widths that provide adequate field of vision for desk chores and other near work.

Multifocal lenses may also be categorized according to whether the line or lines dividing the segments are visible or invisible. An **invisible** bifocal lens (also sometimes referred to as a *seamless* or *blended* bifocal lens) provides a "softened" or "blended" transitional zone between the segment and the distance portion and displays no observable dividing line (Figure 8.4). This blended transitional zone is merely cosmetic and does not provide any corrective power, which may result in a small area of blur or distortion for the bifocal wearer.

A **progressive-addition** multifocal lens also provides a seamless appearance, but does so by progressively adding optical power in a transitional zone, or

FIGURE 8.3

D Segments. (A) Bifocal. (B) Trifocal.

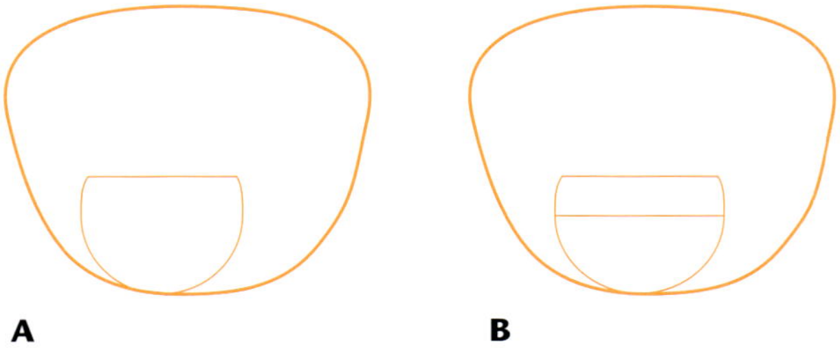

FIGURE 8.4

Invisible bifocal.

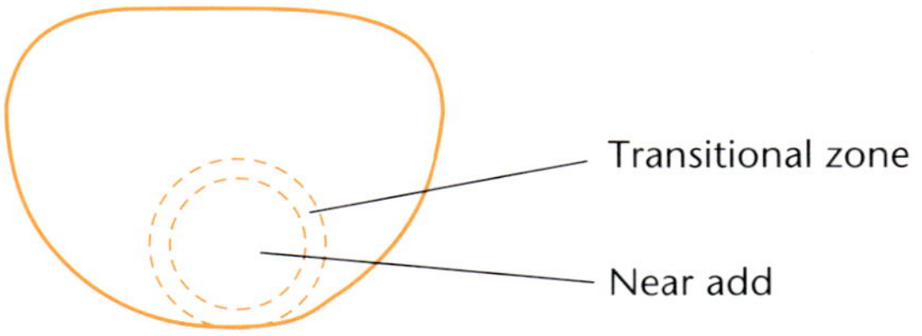

FIGURE 8.5

Progressive-addition multifocal. (1) Distance correction. (2) Corridor of increasing plus power. (3) Maximum plus power of near segment. (4) Zone of significant distortion.

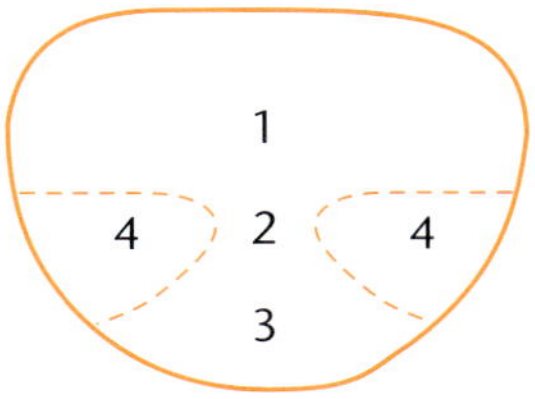

FIGURE 8.6

Double-D segment trifocal.

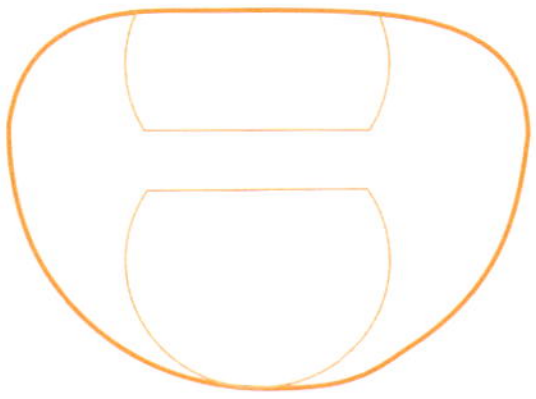

corridor, between the upper distance portions of the lens and the lower near segment. Figure 8.5 shows one possible configuration of a progressive-addition multifocal lens.

Areas of blending and transitional zones or areas adjacent to the near zone in progressive-addition lenses are considered nonoptical areas, which may create distorted or blurred vision for some patients. For this reason, fitting techniques for progressive-addition lenses are more exacting than for invisible or regular bifocals. Some patients consider the cosmetically pleasing seamless effect, as well as the ability to see well at almost any distance, worth the drawbacks of distortion and blur. But for those who complain, the ophthalmologist or optician can try to adjust the frame, remake the lenses, or order replacement lenses from another manufacturer to resolve the patient's problems. If none of these solutions works, the patient may need to use conventional, seamed multifocal spectacles.

The choice of a particular type and configuration of multifocal correction often depends on the patient's work or avocational interests. For example, a house painter, auto mechanic, or other tradesperson may need to see through the middle of a lens for distance, through the bottom for near, and through the top for intermediate overhead work at arm's length. The solution for this type of problem might be a **double-D segment** multifocal lens, with the distance correction in the middle of the lens, a traditional near-power D segment at the bottom, and an intermediate-power inverted D segment at the top of the lens (Figure 8.6) so that the wearer can see a ceiling or a portion of an automobile undercarriage at arm's length while looking up.

Another special need might be that of a choir director, who requires distance vision to direct the choir, intermediate vision to view a music stand, and no near correction. In this case, the bifocal would provide distance vision and a segment to correct for intermediate vision only.

TYPES OF LENS MATERIALS

Patients requiring eyeglasses have many lens materials to choose from today. Each material has its own refractive index, which is the ratio of the speed of light in a vacuum to that in the given material. The closer the index of refraction is to 1.0 (the refractive index of air), the less the material or medium bends, or refracts, the light passing through. The index of refraction of the particular material determines the thickness of the lens made from the material. The higher the index of refraction, the thinner the lens. Examples of common lens materials (and their respective indices of refraction) include plastic, also known as CR-39 (1.49); hi-index plastic (1.54 to 1.60); crown glass (1.52); flint glass (1.65); hi-index glass (1.9); and polycarbonate (1.59).

Plastic lenses are about half the weight of glass lenses, are highly resistant to impact (breakage) and, when manufactured at a center thickness of 3.0 mm, qualify as safety lenses without the special hardening treatments required for glass. However, glass lenses have a thinner profile and scratch less easily than plastic, and they protect the eye from ultraviolet light better than untreated plastic lenses can.

Plastic lenses are usually preferred to glass because plastic weighs less and can be tinted in a wider array of colors. Hi-index plastic particularly has gained in popularity because of its comparable thickness to glass.

The easiest way to determine whether a lens is plastic or glass is to tap gently on the lens with a fingernail. Plastic lenses produce a muted sound, while glass lenses have a more solid "ding" when tapped. In the specific case of a flat-top multifocal plastic lens, a distinct edge can be felt at the junction between the distance portion and the near segment of the lens, whereas a flat-top multifocal glass lens is smooth.

Lens Safety Standards and Treatments

The American National Standards Institute (ANSI) has determined standards for the quality control of eyeglass manufacturing. The latest specification, ANSI Z80.1 1987 Standards, requires that all prescription safety, occupational protective lenses have a minimum edge thickness or center thickness of 3.0 mm. Eyeglasses designated as dress-thickness or impact-resistant dress eyewear lenses must have a center thickness of 2.0 mm and an edge thickness of not less than 1.0 mm at the thinnest point on each lens. ANSI also provides quality control standards for the optician, that is, how much a manufactured lens may deviate from a doctor's refractive prescription (in sphere, cylinder, cylinder axis, prism, and so on).

Glass lenses, unlike plastic ones, must undergo treatment to ensure they can resist breakage. Glass lenses can be hardened by a chemical process or by heat. Chemical treatments have been favored in the last 15 or so years because they have been shown to be far superior to thermal procedures in the manufacture of impact-resistant lenses. Plastic lenses do not require a hardening process for impact resistance because, by its nature, the plastic material is already impact-resistant.

FIGURE 8.7

Wraparound goggles for a variety of sports.

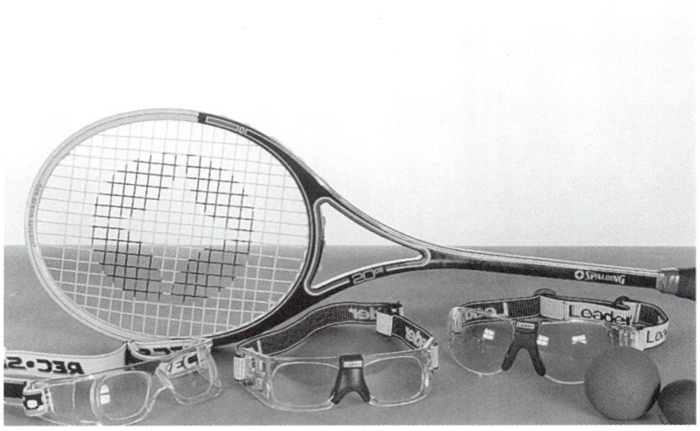

No eyeglass lens is unbreakable. Nevertheless, polycarbonate has become the material of choice for safety lenses because of its resistance to shattering. Polycarbonate materials were used in the face shields of headgear for astronauts, motorcyclists, and firefighters long before these compounds became available for use in eyeglass lenses. Most ophthalmic professionals recommend polycarbonate lenses for sports use because they are virtually unbreakable.

Sports enthusiasts who engage in potentially high-impact activities like tennis, racquetball, and squash should wear protective eyeglasses or shields (Figure 8.7). Special wraparound sports eyewear is available today. Individuals who do not require prescription eyewear should also protect their eyes with nonprescription lenses in the wraparound type of frame during certain sports activities.

Lens Treatments, Tints, and Coatings

Special lens treatments, tints, and coatings aid eyeglass wearers in normal daily activities or in particular situations. **Photochromic** lenses are made of crown glass that is specially manufactured to be sensitive to ultraviolet light (sunlight). These lenses darken when the wearer is in sunlight, but they return to a lightened state when the wearer moves indoors. Photochromic eyeglass lenses are useful for people who alternate

FIGURE 8.8

Relationship of the optical center of the eyeglass lens to the pupil.

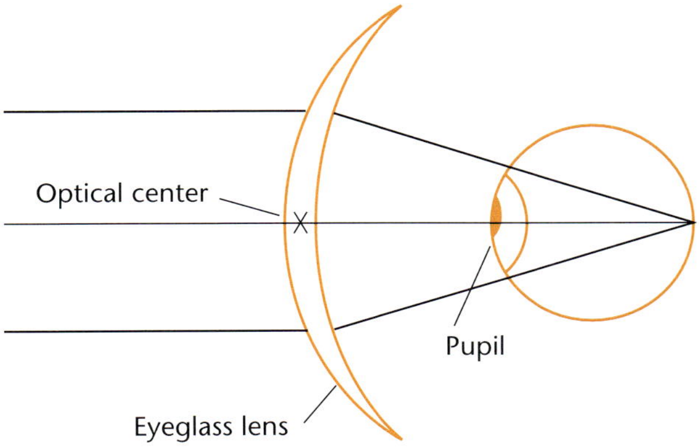

FIGURE 8.9

Relationship of binocular and monocular measurements for interpupillary distance.

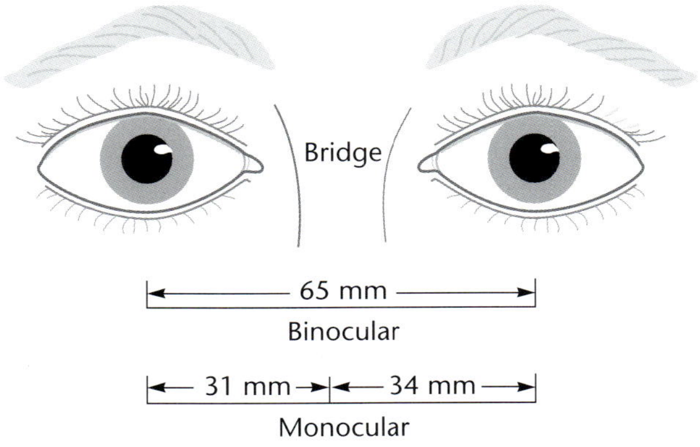

between being outdoors and indoors frequently. **Polarized** lenses, made of specially manufactured plastic, glass, or photochromic glass, help those active in snow or water sports by reducing glare, brightness, and ultraviolet light transmission.

Glass lenses screen out a large percentage of ultraviolet light due to the nature of glass itself. However, plastic lenses will not protect the eye from harmful ultraviolet rays unless these lenses undergo special treatment. Many ophthalmologists recommend a colorless ultraviolet coating for all eyeglass lenses, tinted or not. Most color tints available for eyeglasses today are simply decorative and do not function to screen out ultraviolet radiation, although some may help reduce glare problems for persons under fluorescent lighting. Cosmetic tints also change color perception slightly, which might be a drawback for some individuals.

Both glass and plastic eyeglass lenses may be coated to help make them scratch-resistant or to reduce reflection. Other special coatings are used to reduce infrared light transmission (mirror coatings) and ease cathode-ray tube (CRT) viewing for those working with computer video monitors.

MEASUREMENTS IN FITTING EYEGLASSES

For eyeglasses to be effective, patients must feel satisfied with the prescription and the overall fit of the lenses on the face. Eyeglasses that fit improperly may cause vision problems. To help determine the source of a patient's dissatisfaction or discomfort with eyeglasses, ophthalmic medical assistants may need to measure interpupillary distance, vertex distance, and the base curves of the lenses.

Interpupillary distance (abbreviated IPD or PD) is the distance from the center of the pupil of one eye to the center of the pupil of the other eye. IPD is important to the laboratory technician who makes eyeglass lenses because it indicates where to place the ground optical centers in the finished lenses so that they lie directly in front of the patient's pupils. The **optical center** of a lens denotes the point of optimal vision; it is the single point through which light may pass without being bent or changed (Figure 8.8).

The **vertex distance** is the distance from the back surface of an eyeglass lens to the front surface of the patient's cornea. This measurement can be an important factor in making eyeglasses with powers greater than plus or minus 5 diopters, because at higher powers the distance from the eye can change the effective power of a lens. The **base curve** is the curve of the lens surface, usually the outer or front side of the lens, from which the other curves necessary for sight correction are calculated.

Interpupillary Distance

Interpupillary distance, the distance between the pupils, is measured in millimeters. This measurement should be obtained both at near and at distance for each patient. Both a *binocular* measurement (a single recording of the total distance from pupil to pupil) and a *monocular* measurement (the individual distance from the center of the bridge of the nose to the center of each pupil) should be recorded (Figure 8.9).

In **orthophoric** (normal) patients, the eyes look straight ahead when they focus on an object directly in front of them. Eyes that are straight in the primary gaze (straight ahead) will have virtually parallel axes when they fixate on a distant object. However, when the same pair of eyes focuses on a near object, the eyes converge (turn in slightly) to allow both foveas to fixate the object. Because of this convergence, the near IPD measurement will be less than the distance IPD.

The distance IPD measurement is required to manufacture all eyeglasses, both single-vision and multifocal. The near IPD measurement is required when single-vision or multifocal eyeglasses are prescribed for reading or other close-up activities. The accurate measurement of both distance and near IPD ensures the appropriate placement of the optical centers of the eyeglass lenses. If the **distance between optical centers (DBC)** does not correspond to the patient's IPD, the patient can experience double vision. Therefore, the ophthalmic medical assistant should verify the correct IPD and DBC for all eyeglasses whether they are new prescriptions or eyeglasses brought in by patients with vision complaints.

Several methods exist for measuring distance or near IPD. In addition, either binocular or monocular measurements may be chosen. Monocular measurement of IPD is considered more accurate than binocular measurement because the monocular recording takes into consideration any facial asymmetry that might be present (see Figure 8.9).

A binocular distance IPD requires just one pupil-to-pupil measurement made with a millimeter ruler.

Table 8.1 Monocular Distance IPD With Corresponding Average Near IPD (mm)

Distance	*Near*	*Distance*	*Near*
24.75	23.00	31.00	29.00
25.25	23.50	31.50	29.50
25.75	24.00	32.00	30.00
26.25	24.50	32.75	30.50
26.75	25.00	33.25	31.00
27.25	25.50	33.75	31.50
27.75	26.00	34.25	32.00
28.50	26.50	34.75	32.50
29.00	27.00	35.25	33.00
29.50	27.50	36.00	33.50
30.00	28.00	36.50	34.00
30.50	28.50	37.00	34.50

For a monocular distance IPD measurement, the distances between each pupil and the bridge of the nose are measured separately and the results are added together to yield a single measurement. Simple and accurate monocular IPD measurements may be made with a specially calibrated ruler and a penlight. Specific instructions for both of these distance IPD measuring techniques are presented in the boxes "Measuring Binocular Distance IPD" on page 133 and "Measuring Monocular Distance IPD"on page 134. IPD measurements can also be made with a corneal reflection pupilometer, discussed later.

Both binocular and monocular near IPD may be measured or calculated. Table 8.1 presents the approximate near IPDs corresponding to a range of common monocular distance IPDs. Measuring the binocular or monocular near IPD requires both the millimeter ruler and the penlight. The box "Measuring Binocular Near IPD" on page 134 contains step-by-step instructions for this technique. The monocular measuring technique for near IPD is not presented here because it requires more experience and skill than would be expected of an assistant.

Errors in Measuring IPD

The accurate measurement of both distance and near IPD ensures that the optical centers of the patient's eyeglass lenses are correctly placed in front of the patient's pupils. If the distance between optical centers (DBC) does not correspond to the measured IPD, an optical distortion known as **prismatic effect** may occur. Prismatic effect causes incoming light rays to deviate inappropriately when they strike the lens (Figure 8.10), leading to eye discomfort or distorted or double vision for the lens wearer. The direction of the prismatic effect can vary depending on whether a plus-power lens or minus-power lens is involved and on whether the DBC of the lens is wider or narrower than the IPD.

Several common errors can occur when using the millimeter ruler to measure distance and near IPD. Some errors in measurement relate to a patient's strabismus or asymmetric face. The most common cause of error in assessing IPD is *parallax*, an optical distortion that occurs when the measurer's and the patient's lines of sight are not parallel. Parallax can result in the measured IPD being significantly different from the patient's actual IPD. It can result from the measurer standing closer to the patient than 14 inches; from head movement by the measurer or patient; from

MEASURING BINOCULAR DISTANCE IPD

Gauging the precise center of a patient's pupils can be difficult, especially if the pupils are large. A reasonably accurate measurement can be obtained by measuring from the temporal limbus of one eye to the nasal limbus of the other eye.

1. Position yourself about 16 inches in front of the patient. Make sure your eyes are level with the patient's eyes.
2. Close your right eye and ask the patient to look at your left eye.
3. Rest the millimeter ruler lightly on the bridge of the patient's nose.
4. Line up the zero point on the temporal limbus of the patient's right eye (Figure A).
5. Holding the ruler in this position, close your left eye and open your right eye. Have the patient fixate on your right eye.
6. Observe the number on the millimeter ruler that is directly under the nasal limbus of the patient's left eye (Figure B).
7. Close your right eye, open your left eye, and check the zero point of the ruler, making sure it is at the temporal limbus of the patient's right eye.
8. Check the measurement on the ruler for the patient's left eye and record it on the patient's chart or form as appropriate.

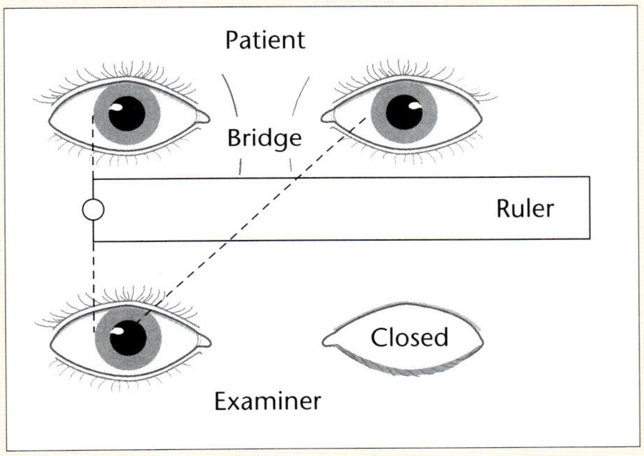

Figure A

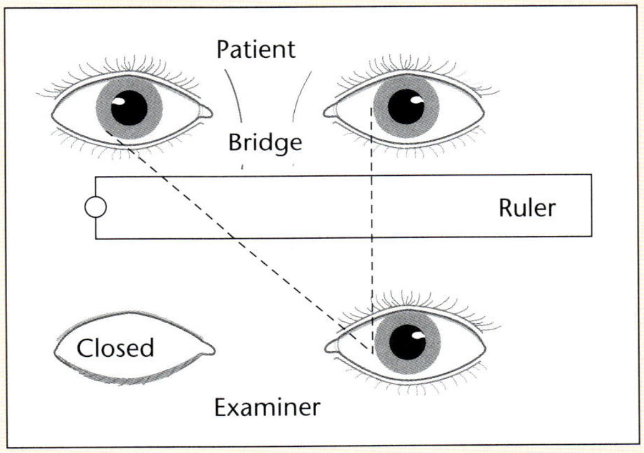

Figure B

FIGURE 8.10

Prismatic effect in a minus-power lens for which the distance between optical centers (DBC) is narrower than the interpupillary distance (IPD).

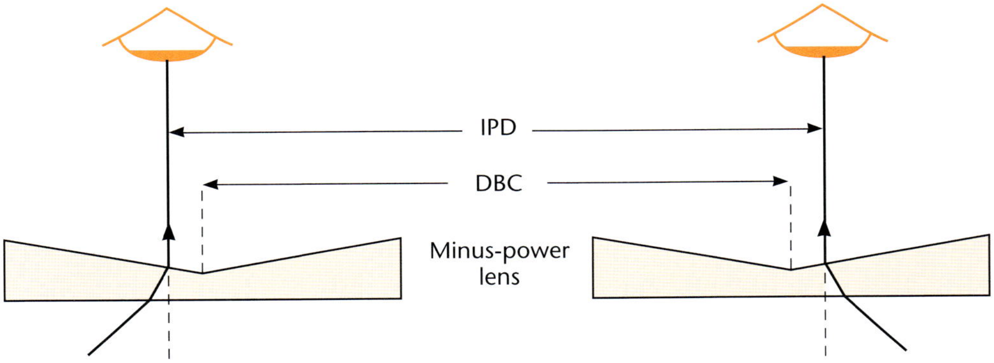

MEASURING MONOCULAR DISTANCE IPD

1. Position yourself 14 to 16 inches in front of the patient. Make sure your eyes are level with the patient's eyes. Hold the millimeter ruler lightly over the bridge of the patient's nose.

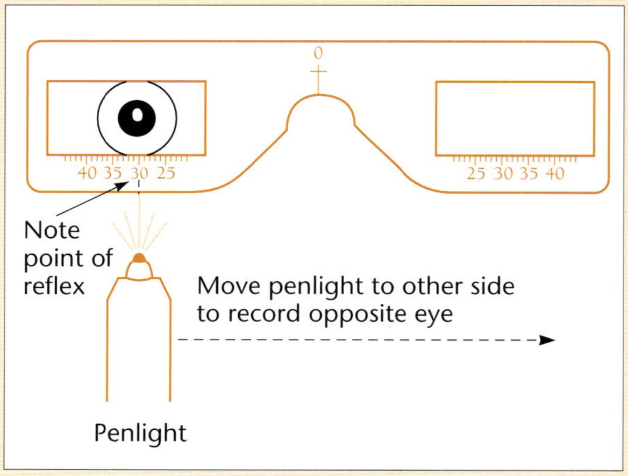

2. Hold a penlight under your left eye, aiming the light at the patient's eye. Note the position of the spot of light reflection called the *corneal reflex* on the patient's right eye (see the figure), and record the number on the ruler just below the reflex. This represents the number of millimeters from the patient's right corneal reflex to the center of the bridge of the nose.
3. Hold the penlight under your right eye, aiming the light at the patient's eye. Observe the corneal reflex on the patient's left eye. Record the number of millimeters from the left corneal reflex to the center of the bridge of the nose.
4. Add the two numbers together and record the sum on the patient's chart or form as appropriate.

MEASURING BINOCULAR NEAR IPD

1. Place your dominant eye in front of the patient's nose at the patient's near working distance, which is usually 14 to 16 inches.
2. Close your other eye and have the patient fixate on your open eye (your dominant eye).
3. Rest the millimeter ruler lightly on the bridge of the patient's nose and line up the zero point at the center of the patient's right pupil.
4. Record the reading from the ruler marking at the center of the patient's left pupil.
5. Hold the penlight directly under your right eye and shine the light toward the patient's nose. A crisp corneal reflection on both eyes will be seen. This may help you in making these measurements because the light reflex is the center of the cornea (and *almost* the center of the pupil), and you can determine a reading on the millimeter scale by reading from the ruler at the corneal reflex.

improper eye fixation by the patient during the measurement; or from the examiner's line of sight being higher or lower than the patient's.

Special instruments, such as the Essilor Pupilometer and other metering devices, are used to measure IPD (Figure 8.11). Opticians use them routinely because these meters correct for parallax error. In addition, the instruments provide a monocular reading that avoids errors due to facial asymmetry or strabismus. Because the operation of each instrument differs, ophthalmic medical assistants should read in detail the user's manual for the particular instrument available in their practice and request practical instruction in its use from the ophthalmologist or a senior staff assistant.

Vertex Distance

The distance between the back of an eyeglass lens and the front of the eyeglass wearer's eye is the vertex distance (Figure 8.12). A vertex distance of 13.5 mm is considered average, but vertex distance can range from 5 mm to more than 26 mm. The most effective fit for eyeglasses usually is obtained by fitting the frame as close to the eye as possible without the eyelashes touching the lenses.

Positioning a patient's eyeglasses at a vertex distance other than that used during refractometry will change the effective power of the lenses. The amount of change depends on the power of the lens. For low-powered lenses, the patient will not notice a difference in vision correction. But for high-powered lenses, a small alteration in vertex distance will make a considerable and noticeable change in the effective power of both the spherical and the cylindrical components of the lens. For example, if a patient's refractive prescription is less than or equal to minus or plus 5 diopters, an accurate assessment of vertex distance is not required to ensure proper eyeglass prescription. But if the prescription calls for more than minus or plus 5 diopters, the vertex distance should be measured during refractometry to avoid refraction errors that could lead to vision difficulties with the eyeglasses. When recording the ophthalmologist's refractive prescription for a patient, the ophthalmic medical assistant should always include a vertex distance on lens powers greater than plus or minus 5 diopters. A specially designed instrument called a **distometer** is used to measure vertex distance accurately. Instructions for measuring vertex distance appear in the box "Using a Distometer" on page 136.

FIGURE 8.11

Essilor Pupilometer used to measure interpupillary distance.

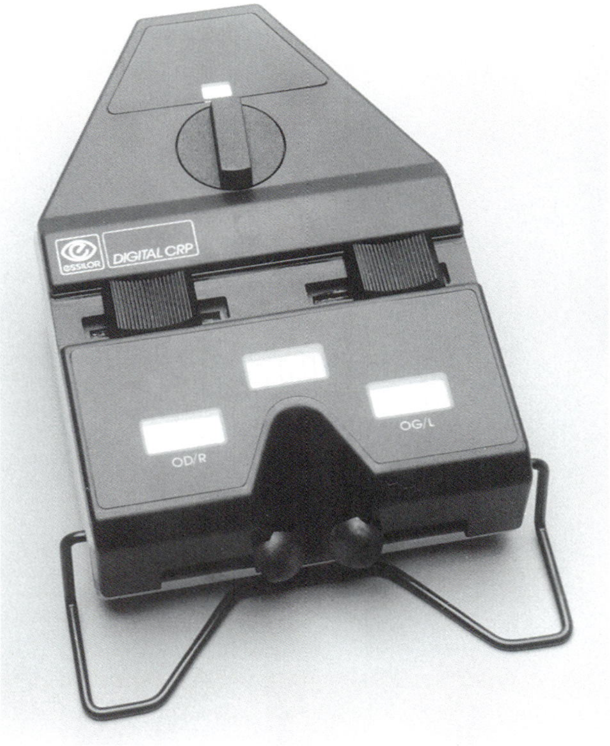

FIGURE 8.12

V = vertex distance.

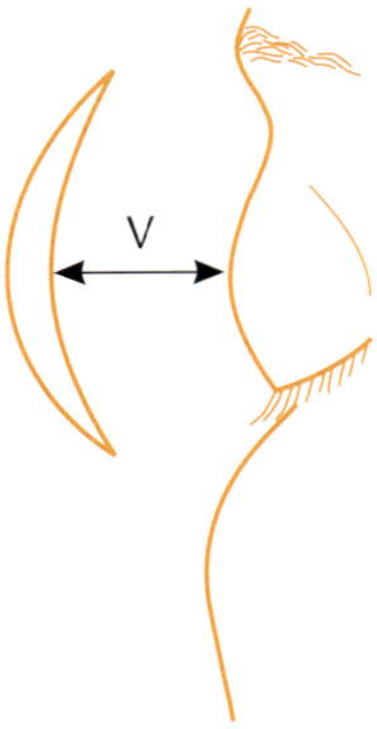

Base Curve

The base curve of a lens is the original single curve on the front or back surface of a lens "blank" supplied by a manufacturer. Using this single curve as a basis for measurement, the laboratory technician grinds additional curves on the lens surfaces to achieve the final power and refractive correction of the lens. The power of a lens equals the algebraic difference between the power of the front curve and that of the back curve, and many different combinations of base curves and other curves can be used to arrive at the same power. Although base curve can exist on either the front or the back surface of a lens, most single-vision lenses have a base curve on the front surface.

Patients become accustomed to wearing lenses ground with a particular base curve. Changing the base curve when a new pair of lenses is prescribed can cause the patient discomfort, ranging from a perception of visual distortion to dizziness and nausea. Thus, when ordering replacement lenses or supplying the patient with a second pair of glasses, the optician must duplicate the base curves for both pairs of eyeglasses to ensure that the patient can comfortably

USING A DISTOMETER

1. Ask the patient to close both eyes.
2. Gently rest the fixed arm of the distometer caliper on the closed eyelid and carefully place the movable caliper arm against the back surface of the trial lens or eyeglass lens (see the figure).
3. Record the separation distance between these two surfaces from the millimeter scale on the distometer. (Note: This scale allows for an average eyelid thickness.)

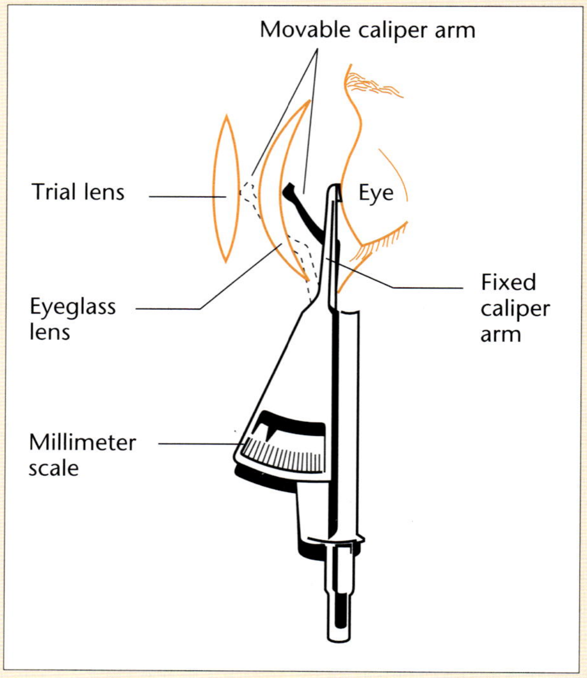

USING A GENEVA LENS CLOCK

1. Place the front surface of a single-vision lens against the pins in the 180° meridian (see the figure).

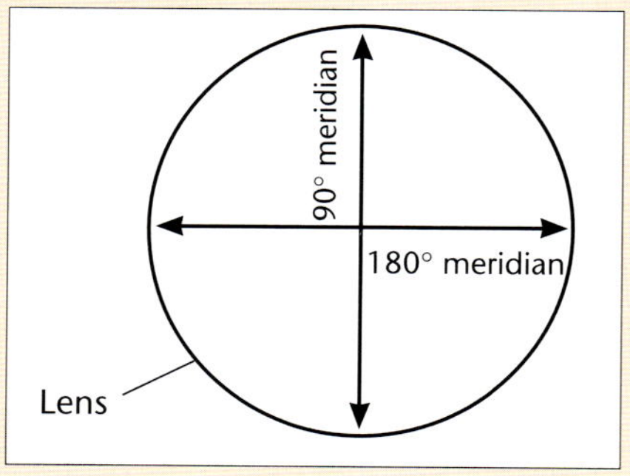

2. Note the position of the pointer on the clock dial and record this number. Remember: The red scale indicates a concave (minus) surface; the black, a convex (plus) surface.
3. Rotate either the lens clock or the lens to the 90° meridian.
   a. If the reading remains constant, the reading noted in step 2 is the base curve.
   b. If the reading changes on rotation, the lens surface has a cylindrical component. The difference between the lower and the higher readings represents the amount of cylinder present. The weaker, or lesser, number of the two measured on the front surface is the base curve.

Note: The orientation of the three contact points on the lens clock at the maximum and minimum readings corresponds to the meridians of lens power.

wear the second pair. The ophthalmic medical assistant may be required to measure base curves of lenses to assure that new lenses have been ground correctly or to help determine the source of a patient's visual complaints.

The **Geneva lens clock** is the instrument used to measure the base curve of an eyeglass lens. The lens clock is calibrated in diopters and has three blunt pins at its foot, the outer two fixed and the central one movable (Figure 8.13). When the pins are held against

FIGURE 8.13

The Geneva lens clock for measuring the base curve of a lens.

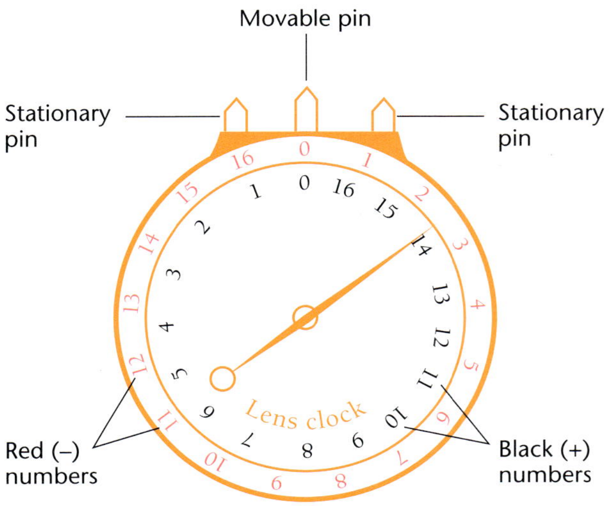

FIGURE 8.14

Placement of the Geneva lens clock onto a multifocal lens. (A) Incorrect placement. (B) Correct placement.

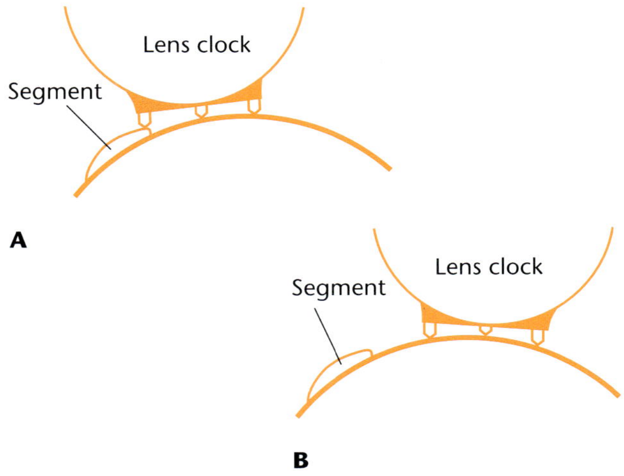

FIGURE 8.15

Anatomy of an eyeglass frame. (A) Front view of frame. (B) Side view temple piece. (C) Top view of frame front.

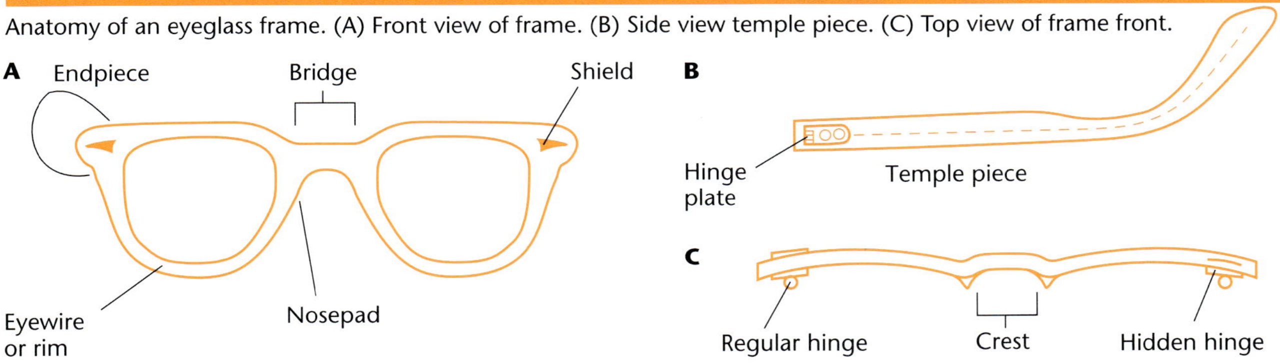

a flat surface, the indicator hand of the lens clock points to zero. When the instrument is placed against a concave lens surface, the indicator will point to minus (–), or red, numbers; placed against a convex lens surface, the indicator will point to the plus (+), or black, number scale. When measuring a multifocal lens, always keep the pins of the lens clock away from the multifocal segment; if the pins impinge on the multifocal segment, an error in base curve measurement could result (Figure 8.14). The procedure for measuring base curve is outlined in the box "Using a Geneva Lens Clock."

FITTING OF EYEGLASS FRAMES

Eyeglass frames come in a variety of sizes, shapes, styles, and materials, all of which have become influenced by fashion as well as the personal preferences of patients. Naturally, most patients try to choose frames that they feel are becoming to their appearance. However, opticians, ophthalmic medical assistants, and others who help patients choose frames and wear them comfortably also must consider frames from the aspect of their tilt and curve in relationship to the wearer's face, and their overall size and shape (both of which can affect proper peripheral vision), as well as their comfortable fit. Figure 8.15 shows the principal parts of a typical frame.

The **pantoscopic angle** of an eyeglass frame is the angle by which the frame front deviates from the vertical plane when the glasses are worn on the face. The pantoscopic angle is estimated by viewing the eyeglasses on the face from the side (Figure 8.16). The lower rims of the frame front normally are closer

FIGURE 8.16

Pantoscopic angle estimated by viewing the eyeglasses on the face from the side.

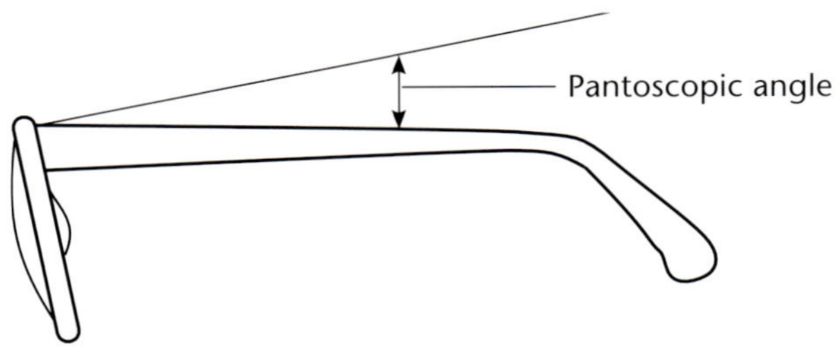

to the cheeks than are the upper rims. A usual pantoscopic angle ranges from 4° to 18° (the average pantoscopic angle is 15°), although an individual with protruding eyebrows may exceed this range. The term **retroscopic tilt** is used to describe eyeglasses that are adjusted so that the lower rims tilt away from the face; this happens only rarely by design but can occur in error.

A proper pantoscopic angle allows the eye to rotate downward from the distance gaze to the near gaze while maintaining a similar vertex distance. Patients can have visual problems that may prompt an office visit if a retroscopic tilt is present or if the pantoscopic angle is incorrect; patients with moderate cylinder powers and above-average refractive errors have more problems and notice this improper tilt.

Some patients' choice of frame sizes and shapes may be restricted because of their lens prescriptions. If the eyeglass prescription is moderate to high (that is, approximately 3 diopters or more of myopia or hyperopia), frame size and shape play a significant role in altering peripheral vision. This problem primarily relates to the increase in vertex distance from the center of the lens to the edge of the lens. For larger lenses, the increase in vertex distance at the edge of the lens compared to the center may dramatically change both the spherical and the cylindrical components of the optical prescription. Moreover, the farther from the center of the lens, the greater the optical distortion. Large lenses may be fashionable, but they may cause significant optical aberration in the peripheral parts of the lens.

Effects on Patient Comfort

A patient who requires eyeglasses will not conscientiously wear them if the frames do not fit well, even though the prescription may be correct. Misaligned frames or improper frame size can cause the following problems:

- Frames slide forward
- Frames fit loosely
- Frames must be positioned awkwardly to see properly
- Frame temples create pressure on the side of the head or at the ears
- Eyelashes or eyebrows touch the lenses

When fitting or adjusting the fit of a pair of eyeglasses, pay special attention to the physical structure of a patient's face. Because most of the weight of the eyeglasses is placed on the bridge of the patient's nose, the weight should be evenly distributed. One ear may be slightly higher than the other ear; therefore, the fit over or behind each ear should be carefully made. The nature of the individual's skin (for example, the degree of oiliness) may cause some types of frames to slip down from the bridge of the nose. No easy formula exists for adjusting a pair of glasses so that the patient will wear them, but thorough observation and listening carefully to what a patient says will allow you to help the patient choose frames appropriately and wear them comfortably.

When checking the fit or assessing other problems, take special care when putting the eyeglasses on the patient or taking them off. Always cover the tips of the temple pieces (also called *temples*) with your fingers until you have moved them past the patient's eyes. This procedure avoids poking the patient in the eye with the pointed ends of the frame temples.

CARE OF EYEGLASSES

Eyeglass lenses and frames, especially those worn daily, are subject to considerable wear and tear. Although most frames and lenses are designed to take a certain amount of abuse, patients can get much longer, more satisfying wear out of their eyeglasses if they receive instructions in proper cleaning and handling.

A variety of cleaning sprays and special cloths exist for cleaning eyeglass lenses. For the most part, however, these products may be needed only if the lenses have been specially treated, such as with antireflection, scratch-resistant, or color coatings. Patients can keep their glasses clean without damaging lens surfaces by using proper cleaning methods and materials. Conventional glass or plastic lenses can be cleaned simply with soap and water, then dried with a soft cloth. All lenses should be cleaned while wet; rubbing a cloth or tissue over dry lenses may drag dirt across the lens surfaces and scratch them.

When appropriate, the ophthalmic medical assistant should instruct patients in the proper method of cleaning their eyeglass lenses. Patients should also be instructed to protect their eyeglasses from impact or pressure by storing them in the eyeglass case when not in use. The assistant may also caution patients that when placing eyeglasses on a surface, they should place the side with the temple pieces down so that the lenses will not be scratched. Plastic lenses are more susceptible to scratching than glass lenses.

FIGURE 8.17

Typical frame screw for a plastic frame.

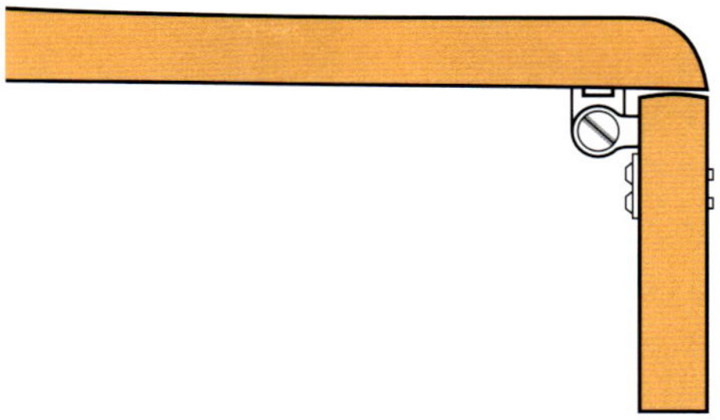

ADJUSTMENT OF EYEGLASSES

Ophthalmic medical assistants are often asked to make minor adjustments to the frames, such as tightening frame screws, measuring optical centers, and, for multifocals, measuring segment heights to ensure that they are properly placed and not a source of patient complaint.

Frame Screws

Plastic frames usually have one screw holding each temple piece to the frame front (Figure 8.17). Most nonrimless metal frames have two screws on each side, one to hold the eyewire (the metal that encircles each lens) together and one to keep the temple piece in place.

Loose eyeglass frame screws are a common problem. To adjust or tighten these screws, a jeweler's or optician's screwdriver and a small bottle of clear nail polish are needed. For instructions, see the box "Adjusting Frame Screws."

ADJUSTING FRAME SCREWS

1. Tighten the screws with a jeweler's or optician's screwdriver so that the temple piece moves freely without binding.
2. Apply a small drop of clear nail polish to the screw head. When the nail polish dries, the screw will not loosen easily.

Optical Centers

The ophthalmic medical assistant may need to check the optical centers of the patient's eyeglass lenses to determine whether the placement of the optical centers matches the measured interpupillary distance. Measuring the optical center or distance between centers (DBC) of eyeglass lenses requires using the marking, or dotting, device on a lensmeter. This procedure is described in the box "Checking Optical Centers" on page 140. (Instructions for operating a lensmeter appear in Chapter 4, "Optics and Refractive States of the Eye.")

Segment Heights

The **segment height** is the distance between the lowest part of the rim and the top of the multifocal lens segment (Figure 8.18). The correct segment height for a multifocal lens has a direct effect on the patient's satisfaction with the eyeglasses. In determining segment heights, remember that each patient has different vision requirements and must be treated individually with respect to these special requirements. Most opticians recommend fitting the top of a bifocal segment level with the patient's lower lid margin, which is the area where the lid touches the eyeball (Figure 8.19). Some patients prefer the bifocal line at a slightly higher or lower level than at the lower lid margin, but the segment height usually will not vary more than 1 or 2 mm higher or lower. Trifocals are usually fit about 7 mm higher than the lower lid margin.

CHECKING OPTICAL CENTERS

1. Place the lens against the lens stop of the lensmeter.
2. Make certain the eyeglass frame sits squarely on the spectacle table.
3. Focus the mires and center them within the focused eyepiece target (see the figure). Use the dotting device to mark the lens while it is held in this position. The center mark (usually of three) is the optical center of the lens. If the lensmeter does not have a marking device, use a nonpermanent marker pen to record the approximate center of the lens.
4. Use a millimeter ruler to measure the distance between the center dots; this measurement should correspond to the patient's distance IPD unless a prism has been prescribed.

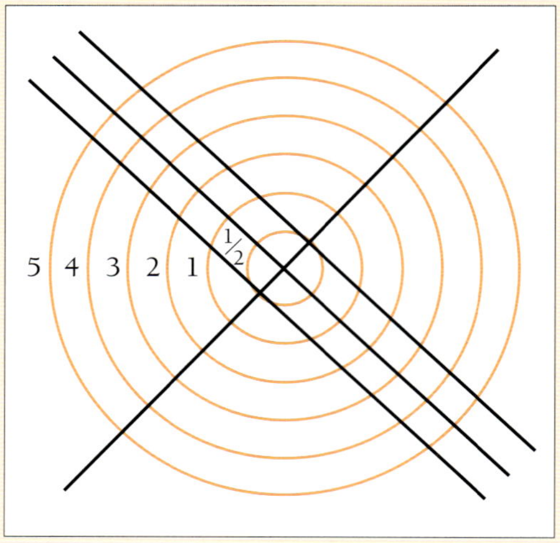

FIGURE 8.18

The segment height is the distance between the lowest part of the rim and the top of the segment. (A) Incorrect measurement. (B) Correct measurement.

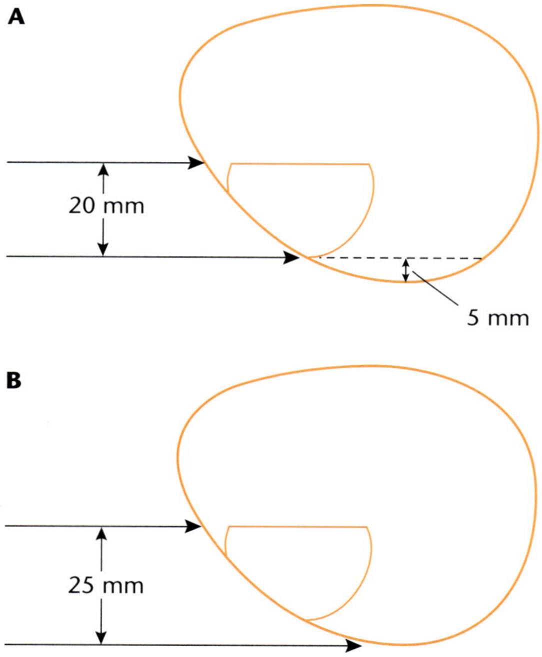

FIGURE 8.19

Placement of bifocal segment.

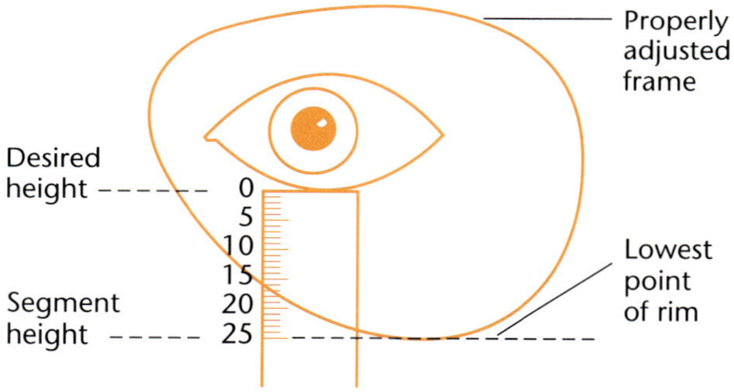

Most opticians recommend fitting progressive-addition lenses according to the individual lens manufacturer's fitting manual. Each progressive-addition lens has a specific optical design, and fitting characteristics will vary. Fitting progressive-add lenses may be very difficult. Sometimes, despite the fact that patient measurements and laboratory quality control are precise, the patient may remain displeased with the eyeglasses. This may be due to the inability of the patient to ignore the areas of distortion inherent in progressive multifocals. Such patients may need to use conventional bifocals or trifocals.

REVIEW QUESTIONS

1. Choose the one lettered description that best matches each type of lens listed.

   ____ bifocal

   ____ trifocal

   ____ progressive-addition

   ____ single-vision

   a. Corrects for one distance
   b. Corrects for two distances
   c. Corrects for three distances
   d. Corrects for two or more distances by increasing optical power in a transitional zone
   e. Corrects for near and intermediate distances only
   f. Corrects for near vision in one eye only

2. Choose the one lettered task that is best associated with each instrument listed.

   ____ lensmeter

   ____ millimeter ruler

   ____ distometer

   ____ Geneva lens clock

   a. Measures interpupillary distance
   b. Determines the optical center of a lens
   c. Determines the pantoscopic angle of a frame
   d. Determines the base curve of a lens
   e. Measures vertex distance
   f. Identifies a plastic lens

3. Prescription safety, occupational protective lenses have a minimum edge or center thickness of

   a. 1.0 mm
   b. 1.5 mm
   c. 2.0 mm
   d. 2.5 mm
   e. 3.0 mm

4. Which lenses require chemical or heat treatment to resist breakage—glass or plastic?

5. Lenses that are treated to darken when exposed to ultraviolet light are described as

   a. Ultraviolet-coated
   b. Photochromic
   c. Safety
   d. Polycarbonate
   e. Heat-treated

6. Define *base curve.*
7. Which color scale on a Geneva lens clock is used when the instrument is placed against a convex surface?
8. The 180° meridian on the front surface of a single-vision lens measures 8 diopters by the Geneva lens clock. Upon rotation to the 90° meridian of the lens, the lens clock registers 6 diopters. What is the base curve of this lens?
9. Define *pantoscopic angle.*
10. Label the parts of the eyeglass frame that are called out in the illustration below.

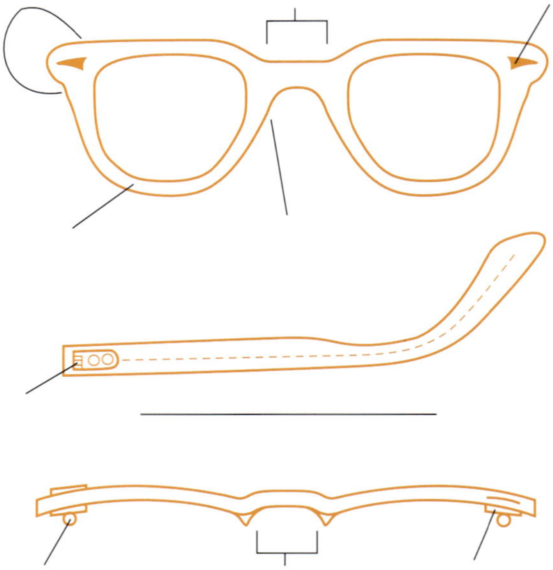

11. Describe the precaution taken to avoid poking a patient when placing eyeglass frames on the patient's face.
12. When the fit of bifocals is checked, the top of the near segment generally should be level with the patient's __________.
13. Label the multifocal lenses listed with the letter corresponding to the correct illustration.

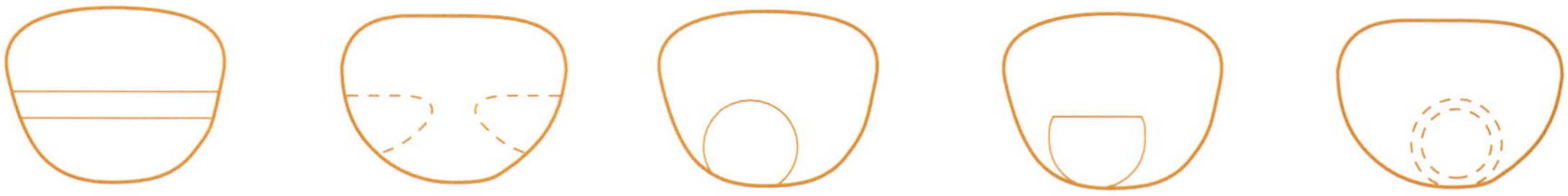

a. b. c. d. e.

____ round-top segment

____ straight-top D segment

____ round-top invisible bifocal

____ progressive-addition bifocal

____ executive trifocal

SUGGESTED ACTIVITIES

1. Schedule a time for your ophthalmologist or a senior staff member to supervise your practice in using the following tools. Use discarded or sample eyeglasses or frames when they are necessary.
   a. Millimeter ruler
   b. Geneva lens clock
   c. Optician's screwdriver
   d. Pupilometer
2. Do the following tasks several times to gain practice:
   a. Measure the segment widths of various multifocal eyeglasses to become familiar with the different multifocal styles.
   b. Measure the segment heights. Note that sometimes they will be dissimilar. Consider why this is so.
   c. Use the Geneva lens clock to measure the base curves of a patient's new and old pair of glasses. Compare these two sets of readings.
   d. Ask those in the office who wear eyeglasses if you may check the tightness of the temples on the frames. With their permission, use the technique described in this chapter to tighten the frame screws.
3. Arrange with several of your coworkers to measure their distance and near interpupillary distance, using the procedures outlined in this chapter. Have your ophthalmologist or senior technician check your work.
4. Arrange with coworkers who wear eyeglasses to measure their vertex distance with a distometer, using the procedure outlined in this chapter.
5. Ask a local optician if you may have samples of old single-vision and multifocal lenses that are chipped, undersized, crooked, or otherwise not useful. Use them to perform the following tasks for practice and learning. Ask your ophthalmologist or senior technician to check your work.
   a. Practice using the lensmeter to dot the various lenses for optical center.
   b. Measure the segment heights of the multifocals with a millimeter ruler.
   c. Use the Geneva lens clock to measure the base curves of all sample lenses.
   d. Tap each lens with your fingernail. Listen to the sound and record which lenses are glass and which are plastic.

SUGGESTED RESOURCES

DiSanto MR: *Technical Options for Professional Service: A Dispensing Manual.* Dayton, OH: Bell Optical Lab; 1994.

Gansen ML: Opticianry. In: Rhode SJ, Ginsberg SP, eds: *Ophthalmic Technology: A Guide for the Eye Care Assistant.* New York: Raven; 1987; chap 21.

Milder B, Rubin ML: *The Fine Art of Prescribing Glasses Without Making a Spectacle of Yourself.* 2nd ed. Gainesville, FL: Triad; 1991.

Opticians Association of America, Guild of Prescription Opticians of America: *Professional Dispensing for Opticianry.* 2nd ed. Newton, MA: Butterworth-Heinemann; 1996.

Physician's Desk Reference for Ophthalmology. Oradell, NJ: Medical Economics Co; updated annually.

9 Patient Interaction, Screening, and Emergencies

The ophthalmic medical assistant is frequently the first professional contact the patient has when telephoning or visiting the ophthalmologist's office. In this role, assistants represent the doctor's office to the patient and therefore are responsible for acting in a manner that is both caring and courteous as well as technically adept. Assistants not only greet patients but also screen patients by asking a specific series of questions to determine the urgency of their need to see the doctor and to schedule a visit appropriately. Assistants also must be able to deal confidently and quickly with patients who call the office with a medical emergency or who experience an emergency during an office visit. In these capacities, assistants are required to be aware of certain ethical and legal concerns to avoid compromising the rights or proper treatment of patients who visit or call.

In the context of caring, professional conduct, this chapter discusses how to greet patients courteously in person and by telephone, screen patients and schedule appointments, process patients referred by other physicians, and handle a variety of emergency situations. While most of the ethical principles discussed in Chapter 1 apply to the situations considered in this chapter, others specific to this chapter's topics are presented here.

PATIENT–ASSISTANT INTERACTION

Patients telephoning or arriving at the ophthalmologist's office often are frightened or apprehensive. In addition to exercising common courtesy in office greetings and telephone conversations, therefore, you should convey your concern for the patient as an individual by talking calmly and quietly and showing genuine compassion, understanding, and, when necessary, reassurance. The ability to gain the patient's trust and respect will aid both assistant and doctor in gathering necessary information for diagnosis and treatment and will help ease the patient's concerns.

Patient Greeting

Whether in person or on the telephone, always address adult patients as Mr, Mrs, Miss, Ms, or according to their preference. When meeting patients in the office, introduce yourself by full name and identify your role in the office (for example, "I am ________ ________, Dr ________'s assistant"). Let patients who seem concerned know that your interaction with them is not delaying their seeing the ophthalmologist but is, in fact, facilitating their meeting with the physician.

The caring and concern that you exhibit over the telephone help put patients at ease and assure them that they will be treated with courtesy and respect. Office personnel who answer the telephone must remember that callers who seem aggressive or even rude may simply be masking fear and worry. Maintaining your composure and assuring these individuals that you understand their situation are the best ways to respond to their anxiety. Chapter 10, "Patients With Special Considerations," presents specific tips for dealing with patients who are worried and concerned.

Although general office procedures may vary from practice to practice, the requirement for good telephone manners applies to all areas of medical and health care. Basic efficient office telephone protocol includes the following:

- Ask the ophthalmologist which callers should be transferred immediately to him or her and under what circumstances.
- When the telephone rings, answer it as promptly as possible.
- Answer the telephone by stating your doctor's name or the name of your association; then identify yourself and ask "How may I help you?"
- To project an attitude of patience and helpfulness, answer the telephone with a cheery, patient (not tense) voice. The individual calling may need a calm person to talk to, and although your face cannot be seen over the telephone, the caller can easily sense your mood by your tone of voice.
- Handle all telephone calls efficiently by forwarding to the correct individual quickly. Ask for a return telephone number in case the call is inadvertently disconnected.
- Try not to put the caller on hold unless it is absolutely necessary. If it *is* necessary, ask if it is permissible and *wait* for the caller's response.
- Write all messages, including names and return telephone numbers, on a pad kept beside the telephone. Ask the callers to spell their names if you are not sure about the spelling.
- Ask the caller to repeat information if you are uncertain about something you have heard.
- At the end of the call, thank the person for calling. End the conversation gently and avoid abruptness.
- Always return a call if you have told the caller you would do so.

PATIENT SCREENING

In many offices, one of the ophthalmic medical assistant's major responsibilities is to perform a preliminary interview with patients to determine the urgency of their situation and to schedule their visit with the ophthalmologist appropriately. This important screening, known as **triage**, ensures that patients with the most serious complaints are seen promptly. Triage most frequently takes place on the telephone when the patient calls the office, but it may apply when a patient appears in the office requesting to see the doctor without calling beforehand. In either case, the basic triage procedure (determining whether a patient's complaint is an emergency, an urgent problem, or a routine situation and scheduling an office visit accordingly) is the same.

The triage situations and procedures presented in this chapter are intended mainly as illustrations and general guidelines; ophthalmic assistants should verify the precise triage situations, steps, and policies followed in their office. Assistants have an important responsibility to perform triage exactly as their ophthalmologist or senior staff instructs or as their office policy dictates, because failure to do so could result in a disservice to the patient's health and vision.

Triage Procedure

The aim of triage is initially to assess and classify patients' signs and symptoms according to their severity and urgency. This process aids the ophthalmic medical assistant in deciding if the patient's difficulty is an emergency or urgent problem, which should be seen relatively soon, or a routine case, which can be seen at a later time.

Triage does not include an in-depth evaluation of the patient's dilemma or a complete medical history. Rather, it is a brief gathering of essential data, beginning with the date and time of the call and the name and telephone number (and possibly the address) of the caller. Thereafter, the urgency for an appointment depends on three factors: the nature, origin, and duration of the patient's complaint or symptom. To determine this, the assistant must ask the patient the following questions:

- What is the basic medical complaint or symptom?
- How did the complaint or symptom originate?
- When did the complaint or symptom start?

As with history-taking procedures, occasionally some prompting is required to elicit a complete answer, and sometimes an answer to a general question leads to more specific questions. To ensure proper scheduling, assistants performing triage must be certain they completely understand what the patient's chief complaint is. It may be necessary to ask patients to restate or rephrase their complaint to obtain this information. The patient's own mental state or sense of emergency should also be taken into consideration when scheduling the visit with the doctor.

In general, the more recent the onset of a symptom, the more urgent the situation. However, when any doubt exists about the nature or urgency of a patient's situation or how to schedule a patient, assistants should either consult the ophthalmologist or allow the patient to speak to the ophthalmologist directly. Sometimes you may find it helpful to speak with family members during triage or have them present during the patient's office visit. They may be able to provide details about the injury or problem that the patient may have overlooked or forgotten. If you do not speak the language of a patient who calls or if you otherwise cannot understand someone's speech, try to identify a family member, friend, or neighbor who can clarify the situation and/or accompany the patient to the office.

Because physical abuse frequently results in eye trauma, as a medicolegal consideration ophthalmic medical assistants should be alert for discrepancies between the report of a traumatic injury and the injury itself, in both children and adults. Any dissimilarities in the details of an injury should be brought to the attention of the ophthalmologist, alone and away from the patient and those accompanying the patient.

Emergency Situation

Ophthalmic **emergencies** are those situations that require immediate action. Assistants who determine that a patient has a medical emergency should advise the patient to come into the office immediately or go to the nearest medical or emergency facility capable of treating ophthalmic problems.

The following situations constitute emergencies:

- Chemical burns: alkali, acid, or organic solvents in the eye (Important detailed instructions for dealing with chemical burns both over the telephone and in the office appear later in this chapter.)
- Sudden, painless, severe loss of vision (This problem suggests an acute vascular occlusion and could cause permanent loss of vision if not treated immediately.)
- Trauma in which the globe has been or is likely to be disrupted or penetrated
- Any trauma that is associated with visual loss or persistent pain
- Severe blunt trauma, such as a forceful blow to the eye with a fist or high-velocity object such as a tennis ball or racquet ball
- A foreign body in the eye or a corneal abrasion caused by a foreign body

- Acute, rapid onset of eye pain or discomfort
- Any emergency referral from another physician

Urgent Situation

The **urgent** situation requires that the patient be seen within 24 hours of contacting the ophthalmologist's office. Some offices define this time period as up to 48 hours. In general, however, patients with urgent conditions should be seen before the next available routine appointment time.

Patients with urgent conditions may report a variety of symptoms, some of which may suggest an emergency condition while others, although not as serious, may nevertheless deserve prompt attention. It can be difficult to distinguish an urgent situation from an emergency. When you have any doubt, the safest course of action is to consult with the ophthalmologist, perhaps with more regularity than you would for an emergency or routine situation. Obviously, erring on the side of safety and completeness is preferred to the possibility of patients losing their vision or their eye because they were not promptly seen by a physician.

The following are generally considered to be urgent situations:

- Subacute loss of vision that has evolved gradually over a period of a few days to a week (Ask the patient whether vision loss has been persistent or intermittent.)
- Sudden onset of diplopia or other distorted vision
- Recent onset of light flashes and floaters
- Acute red eye, with or without discharge (In some patients, such as contact lens wearers, this may be an emergency.)
- Blunt trauma, such as a bump to the eye, that is not associated with vision loss or persistent pain and where penetration of the globe is not likely
- Double vision that has persisted for less than a week
- Photophobia (sensitivity to light)
- Progressively worsening ocular pain
- Loss or breakage of glasses or contact lenses needed for work, driving, or studies (Not all physicians consider losing or breaking glasses urgent.)

Routine Situation

The **routine** difficulty usually includes conditions that have been present for several weeks or more. Patients with routine conditions do not normally have problems that pose an immediate threat to their vision. However, because their condition may cause considerable concern, these patients should be shown an appropriate level of attention. When assessing a routine situation, take the patient's mental state into account. It may suggest that an urgent or emergency visit is more appropriate, even though the medical condition is more routine.

Schedule patients with routine difficulties for the next available routine appointment time, which might be within a few days or a week or two. However, the assistant performing the triage should inform patients to contact the office if their symptoms worsen or if vision becomes impaired before their scheduled office visit.

The following situations may represent routine cases:

- Discomfort after prolonged use of the eyes
- Difficulty with near work or fine print
- Mild ocular irritation, itching, burning
- Tearing in the absence of other symptoms
- Lid twitching or fluttering
- Mucous discharge from the eye
- Mild redness of the eye not accompanied by other symptoms
- Persistent and unchanged floaters whose cause has been previously determined

Appointment Scheduling

Whether as a part of performing triage or simply filling the role of office receptionist, ophthalmic medical assistants should follow these basic guidelines for scheduling appointments efficiently and courteously:

- Be sure the patient knows the exact location of the office.
- Provide details about parking facilities or access to public transportation if necessary.
- Let patients know if their condition or the tests or treatments they will be receiving require that they be assisted to or from the office by a companion or family member.

- In a multiple-physician office, be sure patients know which physician will be attending to them.
- Remind patients to bring their glasses and/or contact lenses with them. They should also bring all medications they are using, especially those for the eye.
- Advise contact lens patients who need a refitting or a change from hard to soft lenses that they must stop wearing the lenses for an appropriate time prior to an examination. Ask your ophthalmologist for the appropriate recommended time.

If time permits and if you have the information, it is thoughtful to let patients know the approximate length of their visit with the doctor (which would depend on the nature of their complaint). Prepare patients for any possible postexamination side effects if you know of them. For example, if you know that patients will be receiving topical eyedrops that increase light sensitivity or temporarily blur vision, tell them how long the side effect will last and whether they might need to wear sunglasses for a while afterward or might require someone else to drive them home. In determining the precise time for their visit, inform patients of office hours and ask if they have any considerations related to transportation or work or school schedules and whether they have a preference for appointment days or times; accommodate their desires as much as possible.

REFERRED PATIENTS

Each medical practice has specific office procedures for handling patients referred by other physicians. Upon your joining the ophthalmologist's office, you should familiarize yourself with these protocols. Follow these general guidelines when receiving a telephone call from a referring physician or referred patient:

- Obtain the referring physician's name and, if possible, the reason for the referral, especially if a letter from the referring doctor is not available.
- If it is routine in your office after the patient's examination, assure the patient that the referring physician will be informed of the results of the examination and any treatment recommendations.

EMERGENCIES ENCOUNTERED IN THE OFFICE

The assistant's competence in handling an emergency calmly and capably is a skill most appreciated in the ophthalmology office. In general, assistants will encounter two types of ophthalmic emergencies in the office: chemical burn and trauma. Nonophthalmic emergencies that may occur during the patient's office visit include fainting and falling.

In any emergency, if you are uncertain about what to do yourself, lose no time in summoning someone nearby—either the doctor or a senior staff member—who you think will be able to assess the situation and administer appropriate aid. Before an emergency happens, take the time to familiarize yourself with the location of all emergency medications, instruments, and materials kept in the office. After the initial emergency aid, the assistant may be asked to help with the patient's examination. You can also be helpful in reassuring the patient or accompanying family member or friend by explaining what is happening, what can be expected next, and how long each step will take. However, do not waste time that should be spent in providing basic, initial emergency aid.

Chemical Burns

A chemical burn can cause severe eye damage in a very short time. Ophthalmic medical assistants should know whether their office policy allows them to initiate first aid for chemical burn injuries that are true emergencies and what to do when the doctor is out of the office.

Any patient who telephones the office to report a chemical in the eye should be instructed to irrigate (wash out, or flush) the affected eye immediately by holding it open either under a continuous flow of running tap water or in a basin filled with water for at least 15 to 20 minutes *before* coming to the office or proceeding to an emergency facility. Once the patient arrives in the office, chemical burns must be treated *immediately* by irrigating the eye with large amounts of sterile saline solution (if available) or tap water.

An alkali burn, the most destructive type of chemical injury, especially requires prompt irrigation even before the patient comes to the doctor's office. Alkali compounds such as ammonia, calcium hydroxide or lime (which is found in plaster, cement, and whitewash), household ammonia, and agricultural anhydrous ammonia can rapidly penetrate ocular tissues. These substances also may leave particles in the eye, which can cause further damage if they are not completely removed. Alkali burns, because of their destructive nature, may require prolonged irrigation in the office, possibly exceeding 30 minutes.

Acid burns usually result from exploding car batteries, industrial accidents, and household bleach spills and splashes. Although they tend to be less injurious than alkali burns, they nevertheless require thorough, prompt irrigation, too. Irrigation in the office should continue for between 20 and 30 minutes nonstop.

Organic solvents include such common household substances as kerosene, gasoline, alcohol, and cleaning fluids. Although some organic solvents may not be as destructive to the eye as alkali or acid, they nevertheless require both home and office irrigation, as with other chemical injuries.

The ophthalmologist is the best judge of the necessity for irrigation and the length of time it should be performed. Even when irrigation is necessary, care must be exercised, as profuse or excess irrigation can cause damage to the cornea. The ophthalmologist also decides whether a topical anesthetic to numb sensation in the eye may be necessary prior to irrigation in the office. The ophthalmic assistant may be asked to administer the anesthetic drops as well as to perform irrigation. The box "Irrigating the Eye" presents the steps of this office procedure.

Following irrigation, the assistant may be asked to help gather important data, including:

- The patient's visual acuity measurements, when possible
- A summary of the accident (Worker's compensation cases require very specific information, often including time, place, and other information.)
- The name or type of chemical involved—for example, a household cleaning product that contains chemicals such as bleach, ammonia, or lye
- The extent of exposure to the chemical—for example, a large quantity splashed directly into the eye or a small amount of chemical residue transferred from the finger to the eye

Trauma

Because of the seriousness of the possible consequences of trauma, the ophthalmologist takes principal responsibility for assessing and treating patients who appear in the office with eye trauma. However, assistants may be requested to help in the following ways:

- Take the patient's medical history.
- Check visual acuity to establish a baseline measure; this should always be done *unless* further trauma or injury could result from forcefully opening the eyelid or disrupting traumatized tissue.
- Ask questions to help identify the nature of a foreign body if one is suspected and gather details of the accident.

When assisting the doctor with a patient who has a traumatized eye, *never* do the following:

- Unnecessarily touch or handle an eye that has a laceration or rupture
- Apply pressure to the globe while attempting to open the lids
- Administer drops or other medications without authorization from the physician and instruction on the proper methods
- Use a previously opened bottle of eyedrops for a patient who may have a penetrating eye injury (always use a new, unopened, sterile bottle) or touch the dropper to the eye

General Emergency Assistance

Be alert to patients who are in pain, feel faint, need to lie down, or feel nauseated. These symptoms may require immediate aid or may signify an impending emergency. Ophthalmic medical assistants should know or keep prominently posted the emergency numbers of hospitals or clinics or community emergency numbers if not 911. The telephone number of the nearest poison control center should also be immediately available. All assistants also should be able to administer first aid and cardiopulmonary resuscitation (CPR) in an emergency. First aid or CPR may be needed to treat a patient who has fainted or fallen or who develops respiratory distress or other adverse reaction to medication. Ophthalmic medical assistants can and should pursue first aid training and gain CPR certification through local chapters of the American Red Cross or other community service organization.

Learn where the emergency first aid kit for minor injuries is kept in your office. If your office has an emergency cart, know its location. This portable, wheeled

IRRIGATING THE EYE

1. Immediately upon arrival, ask the patient to lie down on a stretcher, sofa, examining table, or a chair with a tilted back.
2. If the ophthalmologist requires and permits and if the patient has no known allergy to anesthetic medication, instill one drop of topical anesthetic solution. (Information about instilling eyedrops appears in Chapter 11, "Basics of Ophthalmic Pharmacology.")
3. Holding a gauze pad to help you keep your grasp, use your gloved fingers to separate the lids of the affected eye. Gently but firmly hold the lids open to counter the spasm and forceful closure of the eye during irrigation. A lid speculum may also be used to hold the lids open.
4. Give the patient a towel to hold against the face to absorb the excess fluid. In addition, you can position a basin next to the patient's face to catch the fluid.
5. Perform irrigation with a bottle of ready-made balanced salt solution. If available, a continuous–rapid-drip bottle (suspended like an intravenous drip) is easier because you don't have to keep squeezing the bottle; you just have to direct the stream into the patient's eye. Direct the irrigating stream away from the nose to avoid contaminating the other eye.
6. You may need to evert (turn out) the upper lid while irrigating to wash away particles of chemical that may have become lodged there. To evert the lid:
   a. With the thumb and forefinger of one gloved hand, grasp the lashes of the upper lid and pull it out and down slightly (Figure A).
   b. Using your other hand, place the stick portion of a cotton-tipped applicator horizontally on the upper eyelid, approximately 1/2 inch above the margin of the eyelid (Figure B).
   c. Rotate the lid up and over the applicator stick to expose the conjunctival surface (Figure C).

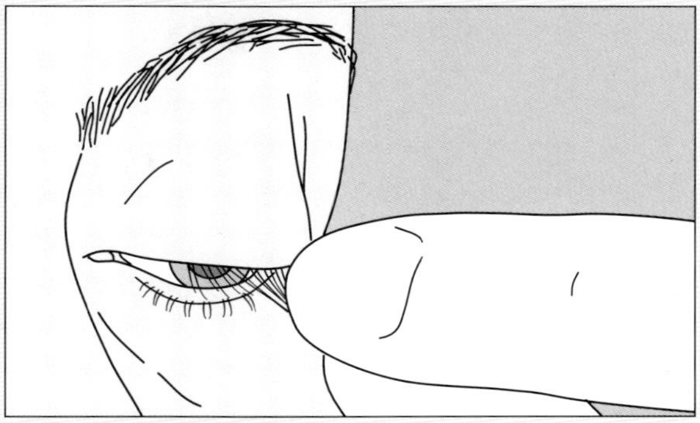

Figure A

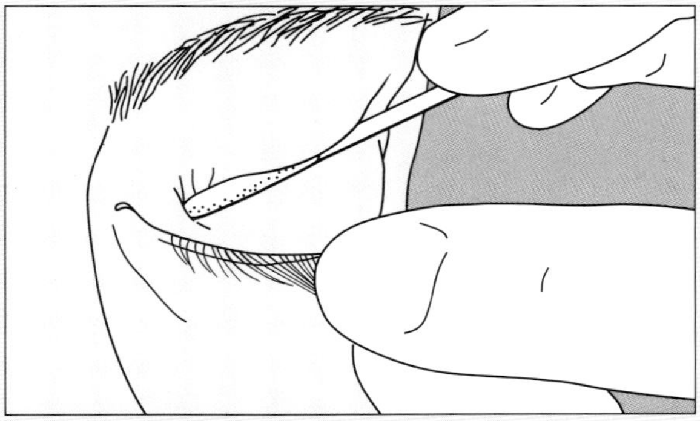

Figure B

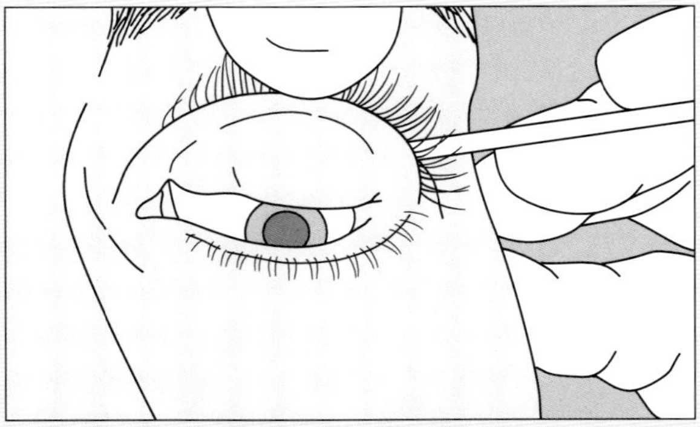

Figure C

7. After irrigation has been completed, patch the eye if you have been requested to do so. (Information about patching the eye appears in Chapter 13, "Minor Surgical Assisting in the Office.")

ASSISTING A PATIENT WHO FEELS FAINT

1. If possible, get the patient's head below the heart; if the patient is sitting, do this by bending the patient's head forward and down toward the knees (see the figure).
2. Loosen the patient's collar or tight clothing.
3. Break the capsule of smelling salts or ammonia from the first aid kit or emergency cart and hold it under the patient's nose to revive the patient.
4. Insist the patient remain seated until the faintness has completely disappeared; be prepared to steady patients when they stand.
5. Reassure the patient, who may be disoriented or embarrassed by the fainting incident.
6. Notify the doctor of the patient's fainting episode.

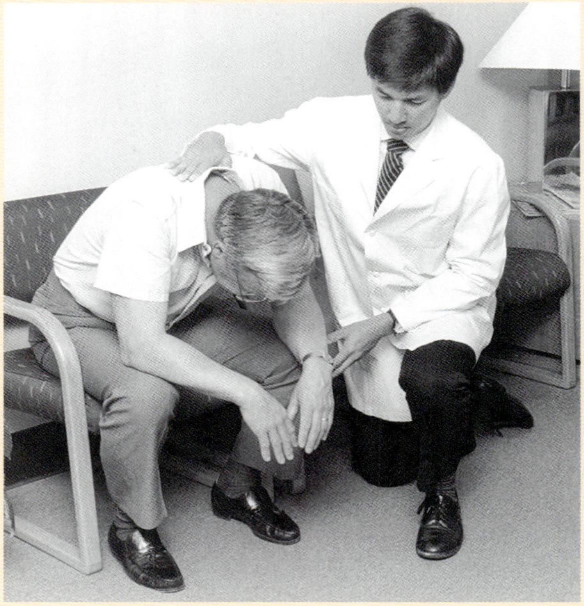

FIGURE 9.1

An office emergency cart.

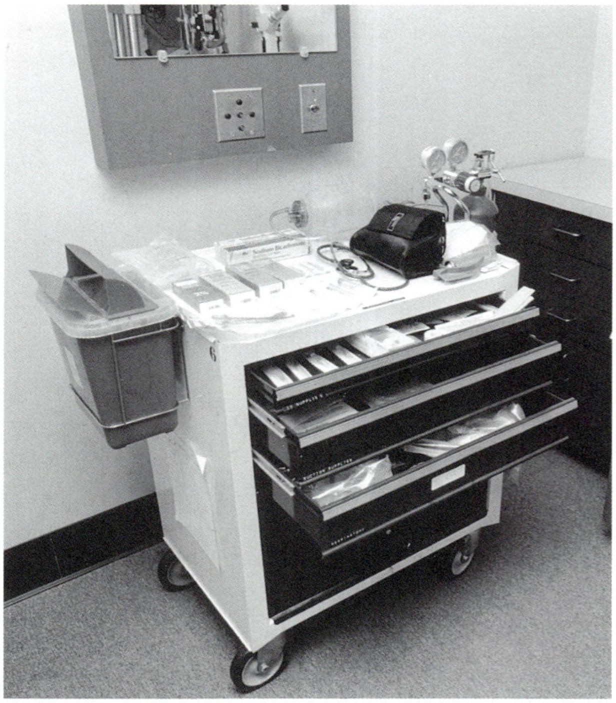

device usually contains oxygen, IV glucose, and medications, such as epinephrine or adrenalin, used to revive a patient (Figure 9.1). The cart may also include cortisone, which may be required to manage a severe allergic reaction, intravenous syringes, and CPR instructions. In addition, some offices keep a supply of juice on hand to give to patients with diabetes who experience unexpected low blood sugar. The box "Assisting a Patient Who Feels Faint" presents steps to take in this emergency situation.

Guidelines for Handling a Patient Fall

- Notify the doctor or other staff of the fall immediately.
- If you witness the fall or if the patient is on the floor when you arrive on the scene, do not move the patient until the doctor has assessed the patient for obvious injury.
- If you do not witness the fall and the patient has since become able to stand, do not allow the patient to leave the office until the doctor has assessed the patient for obvious injury.

Hospital Admission

Ophthalmic medical assistants may be called upon to help arrange emergency hospital admission for a patient who is not only ill but also possibly confused, scared, and upset. In addition, you may be asked to contact family members or work associates for the patient. The following tips can help you make the process go smoothly:

- Let the patient know the plan of action; repeat it if necessary.
- Provide the patient with written directions to the hospital.
- Write the name of the ophthalmologist, the office address, and phone number for the patient to keep on hand for admission to the hospital.
- If the patient is alone and proceeding immediately to the hospital, ask for (and write down) the name of the nearest family member or friend to notify.

REVIEW QUESTIONS

1. Define *triage*.
2. What three basic questions should be answered during the triage process?
3. Name the three main types of substances that may cause a chemical burn in the eye.
4. What is the first instruction to be given to a patient calling to report a chemical burn to the eye?
5. Which of the following might probably be scheduled as routine situations? (More than one response may be correct.)
   a. Photophobia
   b. Progressively worsening ocular pain
   c. Mucous discharge from the eye
   d. Difficulty with near work or fine print
   e. Sudden onset of diplopia or other distorted vision
6. What is the first step to take in assisting a patient who feels faint?

Patient Screening Exercises

Complete the following patient screening exercises, which are intended to help you learn to clarify the patient's symptoms systematically.

1. A 54-year-old office worker calls complaining of blurred vision. Select from the questions listed below all those that would be most appropriate in screening this call.
   a. Do you have a history of hypertension?
   b. How long have your symptoms been present?
   c. Was your vision change rapid or gradual?
   d. Do you see well at night?
   e. Are both eyes involved?

f. Has your vision decreased or worsened?

g. Do you have a family history of cataracts?

h. Do you have other eye problems of recent onset?

2. A 22-year-old woman calls to say she has splashed a cleaning solution in her eye. Select from the questions listed below all those that would be most appropriate in screening this call.

a. Have you flushed your eye with running water for at least 15 minutes?

b. Were you wearing glasses?

c. When did the accident occur?

d. Is your vision impaired?

e. Do you know what the chemical was?

f. Do you have glaucoma?

g. Are your eyes tearing?

h. Which eye was involved?

i. Do you have transportation to the doctor's office available?

3. A 67-year-old patient calls to complain that his eyes are burning. Select from the questions listed below all those that would be most appropriate in screening this call.

a. Do you use reading glasses?

b. How long have your eyes burned?

c. When do your eyes burn the most?

d. Do you have cataracts?

e. Are your eyes red?

f. Do other symptoms accompany the burning?

g. Are you seeing double?

h. Does anything you do relieve the burning?

4. A 73-year-old patient calls to report episodes of transient visual loss (vision that seems to come and go). Select from the questions listed below all those that would be most appropriate in screening this call.

a. When did the episodes of visual loss begin?

b. Is the visual loss in one eye or both?

c. Do you have any tearing or discharge?

d. For how long is your vision impaired when the losses occur?

e. Do you have other symptoms preceding or occurring with the episodes of visual loss?

f. Is there a family history of blindness?

g. Do you have headaches?

SUGGESTED ACTIVITIES

1. Review the triage and emergency procedure guidelines presented in this chapter with your ophthalmologist or senior staff member. Determine in what ways your office's protocol is similar or different.
2. Discuss with the ophthalmologist and the office manager how appointments are made in your office, especially covering how emergency appointments are handled.
3. Tour your office in the company of a senior staff member to learn where emergency supplies are kept and how to use them.
4. Set up a time to role-play some patient screening and emergency exercises (handling an emergency phone call, performing eye irrigation, and the like) with experienced members of the office staff. Discuss your performance together afterward.

SUGGESTED RESOURCES

Davis CM: *Patient Practitioner Interaction: An Experiential Manual for Developing the Art of Health Care.* 3rd ed. Thorofare, NJ: Slack; 1998.

Herrin MP: *Ophthalmic Examination and Basic Skills.* Thorofare, NJ; Slack; 1990; chap 11.

Nemeth SC, Shea CA: *Medical Sciences for the Ophthalmic Assistant.* Thorofare, NJ: Slack; 1991.

Purtilo R: *Health Professionals and Patient Interaction.* 5th ed. Philadelphia: WB Saunders Co; 1996.

Stein HA, Slatt BJ, Stein RM: *The Ophthalmic Assistant: A Guide for Ophthalmic Medical Personnel.* 7th ed. St Louis: Mosby; 2000.

10

Patients With Special Considerations

Ophthalmic medical assistants have an important role in assuring that patients are satisfied with their eye care. Often, the way a patient is treated in the physician's office is as important to that individual as the medical care itself. The ophthalmic medical assistant who can communicate with all patients in a compassionate and polite manner truly serves the profession. Grouping patients in neat categories is neither proper nor possible. However, assistants do encounter patients who require extra care or attention because of their age, health condition, or life situation. Being aware of what to expect and which common complaints may be associated with certain conditions will help you perform your professional duties better.

This chapter will aid you in understanding patients' feelings and in learning how to assist patients with the following special considerations: disruptive patients, visually impaired or blind patients, infants and young children, elderly patients, physically handicapped patients, and patients with diabetes. In this chapter, you will learn to recognize the stresses and difficulties all patients can experience and the importance of offering understanding, care, and compassion to everyone. You will also learn to provide the special assistance and perform the special testing or care some patients require because of their situation or disability.

ALL PATIENTS CONSIDERED

By considering all patients as individuals and attempting to understand and anticipate their needs, you can make each patient's office experience more pleasant and aid the ophthalmologist in effective treatment. Considering patients as individuals requires that you view patients as people, not as diseases. In any conversation, whether in the presence of patients or not, always discuss their problem or condition in terms of the individual: "Mrs _____, our patient with the cataract," not "the cataract in examining room 3"; "Mr _____, who has his eyelid sutured," not "the lid suture we did last week."

Do not avoid patients who do not speak your language or who have physical disabilities. Try to overcome any personal discomfort or embarrassment you feel and give these individuals the same quality of attention you would give to any other patient.

Patients and Their Families

Many times a family member will accompany the patient for the office visit, either out of concern or in the capacity of a helper, especially in the case of an elderly patient or a patient with visual or other physical disabilities. These family members are often greatly concerned about the patient's condition and may ask for specific information about the patient. In such situations, the ophthalmic medical assistant must be sensitive to the patient who may not want medical information shared with relatives and respect the patient's right to confidentiality and privacy. When relatives question you, politely inform them that you are not permitted to share such information with anyone but the patient. If they insist, refer their questions to the doctor.

By the same token, try to accommodate family members who may not want to voice their concerns in front of the patient but may want an opportunity to talk with the doctor in private. You can suggest a later time to call the doctor or have the doctor call them.

Office Waiting Periods

Waiting for any reason can be frustrating, but it can be especially so for patients, who may be anxious about their illness and fearful about an upcoming procedure or diagnosis. Because ophthalmic medical assistants frequently help manage the daily flow of patients through the office, they often are required to communicate with patients if an unusually long delay occurs. Most people are understanding about such delays, especially if they have received a logical explanation of the circumstances and do not feel they have been forgotten.

The following guidelines can help avoid waiting-room situations that tend to distress patients:

- Be sensitive to the valuable time a patient may have lost in waiting excessively for an examination. Assure patients that you do think their time is important.
- Whenever possible, tell patients when the doctor will actually see them or how long a test might take.
- Tell patients how long you will be gone when you leave them alone in the examination room or waiting area.
- If one patient must be seen out of turn ahead of others, explain the situation to those who are waiting in a way that helps them understand and accept the occurrence.
- If a child becomes fussy, try to have the doctor see the family quickly or suggest they take a walk and come back in a specific amount of time. If the family is seen ahead of others, explain the situation to those waiting and ask for their understanding. Many offices have a small play area or keep books and toys to occupy children.
- Be alert to patients who say they feel sick or are in pain. They may need to be seen by the doctor promptly or be rescheduled.
- If an appointment time is excessively delayed, offer to reschedule an appointment or invite the patient to use the telephone to call home or work.
- Patients who are in the office for more than one type of procedure or examination may be required to wait for periods between tests. Be sure these patients know what to expect and why and how long they will be waiting. Do not assume that anyone else has explained anything to them.

DISRUPTIVE PATIENTS

The sheer stress of illness, fear of an unknown diagnosis or procedure, a previous bad experience in a doctor's office, or just the office wait occasionally can make some patients speak loudly and become irritable, hostile, or disruptive. Patients scheduled for office surgery may be anxious, fearful, and impatient, which can cause them to overreact to a comment or question. Some patients may also react this way if they are just overwhelmed by problems, whether associated with their medical condition or with an unrelated situation, such as a financial or family problem. Unfortunately, you may be the person on whom the patient decides to vent anger or frustration.

Ophthalmic medical assistants should be aware of the reasons for these kinds of patient reactions and resist the temptation to react impatiently or angrily to a distressed patient. All patients, no matter what their situation, deserve your compassion and understanding. The following guidelines can help you deal with patients who are irate or disruptive:

- Take the patient out of the reception area or waiting room to avoid upsetting other patients.
- Listen to the patient. Often your caring attention alone will defuse the patient's anger, and listening may help you understand the origin of the patient's hostility.
- Try to identify the problem or perceived problem by restating or paraphrasing what the patient has said to you.
- Offer explanations and alternative solutions.
- Apologize when appropriate, even if you believe the patient is unreasonable or wrong. An apology is often sufficient to defuse anger.
- Never argue and never respond aggressively or offensively.

Aggressive, hostile, angry patients may be individuals who cannot work out feelings with their family or friends. They may be overwhelmed or feel they are a burden to those around them. Talking with someone such as the ophthalmic medical assistant, who knows and understands their medical circumstances but is removed from the daily situation, can be a comfort.

During your encounter with an irate or hostile patient, you may learn of some nonmedical reason for the behavior. While respecting the patient's confidences and right to privacy, the ophthalmic medical assistant may be able to alert the doctor that the particular patient has a troubling nonmedical difficulty. It may then be appropriate for the doctor to refer the patient to a social service agency or support group for help.

VISUALLY IMPAIRED OR BLIND PATIENTS

Loss of vision or the fear of vision loss can totally change a person's life and be a devastating experience at any age. People who lose sight later in life still relate to the world as sighted persons and require visual information. They want to know what people and their surroundings look like. Providing this information is an important aspect of assisting patients with visual impairments.

People with unimpaired vision sometimes erroneously categorize all persons with visual impairments as blind. They also may assume persons who are blind to be in complete darkness when, in fact, only 10% of all "legally blind" persons are totally without sight. **Legal blindness** is often defined as a best-corrected visual acuity of 20/200 or less or as a visual field reduced to 20° or less in the better-seeing eye. It is of utmost importance that those who work with people with visual impairments appreciate the great differences in an individual's degree of deficit and the varying abilities of those with visual impairments to cope and maneuver in the "sighted world." Any of the following common deficits, either singly or in combination, can impair vision: no peripheral vision but good central vision, no central vision, less than 20/200 visual acuity, only portions of the visual field perceived, light perception only, no light perception, or fluctuations in vision.

The ophthalmic medical assistant should be careful not to treat visually impaired or blind patients as if they were deaf or mentally defective. Although visually impaired and blind patients may not see as well as others, they usually hear, speak, and think as well as the average individual. Patients with poor vision often rely on their hearing to understand activity around them. Be careful not to startle these patients, which can happen unintentionally if you approach them noiselessly in a carpeted room. Try always to face these patients and use their name when speaking to them, or gently touch their elbow when speaking to them. It is never appropriate to shout at any patient.

Patient Greeting and History-Taking

When first encountering a patient who is visually impaired or blind, approach the patient, introduce yourself, and use the patient's name as well as your own; for example: "Hello, Mr _____. My name is _____ _____ and I work with Dr _____, who will be examining you today. Let's go on back to the examining room now." Or "Hello, Ms _____. I'm _____ _____; I saw you last time you were in. Are you ready to get started?" A smile may not be seen, but it can be "heard" when you speak in a friendly, cheerful manner. Another important point is to speak directly to the patient, not to an accompanying companion or, worse, to others in the waiting room.

Look for an extended hand to shake but do not make a point of insisting on a handshake if none is offered. Do not stumble over expressions like "How nice to *see* you!" or "I look forward to *seeing* you again soon." Generally, you may be more apologetic or overly sensitive about the use of such words than is the person you are addressing.

Ask the patient whether the accompanying family members or friends should be invited to come along to the examining room. Some patients welcome the company, but others prefer to be alone with the doctor during the examination so they can ask their own questions. You can help smooth over any awkwardness by telling the family you will call them in when the testing is over and the doctor is ready to talk to everyone. When you arrive at the examining room, introduce the patient to the people who are in the room as you enter as well as those who enter later.

Some special questions are usually included when taking the history of a patient with low vision. These include questions to ascertain the onset of visual loss; the patient's use of low vision aids; any problems or goals related to the low vision; and the nature of any home, family, or community support that the patient may have. A functional history includes questions about the patient's ability to perform a variety of specific daily living activities, everyday near-vision and distance-vision tasks such as reading a newspaper, mending, watching television, or reading an overhead menu at a fast-food restaurant. Also included are questions about the patient's orientation and mobility skills, such as the ability to ambulate within the home and yard, or to go to and maneuver within a grocery store. Such a functional history is useful to help document progressive visual loss. It reveals how the patient is using his or her remaining vision and what accommodations the patient is making to the low vision. It also allows the patient to relate fears and concerns that may not be communicated during routine eye care.

PATIENT ASSISTANCE

If you have been able to observe how the patient navigated into the office or in the waiting room, you may know what kind of help, if any, the person needs in maneuvering around the office. If you have not noted this, offer assistance as unobtrusively as possible. Do not push yourself on patients or hurry them along.

When guiding a patient with a visual impairment, you may find it useful to ask gentle questions such as "Would you like some assistance?" or "Would you like to take my arm?" Patients who want to take your arm will usually do so above the elbow or around your lower arm. The patient may prefer to walk slightly behind you, which allows you to guide them and enables the patient to anticipate your directional changes. You can keep your arm relaxed and at your side unless the patient has balance problems and needs support in addition to guidance (Figure 10.1). Never push or pull visually impaired patients, even gently.

Think ahead and remove unnecessary chairs or obstacles in the hallway to avoid any embarrassment or accident to the patient who might bump into something. Verbally describe the path you will be taking to the patient: "We will be turning right and going along a narrow corridor" or "The chair is just to the left of the door; I'll put your hand on the armrest (or the back of the chair) so you can seat yourself." If you are called away while guiding a patient to a room, do not leave the patient stranded in the hallway. Either proceed to a room with the patient or have another member of the office staff take over for you.

When interacting with any patients who have severe visual impairment, give verbal information whenever possible. For example, you can say "I am reading through your chart and also making some notes" or "I will leave you alone in the room now while you wait for Dr_____. She should be about 10 minutes" or "Dr_____ is not quite ready to see you. I'd like you to come with me to another waiting area

FIGURE 10.1

Guiding a visually impaired patient.

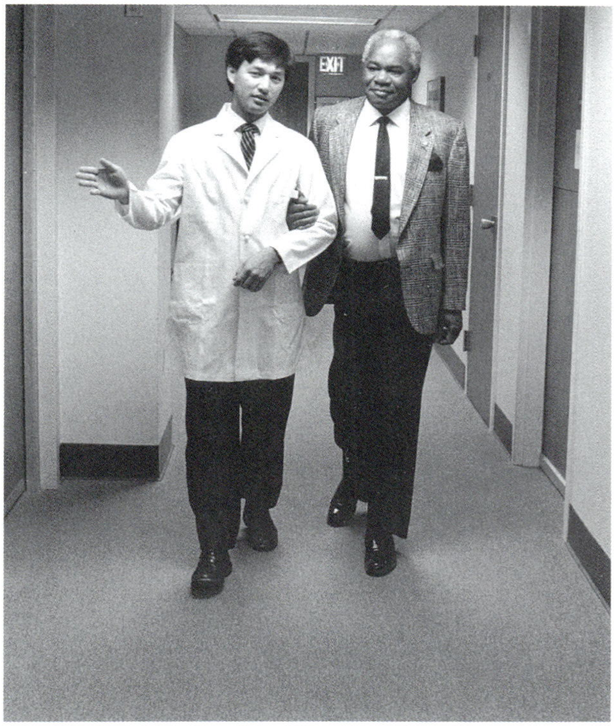

while your pupils are dilating." Tell the patient what is planned: "This next test will take about 20 minutes." If you must leave the patient, do not just quietly leave the patient alone. Instead say "It was nice talking with you. I have to go now."

Visual Acuity Assessment

The term *legal blindness* can be misleading, carries an unfortunate stigma, and offers little information about how the individual functions. One person who is visually impaired may work, study, and function in society, while another may be totally handicapped and dependent on others.

Patients with severe low vision may be referred to a low-vision specialist. However, the ophthalmic medical assistant may first be required to estimate visual acuity. To begin, perform the visual acuity test using the standard Snellen chart and procedure (see Chapter 5, "Comprehensive Medical Eye Examination"). If the patient cannot see the largest (20/200) Snellen letter from the standard distance, ask the patient to move toward the chart or move a portable chart toward the patient yourself until the largest optotype can be seen.

In the visual acuity record, the numerator will then indicate the distance from the chart and the denominator, the largest line seen; for example, 10/200 means the patient could see the 200 optotype at 10 feet; 5/200 means the patient was tested at 5 feet. If a patient cannot see the largest Snellen letters at 3 feet, test the patient's ability to see and count fingers, detect hand movements, or perceive light, as described in the box "Performing a Low-Vision Test" on page 162. However, standard testing distances and performance procedures may differ between ophthalmology offices. Be sure to check the preferred procedure used in your office for testing the visual acuity of patients with visual impairment.

INFANTS AND YOUNG CHILDREN

In physical development, behavior, and needs, children differ greatly from adults. They should be approached and examined in a different manner than adult patients. When assisting and testing children, be aware of their short attention spans and be understanding of their keen interest in exploring everything around them. You should be prepared to protect any valuable instruments and lenses in the examination room that may be within a child's inquisitive reach. Offer a toy as an alternative to the instrument.

Parents want and need to understand their child's condition and to help the child comply with the treatment that the doctor prescribes. Their needs and those of the child must be met in order to have a successful and worthwhile visual examination that yields useful information.

Patient Greeting

Introduce yourself to the child as well as to the accompanying adult. For children older than 3, you might ask who they brought along with them today, but do not assume it is a parent. Explain who you are and what you will be doing both to the adult and, in simpler terms, to the child.

Be flexible enough to change the order of your examination. You might wish to start with taking a medical history, but you may find this procedure bores children, causing them to become inattentive or uncooperative for the duration of the examination. Be

PERFORMING A LOW-VISION TEST

Test and record the visual acuity in each eye separately, beginning with the right eye. Make sure that the eye not being tested is well covered.

1. Starting at a distance of 5 feet, hold up fingers of one hand and ask the patient to count them. Record the distance at which counting is done accurately; for example, CF 3 ft.
2. If the patient cannot count fingers, move your hand horizontally or vertically before the patient at a distance of 3 feet. Record the distance at which the patient reported seeing your hand movement; for example, HM 2 ft.
3. If the patient cannot detect your hand motion, shine a penlight toward the patient's face from 15 inches and turn it on and off to determine if light perception is present. If the patient cannot see the penlight, use the indirect ophthalmoscope on its brightest setting and try again (be sure the fellow eye is completely occluded). If the patient cannot see the light, record the response as NLP (no light perception). If the patient can see the light, record the response as LP (light perception). No record of distance is required. Some ophthalmologists distinguish "bare light perception" as vision that cannot perceive a penlight but can perceive an extremely bright light such as that from an indirect ophthalmoscope or a slit lamp.
4. If the patient perceives the penlight, shine the light from different fields of gaze with the patient looking straight and the nontested eye occluded. If the patient can see light from different directions, record the patient's vision as LP with projection.

prepared to obtain pieces of the child's medical history throughout the examination or during testing. Explain this approach to accompanying adults, so that they do not feel you are ignoring them or are disorganized in your history-taking.

Patient Positioning

Be sure the child is comfortable. Some small children may be more comfortable on the adult's lap, while others will feel important if they can sit alone in the chair (Figure 10.2). Ask children what they prefer, then respect the answer. Adults can be requested to hold infants and babies in the lap, over the shoulder in the burping position, or in some other way that both facilitates the examination and keeps the child quiet and comfortable.

A **papoose board** may be needed to immobilize an infant during an ophthalmologic evaluation, and the ophthalmic medical assistant may be asked to help with it. Basically, the papoose board is a padded board with Velcro straps that fasten around the baby,

FIGURE 10.2

A child may prefer to sit alone for the examination, rather than on an adult's lap.

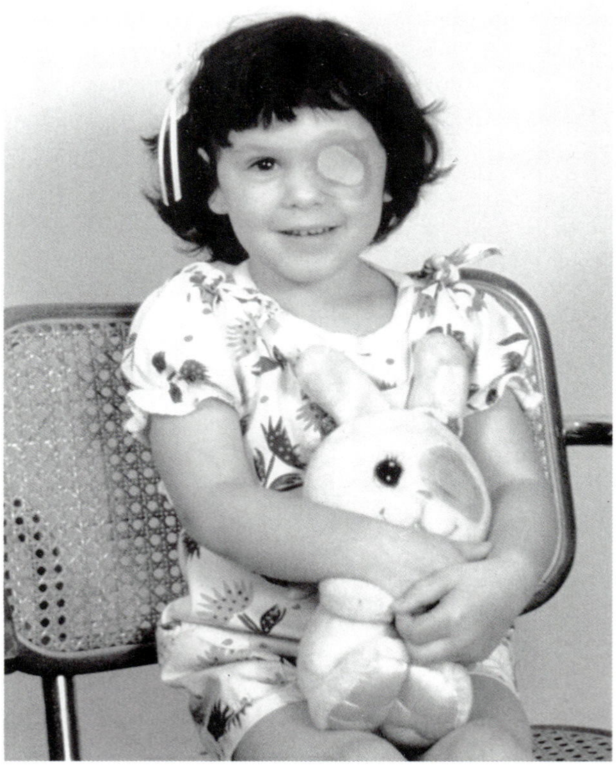

TESTING AN INFANT'S VISUAL ABILITY

1. Seat the infant on the adult's lap.
2. Select an object that stimulates sight only, such as a hand-held spinning top or a sparkler-type toy.
3. Hold the object about 1 to 2 feet from the baby's face and slowly move it horizontally to the left, then to the right (see the figure). Watch the infant's eyes for fixation eye movements.
4. If you discern no visual response, repeat step 3 in a darkened room with a small penlight.

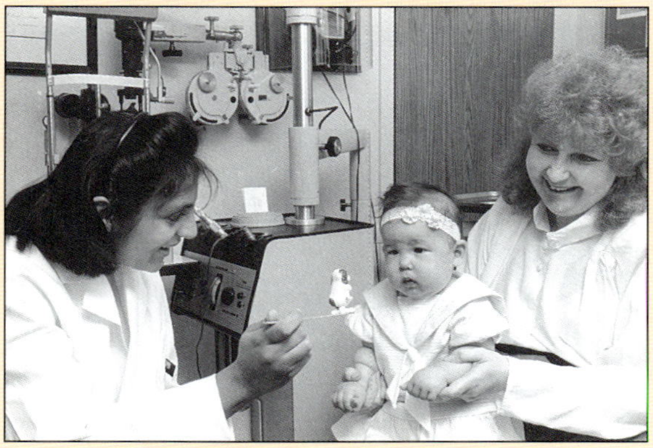

holding arms and legs still and out of the way. The board is then placed on a stretcher.

Alternatives to a papoose board include the use of sheeting wrapped around the infant's arms and legs in mummy fashion or placement of the infant on the adult's lap with the head on the adult's knees and legs around the adult's waist. The adult holds the baby's arms outstretched and snugly against the baby's own head. The infant thus feels the warmth and security of the adult.

Visual Acuity and Ability Testing

Visual acuity can be measured in toddlers and older children. However, infants and handicapped children, such as those with Down syndrome or cerebral palsy, frequently do not have the verbal and motor skills required to participate in a routine visual examination. For these children, it may only be possible for you to assess their general visual function by observing their behavior as it appears to relate to visual stimuli or tasks.

Assessing visual function in infants, in children with mental or physical disabilities, and in children with severe visual impairment is difficult even for the most experienced examiner. The ophthalmic medical assistant will probably not be asked to make such an assessment alone, but may be asked to help with a child who is being evaluated. Checking visual function or acuity can be divided into examination groupings such as infants, toddlers, and school-age children if one keeps the categories flexible and does not adhere to strict age limits.

Infants

Infants do not undergo testing for visual acuity but rather for visual function, which is considered the ability to fixate a visual object and to follow the movement of that object with the eyes. Most babies without visual impairment display this capacity to "fix and follow" by age 2 months.

The box "Testing an Infant's Visual Ability" provides step-by-step instructions for performing this procedure. When testing an infant, keep the following guidelines in mind:

- Many infants do not want a stranger nearby or their head touched by someone they do not recognize. Always approach babies slowly to avoid frightening them.
- Generally, the younger the patient, the less precisely you can estimate visual acuity; therefore, ask the accompanying adults how they think the child sees. Ask for examples of the baby's visual behavior, such as the ability to reach for toys or recognize familiar faces.
- Check for a difference in the baby's response when either eye is covered. Some infants will object to the examination only when the better-seeing eye is covered.

FIGURE 10.3

Charts for testing the visual acuity of toddlers and children. (A) Allen chart. (B) E chart.

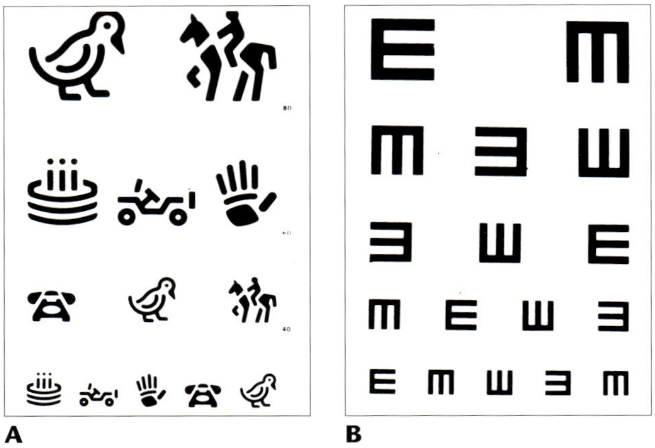

Toddlers and School-Age Children

When joining the staff, ophthalmic medical assistants should learn the office protocol for working with young patients. Try to determine which charts and testing routines are preferred, whether you should check acuity with and without glasses, and whether you should check both distance and near vision.

Toddlers and school-age children are tested for visual acuity with standard charts. Children in these age groups present some special challenges, however. Children play: they peek, they guess with a straight face just as if they were reading the chart, they memorize with lightning speed, they can suddenly become very shy and uncooperative, and they often need extra encouragement.

Toddlers as well as school-age children thrive on praise; they need to be told that they are doing a good job and that it is all right when they do not know the answer to a specific question or cannot see something. It is especially important that you tell them they are doing a good job not only when they answer correctly, but also when they are trying hard and cooperating—even if they cannot see or they make an error. Some children will need a reward such as letting them look at a little toy following each part of the exam.

A principal goal is to assess visual acuity without intimidating the child. Allow the child to read from right to left or confuse common letters. You are not being asked to teach letter recognition, to diagnose reading problems, or to administer an intelligence test.

During your testing of a toddler's or school-age child's visual acuity, make a note of any unusual head positions, jiggling eye movements (nystagmus), excessive squinting, or closing one eye when both eyes should be opened.

Charts Used to Test Children

The following charts are most often used to test the visual acuity of toddlers and school-age children:

- Standard Snellen charts for children who know the alphabet or numbers
- Charts with silhouetted pictures to identify, called Allen charts (Figure 10.3A)
- The tumbling E or E game chart, which shows the capital letter E turned on its various edges (Figure 10.3B); the child points the hand in the direction that the spokes of the E are pointing for the letter you indicate
- Letter-matching tests, in which you point to one of several letters on a chart and the child selects the matching letter from a hand-held card (HOTV-type test); children do not need to know letters in order to be able to match the shapes in this test
- Teller Acuity Cards, which test infants' and preverbal children's visual acuity by means of gratings (vertical black-and-white stripes)

All of these visual acuity testing charts have advantages and disadvantages. As you become experienced in conducting visual acuity examinations, the ophthalmologist or senior staff assistant who helps with your training can give you specific instructions in using these specialized charts with children and recording the visual acuity measurements.

Tips for Testing Toddlers

Some toddlers do better with number charts; others seem to prefer letter charts. If a child seems hesitant with one kind, try the other. Do not be surprised if children seem to have difficulty identifying images on an Allen picture chart. Some of the images are so schematic and old-fashioned that many are not readily recognizable today.

The E game can present problems unrelated to visual ability. Preschoolers may not readily understand that a letter or a symbol turned in other directions is a "new" letter; they frequently interpret an E that is upside down and an E on its side as the same. They may be able to point up and down but often cannot twist their hands to demonstrate fingers pointing right or left. In this case, you might try testing using just the up and down E.

Tips for Testing School-Age Children

When working with children in general, do not assume that at a given age all children are able to recognize and name letters of the alphabet. If embarrassed, they may become very shy and not cooperate at all. It is preferable to ask "Do you know some letters?" rather than "Can you read?" It is not uncommon for children to struggle over the word OFLCT because you have asked them to "read" the chart. Until you tell them to say each letter separately, they may not understand that this is what you really wish them to do. Some children will say they know the letters and, when shown the line, will brightly say "A,B,C,D,E" instead of naming the letters on the chart.

Be sensitive about embarrassing children who stumble when trying to read a chart. Some 2-year-olds know and read letters but some 8-year-olds do not. When children act timid in the beginning or reach a line that is smaller than they feel confident to try, you can begin to do it together by each saying a letter in turn along the line. This sort of game often gets the child started. When a letter is said incorrectly, you can skip it and check it later.

Often children stop at the "small" 20/30 line at the bottom of a chart projected on a screen, but if you isolate that line they can read it easily. If you make it the top or biggest of several smaller lines, they often do not hesitate in identifying the letters.

Do not be too concerned if the letters are read in a scattered order or from right to left. Allow errors if consistently stated; for example, the child may repeatedly call a V an A or a P a B. When examining children in these age groups for visual acuity, do not give up: be creative.

ELDERLY PATIENTS

It is important not to draw conclusions about patients based on their age alone or their medical condition. However, elderly patients seen in the ophthalmology office often have special age-related health problems and emotional needs, which ophthalmic medical assistants should consider. An elderly person may be particularly worried about declining health and may notice or complain about subtle changes in vision. Examiners should not overlook or downplay these observations. Make note of the symptoms so that the doctor can follow up.

In elderly patients as well as in others, worry may take the form of crossness, unreasonable blaming of others, or anxiety. The ophthalmic medical assistant needs to treat elderly patients with special consideration, keeping in mind the following:

- Healing may be slower.
- Understanding may be slower.
- Apprehension about their condition may be greater than with younger patients. Some elderly patients fear impending blindness, even with relatively minor eye problems.
- Not only visual acuity may be affected by eye diseases but color perception and low-contrast vision as well.
- Many elderly people live alone, so a small change in objective acuity may cause a big change in functional ability; for example, changing from 20/30 to 20/40 may seem trivial, but it may make the difference between being able to read the newspaper or the label on a medication container easily and having difficulty in doing so.
- Having to give up shopping alone, driving, or other independent activities because of declining ability can be a very difficult adjustment.

Age-Related Vision Changes

Many changes in vision in elderly patients come as a result of physical changes in the eye itself. With age, the lens gradually yellows, resulting in some difficulty with color discrimination. It also becomes increasingly rigid and opaque, resulting in a significant loss of accommodative ability. The patient may be unable to shift focus from distance to near or to read clearly at near and intermediate distances with or without corrective lenses.

When ophthalmic medical assistants know and understand the problems faced daily by elderly patients, they can become more sensitive to these individuals. This sensitivity and caring will also help you to take a more complete, accurate medical history. Common complaints and ophthalmic entities of the elderly include

- Floaters
- Watery, dry, or itchy eyes
- Difficulty seeing when going down stairs
- Decreased vision at night
- Decreased contrast sensitivity
- Difficulty with glare
- Extra time needed to adjust when entering a darkened room
- More light needed to read yet have problems with glare
- Diminished color discrimination, especially blues and greens
- Changes in visual ability related to cataract (present in some degree in 95% of people over age 65), glaucoma, or diabetes

The special needs of elderly patients can be multifaceted. Some elderly patients may have one or more chronic illnesses or limitations on their ability to maneuver easily through their daily activities. Their current visual loss may be just the latest event to occur among other medical concerns.

Some elderly patients also have loss of hearing, which can compound their sense of isolation. Speak slowly and distinctly to patients who have difficulty in hearing. Face such patients squarely and allow them to see your lips so they can obtain extra clues to what you are saying. It is rarely necessary to raise your voice excessively and never necessary to shout.

Many elderly people who are "partially sighted" do not get around as well as younger, more severely visually impaired individuals who may be in better general health, have a broader support system, and are more optimistic. However, no one can predict a patient's reaction based on age. A sudden loss of vision for one patient may be far more devastating than a slowly progressive one for another.

Some older persons mistakenly believe they should "preserve" their eyes by not "using them up." Tell them it is not possible to use up the eyes, even if a visual abnormality exists. Encourage them not to sit in the dark, not to give up hobbies, and to continue reading or doing other near work. By participating in living as fully as possible, they can continue to have a good quality of life.

Visual Acuity Testing

As with most adult patients, visual acuity in elderly persons is tested using a standard Snellen chart and procedure (see Chapter 5, "Comprehensive Medical Eye Examination"). When distance acuity is less than 20/200, you usually would have the patient walk toward the chart. With elderly patients, however, consider their ability to get in and out of the examining chair; instead, move the chart toward the patient if possible.

Check the near acuity of elderly patients even if distance acuity is poor. The importance of near vision in this age group cannot be overestimated. Reading, needlework, or arts and crafts may be the person's major, if not only, independent activity and source of enjoyment. It is particularly important to adjust the near vision test appropriately to avoid glare, which can be a noticeable problem for patients in the initial stages of cataract formation. Glare presents a paradox for the elderly person, who may benefit from additional lighting for reading but at the same time may be bothered by the glare it creates. Maintain the standard distance required for a particular test but allow the patient to adjust the tilt of the near card. The ideal situation is to have the highest contrast with the least amount of glare. Good contrast can often be an easier and better solution to comfortable reading than high magnification.

When checking both distance and near visual acuity, remember that the elderly patient may require extra time to search for and locate the letters, especially the patient with macular degeneration. Give these patients coaching and extra prompting as needed. Elderly patients may have a slower reaction time than younger patients, so it is important also to give them some additional time to respond.

If an elderly patient is unable to read a distance or near acuity chart at all, proceed with low-vision testing, as described earlier in this chapter. Elderly patients may also require additional tests of visual abilities, such as contrast-sensitivity and glare testing. These and other specialized vision tests are discussed in Chapter 6, "Adjunctive Tests and Procedures."

PHYSICALLY DISABLED PATIENTS

Ophthalmic medical assistants may expect to help physically disabled patients in wheelchairs during the course of the office visit (Figure 10.4). Sometimes, moving a patient into and out of a wheelchair can be difficult. This occurs especially with patients who have disabling multiple sclerosis, are disabled with rheumatoid arthritis, or need to be belted into the wheelchair for safety. An increasing number of children with cerebral palsy use wheelchairs equipped with straps that hold them upright and communication boards that allow them to "speak" with others.

Always ask patients in wheelchairs or their helpers if the patients can be moved easily from the chair, if they need assistance, or if they can walk to an examination chair. Remember to lock the wheels and to support the chair from behind while the patient is getting in or out or being moved to the examination chair; otherwise, the wheelchair may accidently roll backward.

If possible, it is advisable to have at least one examination area in the office that can accommodate patients in wheelchairs. Having to move patients into and out of wheelchairs can cause these patients undue stress or embarrassment. Under certain circumstances, the ophthalmic medical assistant may be asked to accompany a patient in a wheelchair to the restroom. If you have never helped anyone in and out of a wheelchair in a restroom, you should ask for assistance.

PATIENTS WITH DIABETES

Diabetes mellitus is a chronic disease that inhibits the proper processing of carbohydrate (sugar) in the body. Diabetes can affect many body systems, including the eye (the retina, specifically). The effect of diabetes on the retina is known as *diabetic retinopathy*. Because diabetic retinopathy can lead to visual impairment that requires treatment or may even result in blindness, the ophthalmic medical assistant is likely to encounter patients with diabetes in the ophthalmologist's practice. Patients with diabetes also may have cataracts or glaucoma. Understanding the condition of, and daily problems faced by, patients with diabetes can help the ophthalmic medical assistant consider the comfort and proper care of these patients.

People with diabetes must constantly monitor the level of sugar in their blood, which for some means pricking their finger several times a day to draw blood and using special meters to perform this test (Figure 10.5). Some patients control their blood sugar level by frequent self-administered insulin injections, while others manage by a combination of dietary balance, exercise, and stress reduction. This process for daily health management can create a great amount of stress in and of itself.

FIGURE 10.4

Helping a physically disabled individual during an office visit.

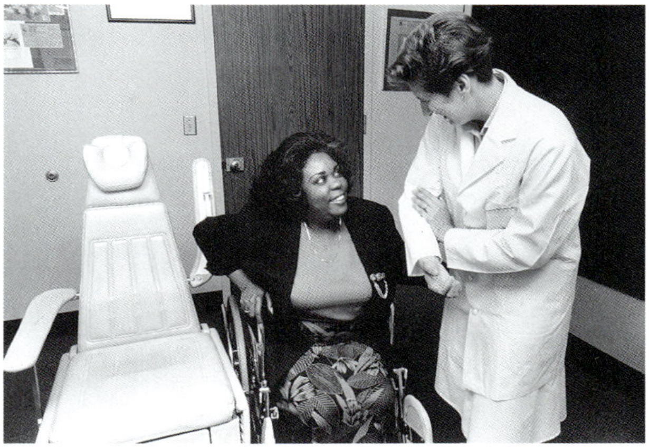

FIGURE 10.5

A patient with diabetes monitoring the level of glucose in the blood.

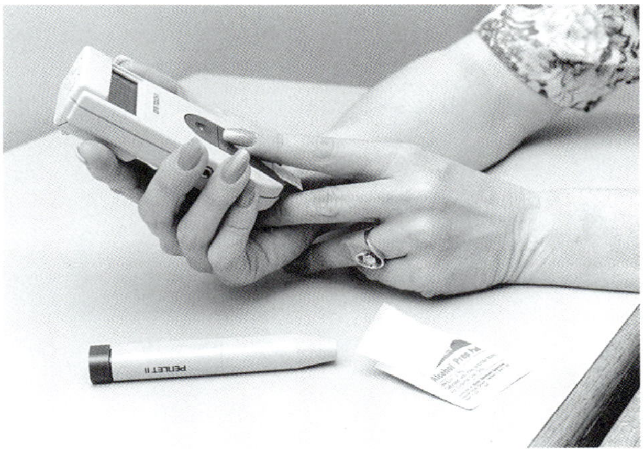

Diabetes-related eye symptoms, such as double vision, visual fluctuations, or sudden loss of vision, coupled with frequent eye examinations or treatments also create stress. Patients may have high blood pressure, kidney problems, nerve disease, and other conditions related to the diabetes in addition to their visual difficulties. They may be undergoing treatments for these various problems, all of which can add stress and anxiety to their lives.

Special Help for Patients With Diabetes

The doctor who treats a patient for diabetes often refers the patient to the ophthalmologist for diagnosis and treatment of related eye conditions. The referring doctor usually forwards the patient's medical history, but the ophthalmologist will also wish to have a baseline ophthalmic and medical history. During this procedure, the ophthalmic medical assistant may expect to record some of the following general complaints, which are associated with diabetes:

- Increased hunger or thirst
- Increased urination
- Sudden weight loss
- Fatigue
- Blurred eyesight
- Numbness or tingling of the hands or feet
- Frequent infections
- Slow healing of cuts and sores
- Impotence

Patients with confirmed or suspected diabetes usually have to undergo lengthy ophthalmologic office procedures, such as fluorescein angiography, ultrasonography, electrophysiologic testing, ophthalmic photography, and laser surgery. Many of these procedures, especially laser surgery, can cause discomfort or pain. Ophthalmic medical assistants often are called upon to inform the patient about what will happen before, during, and after the procedure or test. Therefore, they should understand their office's policy and their role in assisting patients who are scheduled for any of these procedures.

Treatment of a Hypoglycemic Reaction

Ophthalmic medical assistants should be alert to the possibility of a diabetic patient having a hypoglycemic reaction while in the office. **Hypoglycemia** results from low blood sugar levels, which can be caused by the amount of food eaten, exercise engaged in, medications taken, or stress endured. Patients having a hypoglycemic reaction may become weak, sweaty, shaky, or dizzy at first. This initial phase may be followed by numbness of the lips, changes in vision or mood, disorientation, or irritability. Finally, the patient may suffer a seizure or go into a coma.

Ophthalmic medical assistants should be familiar with the office policy for treating a hypoglycemic reaction of a patient in the office. Ask the ophthalmologist or senior staff member to clearly define your role in assisting these patients. Which should you do first: notify the doctor or apply first aid measures? Many patients are prepared to care for themselves if a sudden hypoglycemic episode occurs. Even so, many ophthalmology offices store a quick-acting sugar—such as fruit juice, sugar cubes, or candy—to give the patient immediately or on the patient's request. Then the ophthalmic assistant would notify the doctor of the patient's state.

When scheduling an appointment for a patient with diabetes (especially a patient dependent on insulin), try to choose a time that does not interfere with mealtimes, because many patients must eat at very specific times to ensure a correct blood sugar level. If an unexpected test or wait becomes necessary during the office visit, keep in mind that the waiting patient may need a snack or glass of juice.

REVIEW QUESTIONS

1. The doctor is with a patient who requires unexpected additional examination time. You have apologized to the waiting patients and explained that the doctor will be delayed another 15 minutes, but Mrs Wright now tells you she is concerned about getting home later than she had planned. Which of the following would be the best action for you to take?

   a. Explain the nature of the test the doctor is conducting on the patient presently being seen so that Mrs Wright can appreciate its importance.

   b. Suggest that Mrs Wright take a walk and return in 15 minutes.

   c. Ask Mrs Wright to step into a private part of the office with you and explain that you understand how important her time is to her.

   d. Offer to reschedule Mrs Wright's appointment or allow her to telephone home to say she will be delayed.

   e. Tell Mrs Wright that an emergency has occurred but that she should have to wait only a few more minutes.

2. List at least four examples of common deficits that can impair vision.
3. Describe the two alternative actions to take if you are called away while guiding a visually impaired patient to a room.
4. Write the visual acuity recording for patients who require the Snellen chart to be 8 feet away before they can see the 200 optotype.
5. Name the three principal procedures for determining visual acuity in patients who cannot read the Snellen chart at 3 feet.
6. A papoose board is principally used to
   a. Carry an infant from the waiting room to the examination room
   b. Allow an adult to hold an infant in the lap
   c. Immobilize an infant during an ophthalmologic examination
   d. Give an infant a sense of security during an ophthalmologic examination
   e. Calm a crying infant
7. Visual acuity in elderly patients is first tested using
   a. An Allen chart
   b. The finger-counting procedure
   c. A standard Snellen chart
   d. A near vision card
   e. A letter-matching test
8. In a patient with diabetes, low blood sugar level can cause a reaction known as ________.

SUGGESTED ACTIVITIES

1. With an ophthalmologist or senior staff member in your office, review the office protocol for assisting patients with the special considerations discussed in this chapter. If your office deals with patients who have special considerations other than those mentioned in this chapter, ask for practical tips to help you give these patients any needed special assistance as well.
2. Determine your office's protocol for summoning assistance when you find yourself in a situation with a patient that you cannot or do not know how to handle.
3. Ask an experienced assistant on your office staff to role-play the part of an irate, visually impaired, elderly, or other type of patient so you can practice performing appropriately. Have the experienced assistant critique your verbal and physical behavior in a discussion afterward.
4. To understand the kind of guidance a visually impaired patient might need, ask another assistant to guide you from the office waiting room to an examining room with your eyes shut or blindfolded. Then switch roles and guide your colleague. Afterward, discuss the exercise with the other assistant and with senior staff members.

5. Ask permission to observe specialized visual acuity testing procedures when they are performed with children, patients who are visually impaired, and elderly patients. Take notes and ask questions in a meeting with the ophthalmologist or other examiner later.
6. If your ophthalmology office treats many children, you may wish to watch television programs such as "Mister Rogers" and "Sesame Street" to gain pointers on how to work with youngsters 2 to 6 years old. Stopping by a local store to learn what toys are popular with children of specific ages may help you relate to the young patient.
7. If the ophthalmology practice you work for has a large proportion of elderly patients, consider attending an orientation program at a local senior center to gain an understanding of some aspects of their lives.

SUGGESTED RESOURCES

Buckley S, Burdon M, Cheng H, et al: *Emergency Ophthalmology: A Symptom Based Guide to Diagnosis and Early Management.* London: BMJ Publishing Group; 1997.

Freeman PB, Jose RT: *The Art and Practice of Low Vision.* 2nd ed. Boston: Butterworth-Heinemann; 1997.

Movaghar M, Lawrence MG: *Eye Exam: The Essentials.* Clinical Skills videotape. San Francisco: American Academy of Ophthalmology; 2001.

Low Vision [brochure]. San Francisco: American Academy of Ophthalmology; 1993.

Stein HA, Slatt BJ, Stein RM: *The Ophthalmic Assistant: A Guide for Ophthalmic Medical Personnel.* 7th ed. St Louis: Mosby; 2000.

Wright KW, Spiegel PH: *The Requisites in Ophthalmology: Pediatric Ophthalmology and Strabismus.* St Louis: Mosby; 1999.

11 Basics of Ophthalmic Pharmacology

Pharmacology is the term given to the study of the medicinal use and actions of drugs. Also called *medications,* drugs play an important role in most medical practices. In the ophthalmology office, medications are used chiefly to diagnose and treat diseases and to test for normal eye functions. As part of their duties, beginning ophthalmic medical assistants may call in the doctor's prescription for a specific medication to the pharmacy and may record drug information on the patient's history chart. As they become more familiar with medications used to treat eye disorders, assistants may administer certain kinds of drugs on instruction of the doctor. The experienced assistant, especially one who assists in surgical procedures, may need to set out certain types of medications for the doctor to use during certain procedures. To carry out these responsibilities, assistants should have a basic understanding of drug actions, patient reactions to these agents, and the general types and uses of pharmaceuticals in the ophthalmology practice. In addition, assistants must know how and when to administer medications. Any assistant who administers drugs should also be able to recognize the symptoms of allergic reactions, as well as when such reactions require treatment and how to summon help.

This chapter provides an overview of drug delivery systems and describes the procedures for administering eyedrops and ointments to patients. The chapter also discusses the types, actions, and functions of medications commonly used in the ophthalmology office, with an emphasis on their side effects and allergic reactions and, most important, the first aid procedures required for adverse drug reactions. Throughout the chapter, brand names of drugs are mentioned (in parentheses following the generic names) only for the purpose of familiarizing you with some of the names you will encounter in the office.

DELIVERY SYSTEMS OF DRUGS

Patients receive ophthalmic drugs by three principal methods (Figure 11.1):

1. **Topical**, by which drugs are applied directly to the surface of the eye or surrounding skin
2. **Injectable**, by which drugs are injected with a hypodermic needle into or around the eye or into another part of the body
3. **Oral**, by which drugs are taken by mouth

Topical Systems

Topical drugs include liquid drops in the form of solutions or suspensions, ointments, and special wafers called *inserts* for use on the surface of the eye or eyelids. Topical drug application is the most common type used in the ophthalmologist's office. These agents work well in a wide variety of tests and treatments involving the external and anterior eye structures. Ophthalmic medical assistants often apply topical drugs to patients undergoing eye tests.

Solutions

A drug in **solution** is completely dissolved in an inert liquid called the **vehicle**, such as sterile salt water. Because the normal eye is **hydrophobic** (resists water), a topical solution may also contain a chemical to overcome this natural resistance. The solution may also include a preservative ingredient to prevent bacteria or other organisms from growing during storage. Occasionally, the preservative agent can irritate the eyes of some patients, causing redness, tearing, or pain.

Solutions are used frequently in ophthalmologic practice because they are easy to apply as drops and do not interfere with vision, except, of course, for those drugs that alter vision as part of their desired action, such as medications used to dilate pupils. A prominent disadvantage of solutions is that the drops do not remain in contact with the surface of the eye for long; like tears, the medicinal drops drain through the lacrimal system into the nose and throat. Because solutions drain out of the eye, more frequent application may be required if they are used as a treatment. Solutions also may cause effects in other parts of the body.

FIGURE 11.1

Ophthalmic medications are available in a variety of formulations, including topical drops and ointments, injectable solutions, and oral tablets and liquids.

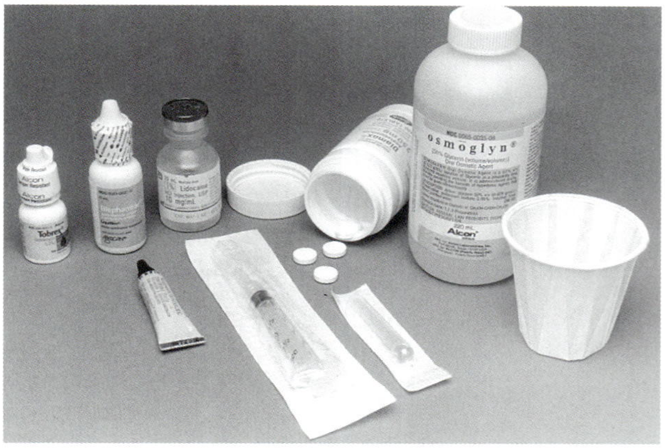

Suspensions

Suspensions are liquid vehicles in which particles of the drug are "suspended." Like solutions, suspensions may contain a preservative ingredient to inhibit the growth of bacteria and other unwanted organisms during storage. Suspensions are also easy to apply as drops and do not interfere with vision unless that is the desired action of the drug. Disadvantages of suspensions are that, like solutions, they do not remain in contact with the eye surface for long and that particles may settle out in the container during storage. If the active drug falls to the bottom of the bottle, it will not be delivered in an adequate amount unless the user shakes the container vigorously before each application. The ophthalmic medical assistant should check each container of medication before use in case it requires this procedure (some labels specify "Shake well before using").

Ointments and Gels

In the form of an **ointment** or **gel**, the drug is dissolved or suspended in an oily or greasy vehicle. The chief advantage of an ointment or gel is that the drug remains in contact with the eye or lid longer than when in liquid solution or in liquid suspension. The greasy character makes the drug less likely to wash away with tears—a useful property in patients with excessive tearing or in crying children. However, ointments and gels may blur vision due to their inherent greasiness (although this effect can be rendered irrelevant by application at bedtime), and they can be difficult to apply correctly.

Inserts

Inserts are drug-containing wafer-like forms that are placed on the conjunctiva, usually under the upper or lower eyelid. Because of their matrix structure, inserts can release medication into the eye slowly. Some inserts can release medications up to a week before requiring replacement. Other inserts are soluble and dissolve over a period of several hours to a day. Soluble drug inserts are a novel drug delivery system that is clinically available but is not in common use.

Advantages of drug inserts include infrequent application (because the wafer delivers a steady, even amount of drug) and a high degree of efficient drug use, coupled with a reduced chance of drug toxicity. Present disadvantages of this type of drug delivery system are that it is expensive; may be difficult to insert, tolerate, or remove; and can become dislodged without the patient realizing it.

Injections

With injections, the drug in solution is introduced into a part of the body by a needle. In ophthalmology, drug injections primarily serve as a means of applying treatment, but they can also be used in some testing or diagnostic procedures. Injections are usually given by a registered nurse or medical doctor.

Four types of injections are available in the practice of ophthalmology:

1. Into the eye (such as intravitreal) or around the eye (periocular, retrobulbar, or subconjunctival)
2. Into a vein (intravenous)
3. Into a muscle (intramuscular)
4. Under the skin (subcutaneous)

The intravenous, intramuscular, and subcutaneous injections are classified as **systemic drug delivery** because the active drug travels through the body's circulatory system before actually reaching the eye.

Oral Systems

Drugs taken orally (by mouth) include tablets, capsules, and liquids. Oral drug intake belongs to the systemic drug delivery category because, as with certain types of injections, the active agent must travel through one or more other body systems before reaching the eye. The practice of ophthalmology uses few oral drugs. However, for patients with certain conditions, such as glaucoma, who cannot tolerate topical agents or whose disorder is not adequately controlled by them, oral drugs fill an important medical need.

ADMINISTRATION OF TOPICAL DRUGS

Many topical ophthalmic drugs are available as a solution, a suspension, or an ointment. The ophthalmic medical assistant commonly aids the ophthalmologist by instilling eyedrops or applying ointments to patients in the office. The box "Administering Eyedrops and Ointments" on pages 174–175 presents step-by-step instructions for this important procedure.

PURPOSES AND ACTIONS OF DRUGS

Ophthalmic drugs may be used as a part of tests to diagnose eye disorders, as a principal treatment of eye conditions, or as an adjunct to surgical eye treatment. In addition to their desired action for each use, drugs of all kinds have certain side effects, some of which can be harmful. Because ophthalmic medical assistants often apply topical drugs or assist in ordering or setting up medications for the doctor to administer, they need to be familiar with the most common types of drugs used in ophthalmic practice and their general uses and actions.

Diagnostic Medications

Medications used to diagnose eye conditions include mydriatics, cycloplegics, dyes, and anesthetics. Most of these are available as topical solutions or suspensions, and some are prepared as ointments. Some of these drugs also produce effects that make them additionally useful in treating certain eye disorders.

Mydriatics

The act of dilating the pupil is called **mydriasis**. Thus, mydriatic drugs cause the pupil to dilate, usually by stimulating the iris dilator muscle. Mydriatic drops are used mainly to facilitate examination of the fundus. During this examination, the more fully dilated pupil allows a greater area of the fundus to be seen with the ophthalmoscope. Occasionally mydriatics may be used to improve the vision of patients with cataracts or

ADMINISTERING EYEDROPS AND OINTMENTS

Preliminaries

1. Have the patient sit or lie down.
2. Wash your hands thoroughly.
3. Check the physician's instructions—what medication and which eye?
4. Select the correct medication and check the expiration date. *Always read the label.* Many ophthalmic medication bottles look alike.
5. If the medication to be used is a suspension, shake the container well to ensure the drug is distributed consistently throughout the liquid.
6. To maintain sterility of the bottle contents, do not allow the inside edge of the bottle cap to contact any surface or object other than the bottle. Avoid touching the bottle tip to the lids, lashes, or surface of the eye.

Instilling Eyedrops

Improperly instilled eyedrops do not reach the eye. The following technique helps ensure optimal drug delivery.

1. Have the patient recline or tilt the head far back. If a patient has difficulty bending the neck back, have him or her recline in the exam chair.
2. Ask the patient to look up, with both eyes open.
3. Use the little finger or ring finger of the hand holding the bottle to gently pull down the skin over the cheekbone, pulling the lower lid down and out. This motion exposes the conjunctival cul-de-sac, creating a cup to catch the drops.
4. Squeeze the bottle gently to expel a drop of medication. Try to direct the drop toward the cul-de-sac, not toward the sensitive surface of the cornea (Figure A).
5. Instruct the patient to close both eyes gently. Use your index finger to apply light pressure over the lacrimal sac for 15–30 seconds. (Figure B). These actions help prevent systemic absorption by reducing the amount of the drug that drains into the lacrimal system, nose, and throat.
6. Wipe any excess drops from the patient's lids with a clean tissue.
7. Record the following information in the patient's chart:
   a. Medication name and strength
   b. Time administered
   c. Which eye received the medication

Applying Ointments

Perform steps 1 through 6 of the section "Preliminaries" earlier in this box. Then continue with steps 1 through 5 below.

1. If the tube of ointment has been opened prior to this use, express 1 inch of ointment onto a fresh cotton ball, gauze, or tissue and discard it.
2. Squeezing the tube lightly and with even pressure, apply the ointment along the conjunctival surface of the lower lid, moving from the inner to the outer canthus (Figure C). Usually ½ to 1 inch of ointment is enough. Avoid touching the tip of the tube to the eye, eyelashes, or skin to prevent contamination of the ointment tube. With a twisting motion, detach the ointment from the tip of the container.
3. Instruct the patient to close the eyes gently.
4. Wipe any excess ointment from the skin with a fresh cotton ball, gauze, or tissue; then discard it properly.
5. Record the application of ointment in the patient's chart, as described in step 7 under "Instilling Eyedrops" above.

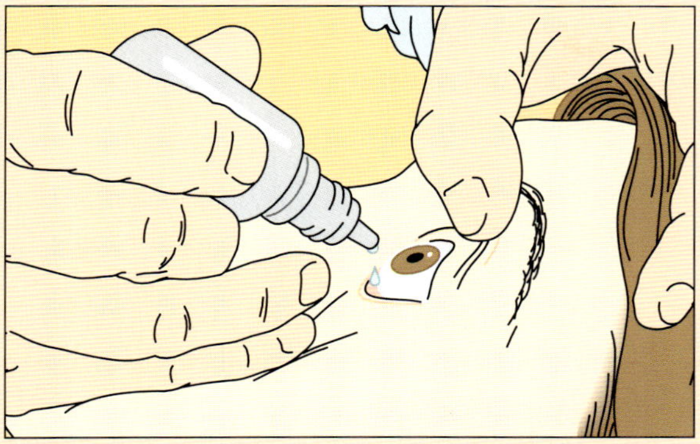

Figure A

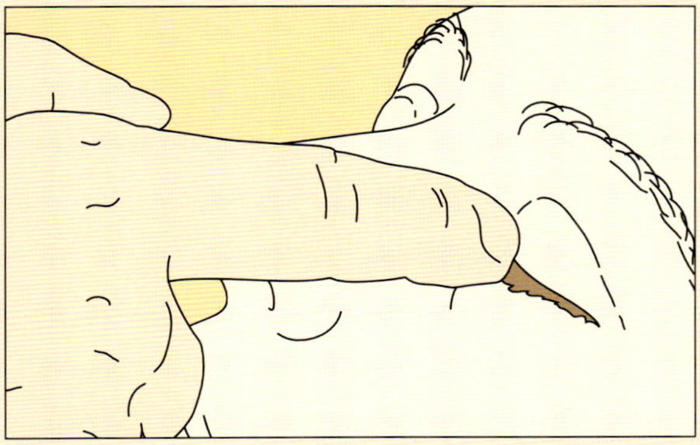

Figure B

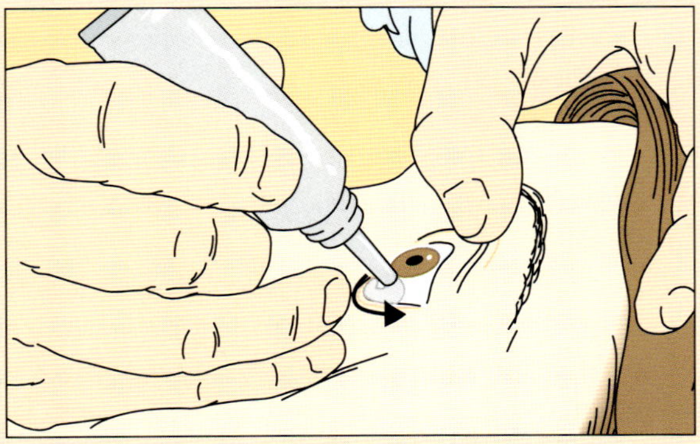

Figure C

other media opacities, but they are usually used to diagnose eye conditions.

Side effects associated with mydriatics include slight stinging on administration, headache, increased blood pressure, photophobia, and (very rarely) death. Because these agents open the pupil, mydriatics may stimulate an attack of angle-closure glaucoma in patients with a narrow anterior chamber angle. The ophthalmologist should check the patient's anterior chamber angle before ordering the use of a mydriatic drug. The most commonly used mydriatic is phenylephrine 2.5% (Neosynephrine, Mydfrin).

Cycloplegics

The term applied to the ability of a drug to paralyze the ciliary muscle temporarily is **cycloplegia**. Cycloplegic drugs essentially paralyze the iris sphincter muscle, causing dilation of the pupil. These agents also limit or prevent accommodation by paralyzing the ciliary muscle, which controls the ability of the lens to expand and contract. Cycloplegic agents differ from mydriatics in that cycloplegics both dilate the pupil and paralyze accommodation, whereas mydriatics only dilate the pupil.

The principal uses of cycloplegics include

- Performing a refraction that requires an absence of accommodation (Cycloplegic refraction is especially important in children, who have a strong accommodation mechanism that frequently interferes with accurate refraction without cycloplegia.)
- Conducting a fundus examination
- Treating uveitis (inflammation of the uveal tract) in some patients
- Treating intraocular inflammation that occurs after surgery

All cycloplegic drugs may sting slightly when administered to the eye. Another important reaction to cycloplegic medication is blurred vision or difficulty seeing at near due to paralysis of accommodation. This altered vision may last from a few hours to days, depending on the type and strength of the drug used. Other major side effects associated with cycloplegics include sensitivity to light, dry mouth, fever, rapid pulse, hallucinations, disorientation, bizarre behavior, and angle-closure glaucoma in patients with a narrow anterior chamber angle.

Cycloplegic drugs may be categorized by the duration of their action. Short-acting compounds are chosen for refraction and retinal examination because their side effects of blurred vision and paralyzed accommodation decrease soon after application. The most common short-acting cycloplegic compounds used in ophthalmology are

- tropicamide 0.5% and 1.0% (Mydriacyl)
- cyclopentolate 1.0% and 2.0% (Cyclogyl)

In children, cyclopentolate is used to obtain an accurate, objective measurement of the eye's refractive error.

Long-acting compounds, which are used for refraction and treatment of uveitis, include

- homatropine 2.0% and 5.0%
- atropine 0.5% and 1.0% (to refract children)
- scopolamine 0.25% (Hyoscine)

Because the bottles of most cycloplegic agents look alike (that is, many have red tops), it is *crucial* that the assistant check the label of the bottle before using, to be sure the correct agent will be instilled.

Dyes

Dyes temporarily stain cells or systems within the eye to outline or highlight defects in their structure or function. Ophthalmologists employ topical dyes in clinical practice chiefly to evaluate the ocular surface. Topical dyes also are used in applanation tonometry and contact lens fitting. Dyes administered by injection may be used to evaluate retinal conditions.

The most common dyes used in ophthalmology are fluorescein, which has fluorescent properties, and rose bengal, a red dye. Both are available for topical use as solutions or as paper strips impregnated with the dye, and both are available under numerous brand names. Fluorescein additionally is available as a solution for injection. Rose bengal stains and highlights degenerating corneal and conjunctival cells, and so is used to test for and diagnose this condition. Fluorescein similarly stains cells, but has other, more complex uses.

For topical testing and diagnostic use, the examiner applies fluorescein drops or a fluorescein-impregnated strip to the eye and exposes the eye to a special cobalt-blue light. Under this lighting condition, the dye fluoresces a bright yellow-green color. In the normal eye, only the tear layer fluoresces, a characteristic that makes the dye useful for applanation tonometry and contact lens fitting. In an abnormal eye, fluorescein can highlight defects in the tear film. It also stains defective or absent corneal epithelium, allowing the doctor to observe and identify corneal epithelial abrasions, infections, and other defects.

When administered intravenously by a doctor or registered nurse, fluorescein courses through the bloodstream to reach the eye. Once there and exposed to cobalt-blue light, the dye highlights retinal structures, especially blood vessels. The doctor may use an ophthalmoscope to observe highlighted defects in the retinal vessels. Fluorescein angiography, a diagnostic photographic procedure described in Chapter 6, "Adjunctive Tests and Procedures," also requires intravenous injection of fluorescein. Used in this way, fluorescein injection is an important adjunct to diagnosing conditions affecting the retinal vessels, such as diabetic retinopathy. Fluorescein given by injection may cause some patients to experience nausea or, rarely, an allergic reaction, although topically applied fluorescein and rose bengal rarely do.

Anesthetics

An **anesthetic** drug causes a temporary deadening of a nerve, which results in loss of feeling in the surrounding tissue and, in some circumstances, paralysis of the affected muscles. Anesthetics used in ophthalmology may be applied as a topical solution or injected. These drugs commonly affect only the eye receiving the medication. Most ophthalmic anesthetics act within a minute or so and have an effect lasting from 10 to 20 minutes for topical anesthetics and hours for some injected types.

Topical anesthetics are most often used to prevent discomfort during diagnostic procedures such as tonometry, gonioscopy, ultrasonography, and other examinations that involve touching the surface of the eye. These agents are also used in cataract surgery and other therapeutic procedures, such as removal of foreign bodies from the eye and sutures from the cornea. On extremely rare occasions, a topical anesthetic may be used to alleviate pain for the few minutes required to diagnose or treat a painful condition. Injectable anesthetics, however, are used more often to perform minor surgery, such as an eyelid procedure and major eye surgery. Although these ophthalmic anesthetics are injected, they still produce only local anesthetic effects; nevertheless, systemic toxicity can occur.

Anesthetics can produce an allergic reaction in a sensitive individual. Topical anesthetics become toxic to the cornea if in contact with the eye for long periods or if used often. They delay the resurfacing of the cornea by the corneal epithelium, which inhibits healing, and they can disrupt the normal stromal architecture, which can cause permanent clouding of the cornea. For these reasons, anesthetics are not used as a treatment except to alleviate pain for a few minutes until definitive therapy can be started.

The ophthalmic medical assistant should caution the patient receiving an ophthalmic anesthetic not to rub the eyes, because the numbed eye could be easily scratched without the patient being aware of it until the anesthesia wears off. Never give a patient a topical anesthetic for home use or use one yourself; blindness could result.

Commonly used topical ophthalmic anesthetics include

- proparacaine 0.5% (Ophthaine, Ophthetic, Alcaine)
- tetracaine 0.5% (Anacel, Pontocaine)
- lidocaine 1.0% to 5.0% (Xylocaine)
- benoxinate plus fluorescein (Fluress)
- proparacaine plus fluorescein (Fluoracaine)

Therapeutic Medications

Medications used to treat certain eye conditions have very specific actions for each individual disorder. Such therapeutic medications are generally prescribed by the doctor for patients to administer themselves. Occasionally, ophthalmic medical assistants may be asked by the physician to either administer such medications to patients or teach patients how to administer the medication to themselves. This class of medications includes miotics and other glaucoma treatments, antimicrobials, antiallergic and anti-inflammatory agents, decongestants, and lubricants.

Miotics

Miotics cause the iris sphincter muscle to contract, producing miosis (pupillary constriction), which leads to a reduction in the light entering the eye. One effect of a small pupil is to increase the patient's depth of field, which may improve vision in a patient with an uncorrected or poorly corrected refractive error. Miotic agents also cause contraction of the ciliary body muscle, which results in increased accommodation and opening of the trabecular drainage system, allowing an increase in aqueous outflow.

Miotics serve chiefly as topical treatment of glaucoma by lowering intraocular pressure and improving the drainage of the aqueous humor through the trabecular meshwork. In addition, certain miotic drugs may occasionally be used to treat accommodative strabismus. Often they are used inside the eye as part of cataract surgery.

Miotics are available for topical application in the form of solutions, gels, and inserts. The major side effects of this class of pharmaceuticals include brow ache, myopia, tearing, cataract, and retinal detachment. With the most potent agents, sweating, salivation, abdominal cramps, and diarrhea can occur. The principal miotic agents used in ophthalmology today are

- pilocarpine
- carbachol
- physostigmine
- echothiophate

These drugs are available in a variety of concentrations and under many brand names.

Other Glaucoma Medications

In addition to miotics, many other medications exist to treat glaucoma, all of which aim to reduce intraocular pressure, although by diverse mechanisms of action. Some glaucoma agents open the outflow pathways of the aqueous humor, others decrease the production of the aqueous humor, and still others work through a combination of both effects. Side effects of glaucoma medications vary with the type and action of the specific drug. These effects can range from an allergic reaction to blurred vision, increased or decreased blood pressure, and emotional or psychological effects.

The major glaucoma medications can be subdivided into categories based on the part of the nervous system or other body system they affect:

1. Adrenergic-blocking agents
   - timolol (Timoptic, Betimol)
   - betaxolol (Betoptic)
   - levobunolol (Betagan)
   - metipranolol (Optipranolol)
   - carteolol (Ocupress)

2. Adrenergic-stimulating agents
   - epinephrine (Eppy, Epinal, Epiphrin, Epitrate)
   - dipivefrin (Propine)
3. Carbonic anhydrase inhibitors: both oral and topical forms
   - acetazolamide (Diamox)
   - brinzolamide (Azopt)
   - methazolamide (Neptazane)
   - dorzolamide (Trusopt)
4. Alpha agonists
   - apraclonidine (Iopidine)
   - brimonidine (Alphagan)
5. Prostaglandin analogs
   - bimatoprost (Lumigan)
   - latanoprost (Xalatan)
   - travoprost (Travatan)
6. Hyperosmotics: oral formulations
   - glycerine (Glyrol)
   - ethyl alcohol
   - isosorbide (Isomotic)
7. Hyperosmotics: injectable formulation
   - mannitol (Osmitrol)

Antimicrobials

Antimicrobials comprise a large variety of agents, including **antibiotics** to treat bacterial infections, **antivirals** for viral infections, and **antifungals** for fungal infections. The ophthalmologist has a great many choices among each type of antimicrobial medication for treatment of a specific eye condition. The side effects of many antimicrobial products are numerous and complex and often influence the doctor's selection of a specific drug. Adverse reactions to antimicrobials include hypersensitivity to the particular drug, digestive system upset, and toxicity to other body systems. First and foremost, however, the doctor chooses an antimicrobial drug based on its ability to counter the specific microbial organism. The ophthalmic medical assistant should become familiar with this broad category of drugs over time by asking questions and reading the package insert that accompanies every drug.

Antibiotics Antibiotics kill or inhibit the growth of bacteria. For ophthalmic use, these drugs exist as topical drops or ointments to treat superficial infections such as blepharitis, bacterial conjunctivitis, and corneal ulcers. Antibiotic solutions can be injected around the eye for severe infections caused by bacterial corneal ulcers or by endophthalmitis. When taken orally or injected systemically, antibiotics serve to treat more serious ophthalmic conditions such as severe endophthalmitis, orbital infections (including orbital cellulitis), and, occasionally, acute dacryocystitis.

Antibiotics in common use in ophthalmology exist in a myriad of formulations and under scores of brand names. An individual antibiotic can be used alone or with one or more other antibiotics. The following are the most common antibiotics an ophthalmic medical assistant would encounter in daily practice:

- bacitracin
- neomycin
- tobramycin
- gentamicin
- sulfonamides
- chloramphenicol
- fluoroquinolones
- fluorinated carboxyquinolone
- ofloxacin
- ciprofloxacin

With the ever-increasing number of new antibiotics available, the ophthalmologist has the option of using combination drugs for treating ocular diseases, and the ophthalmic medical assistant should become familiar with these. These combinations include those composed of different types of antibiotics and those composed of mixtures of antibiotics and corticosteroid preparations. The following are some of the combination drugs commonly used in ophthalmology:

1. Antibiotic combinations
   - neomycin-polymyxin B-gramicidin
   - trimethoprim-polymyxin B
   - polymyxin B-bacitracin
   - polymyxin B-neomycin
2. Antibiotic/steroid combinations
   - neomycin-dexamethasone
   - neomycin-polymyxin B-dexamethasone
   - tobramycin-dexamethasone
   - gentamicin-prednisolone
   - sulfacetamide-prednisolone

- neomycin-polymyxin B-hydrocortisone
- chloramphenicol-polymyxin B-hydrocortisone

Antivirals These agents inhibit the ability of the virus to reproduce itself. Antiviral drugs are used to treat the more serious virus-caused ophthalmic conditions such as the herpes simplex and herpes zoster infections. Some of the antiviral drugs in use in ophthalmology include

- idoxuridine (Herplex)
- vidarabine (Vira-A)
- trifluorothymidine (Viroptic)
- acyclovir (Zovirax)
- valacyclovir hydrochloride (Valtrex)

Antifungals These drugs kill fungi and are therefore used to treat a variety of external ocular fungal infections, such as fungal blepharitis, keratitis, and conjunctivitis, and some internal fungal conditions as well. Antifungals commonly used in ophthalmologic practice include

- nystatin
- amphotericin (extremely toxic)
- pimaricin
- miconazole
- ketoconazole

Antiallergic and Anti-Inflammatory Agents

Corticosteroids are the chief drugs used to treat allergic reactions and inflammations. Corticosteroids, also called simply *steroids*, are hormones derived from the body's adrenal gland or made synthetically. Most corticosteroids are modifications of the hormone cortisone. In the treatment of eye disorders, these hormonal agents act by reducing inflammation and can dramatically decrease swelling, redness, and scarring. Most corticosteroids are applied topically in drop or ointment form to treat conditions involving the eyelid or the anterior segment of the eye. Systemic steroid drugs taken orally are used as therapy for disorders of the posterior segment as well as for acute or severe allergic reactions around the eye or anywhere in the body.

Corticosteroids must be used and administered carefully because of their potentially harmful side effects. The ophthalmic medical assistant should check the patient's medical record for diseases such as hypertension, peptic ulcer, diabetes, and tuberculosis, all of which could worsen through the use of systemic corticosteroids. Side effects of steroid use from topical application can occur, although most of these happen only after weeks to months of treatment. These side effects include glaucoma, bacterial or viral infection, overgrowth of fungi, slower healing, and cataract.

Steroids are sometimes injected around the eye to treat severe inflammation. Side effects are similar to those from topical use. If taken orally for a long period of time, corticosteroids can retard wound healing, cause swelling of the face and eyelids, promote cataract and glaucoma, and lower a patient's resistance to infection.

Topical steroids commonly used in ophthalmology include

- hydrocortisone acetate suspension 0.5% and 2.5%
- hydrocortisone acetate ointment 1.5%
- cortisone acetate suspension 0.5% and 1.5%
- dexamethasone phosphate 0.1% and ointment 0.5%
- prednisolone acetate 0.12% and 1.0% and phosphate 0.5%
- betamethasone solution 0.5%
- fluoromethodone 0.1% and 1.0%
- rimexolone 1.0%
- loteprednol etabonate 0.2% and 0.5%

Commonly used systemic corticosteroids and their tablet doses include

- hydrocortisone 20 mg
- cortisone acetate 25 mg
- prednisone 5 mg
- prednisolone 5 mg
- triamcinolone 4 mg
- dexamethasone 0.75 mg
- betamethasone 0.5 mg

Nonsteroidal Anti-Inflammatory Drugs (NSAIDs)

Because of the severe, unpleasant side effects of corticosteroids, many new nonsteroidal anti-inflammatory medications have been introduced. These medications may be used in the treatment of ocular inflammatory processes and ocular allergies. Commonly used ocular NSAIDs include

- flurbiprofen (Ocufen)
- diclofenac (Voltaren)
- ketorolac tromethamine (Acular)

Decongestants

A **decongestant** acts by constricting the superficial blood vessels in the conjunctiva. Ophthalmologists may prescribe decongestants as a cosmetic aid to reduce the eye redness caused by smoke or smog or to soothe eyes fatigued from driving, reading, or close work. Although this effect is soothing and cosmetic, it does nothing to alleviate the cause of the redness. Side effects related to decongestants include allergy, angle-closure glaucoma (rarely), and rebound, which means the superficial blood vessels become even more congested than before the drug was taken.

Most decongestants used to treat ophthalmologic conditions are available without a doctor's prescription (also known as over-the-counter products), including such brand names as

- Visine
- Murine
- Clear Eyes
- Vasocon

Naphcon is a brand-name prescription decongestant.

Antihistamines

Topical ocular antihistamines provide rapid relief of itching, tearing, and swelling of the conjunctiva and eyelid associated with seasonal or allergic conjunctivitis. Available ocular antihistamines are

- levocabastine (Livostin)
- phenaramine maleate (Naphcon-A, Opcon-A, OcuHist), sold over the counter in combination with the decongestant naphazoline
- olopatadine (Patanol)

Mast Cell Stabilizers

These drugs are effective in reducing the itching, tearing, conjunctival injection, mucous secretion, and corneal complications of seasonal or vernal conjunctivitis. Available mast cell stabilizers include

- cromolyn sodium (Crolom, Opticrom)
- lodoxamide (Alomide)
- nedocromil sodium (Alocril)
- olopatadine (Patanol)
- pemirolast potassium (Alamast)

Lubricants

Lubricants help the patient to maintain an appropriate tear film balance or to keep the external eye moist. When used in solution or ointment form, lubricants protect the eye from dryness. The ophthalmologist prescribes these medications to treat or relieve dry eye conditions, such as keratoconjunctivitis sicca and other tear-deficiency conditions. Side effects of lubricants are allergy to or irritation from the preservative in these agents. Some of the newer lubricant products are preservative-free and thus can be used more frequently than those with preservatives. The lack of preservatives also makes them less likely to cause side effects.

The lubricants used often to treat ophthalmic conditions include numerous artificial tear solutions, most of them over-the-counter. Some common brand names of these products are

- Clerz
- AquaTears
- Tears Plus
- Refresh
- Hypotears
- Tears Naturale
- Celluvisc
- Aquasite
- Ocucoat
- Cellufresh
- Genteal
- Bion Tears

Other Pharmaceuticals

Many other kinds of pharmaceutical products are used as treatment of eye-related conditions and for test procedures. Ophthalmic irrigating solutions comprise a group of sterile solutions of saline and other chemicals intended for flushing the eye or for use during surgical procedures. Osmotics are chemical agents in solution form that, when applied to the eye, employ the process of osmosis to reduce corneal edema by drawing fluid out through the corneal epithelium. Examples of drugs that produce effects used in specialized ophthalmic testing procedures include solutions for diagnosing pupillary conditions and ointments that permit ultrasonic evaluation of the orbit. The ophthalmic medical assistant should become familiar with these agents by continued reading of the large variety of publications and by experience with the actual ophthalmic drugs used in the office or clinic.

Table 11.1 Abbreviations and Symbols Used in Prescriptions

Abbreviation or Symbol	***Meaning***
<	less than
>	greater than
ac	*(ante cibum)* before meals
bid	*(bis in die)* twice a day
dispi	dispense
g	gram
gt, gtt	*(gutta, guttae)* drop, drops
h	*(hora)* hour
hs	*(hora somni)* at bedtime
M *or* Mit	*(mitte)* send
mg	milligram
non rep	*(non repetatur)* do not repeat
OD	*(oculus dexter)* right eye
OS	*(oculus sinister)* left eye
OU	*(oculi uterque)* both eyes, considered separately
pc	*(post cibum)* after meals
po	*(per os)* by mouth, orally
prn	*(pro re nata)* as needed
qd	*(quaque die)* every day
qh	*(quaque hora)* every hour
qid	*(quater in die)* 4 times a day
ql	*(quantum libet)* as much as desired
qqh *or* q4h	*(quaque quarta hora)* every 4 hours
Rx	*(recipe)* prescription
S *or* Sig	*(signa)* label
Sol	solution
tid	*(ter in die)* 3 times a day
tsp	teaspoon
ung	*(unguentum)* ointment

INTERPRETATION OF A PRESCRIPTION

The ophthalmic medical assistant should know how to read the doctor's prescription for medication in order to call it in to the pharmacy when requested and to refer accurately to the medications listed in a patient's medical record. Table 11.1 presents some of the more common symbols and abbreviations (mostly of Latin words or phrases) used by doctors to write prescriptions. The ophthalmic medical assistant should become familiar with them.

FIGURE 11.2

A typical prescription for eye medication.

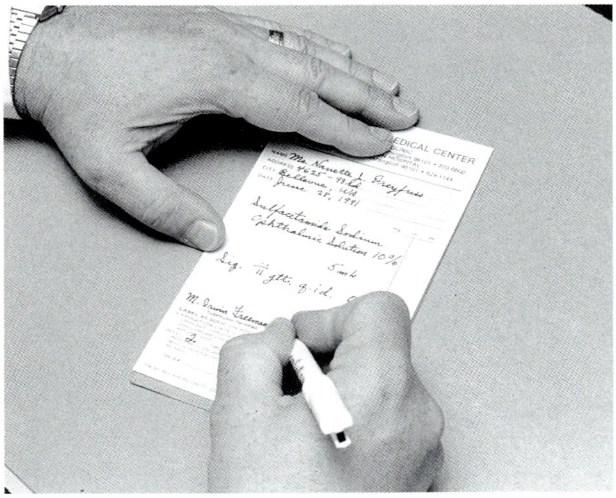

Figure 11.2 illustrates a sample prescription. On a pad printed with the doctor's name, the doctor may include the following information on the medical prescription:

- The patient's name and address, and the date of the prescription
- The name of the drug and its concentration or dose
- The amount of the drug to be given to the patient (the subscription), usually written beside the symbol "M" or "Mit" (for *mitte*, meaning send) or "dispi" (for dispense), which applies to the quantity of drug
- The directions to the pharmacist about what to type on the label of the drug, usually written beside the abbreviation "S" or "Sig," which comes from the Latin *signa* (meaning mark, and thus in English *label*)
- The signature of the doctor
- Sometimes an indication to the pharmacist that the prescription can be refilled; for example, "Repeat × 2"
- Sometimes an indication to the pharmacist that the name of the medication should be typed on the label
- Sometimes the doctor's medical license number and DEA (Drug Enforcement Administration) number, especially if the prescription is for a controlled substance such as a narcotic

GIVING FIRST AID

Tremors or Convulsions

1. Call for the ophthalmologist at once.
2. If the patient has tremors, make sure he is seated so that he won't fall and hurt himself. If the patient is having convulsions, help him lie on the floor, cushioning his head. Never insert anything into the mouth.
3. Loosen any tight clothing.

Respiratory Emergency

1. Call for the ophthalmologist if a patient complains of breathing difficulty.
2. If the patient stops breathing altogether, call for the ophthalmologist and initiate cardiopulmonary resuscitation (CPR).

Prescriptions for some controlled drugs cannot be phoned into the pharmacy by the ophthalmic medical assistant. Additionally, special care should be taken in the office to keep prescription pads in a safe place where they cannot be taken or used by unauthorized individuals.

FIRST AID FOR ACUTE DRUG REACTIONS

Ophthalmic medical assistants should become familiar with the office emergency first aid procedure before assisting in the use of or administering ophthalmic medications. You should ask your doctor or a senior technician for any written procedures or guidelines to deal with such an event.

The ophthalmic medical assistant should be prepared to give general first aid if a patient suffers an acute drug reaction immediately or within a few minutes of receiving an ophthalmic drug. Acute drug reactions include fainting; tremors or convulsions, in which the patient shakes or writhes because the drug has overstimulated the central nervous system; and respiratory emergency, in which the patient complains of difficulty in breathing. Procedures for dealing with a patient who has fainted are given in Chapter 9, "Patient Interaction, Screening, and Emergencies." Instructions for handling tremors or convulsions and respiratory difficulty appear in the box "Giving First Aid."

Acute allergic reaction, one of the most serious drug reactions, requires immediate attention. Patients with such reactions develop an itching skin rash, difficulty in breathing, or a rapid, weak pulse right after receiving the drug. Because prompt medical treatment is needed, the only action for the ophthalmic medical assistant to take in this situation is to call for the ophthalmologist immediately. The doctor may need to give the patient adrenaline or corticosteroid by injection, administer oxygen, or, in severe cases of swelling in the patient's larynx, perform a tracheotomy (surgical cutting of the windpipe).

The ophthalmic medical assistant should know where the following first aid materials are kept and how to make them immediately available to the doctor for an acute allergic reaction:

- oxygen
- epinephrine (injectable)
- diazepam (Valium)
- intravenous cortisone
- smelling salts or spirits of ammonia
- syringes and needles

The assistant should also know where to find materials for flushing an eye and the appropriate procedures for ocular and systemic emergencies in the office (see Chapter 9, "Patient Interaction, Screening, and Emergencies").

REVIEW QUESTIONS

1. List the three principal delivery systems for ophthalmic medications.
2. Name the four principal forms of topical ophthalmic medications.
3. Name three possible types of eye irritations caused by preservatives used in eyedrops.
4. What is the major advantage of drugs dissolved or suspended in ointments or gels over eyedrops?
5. Which eye care professionals usually inject ophthalmic drugs?
6. Place the following steps for instilling eyedrops or applying ointments in the proper order.
   a. Check the doctor's instructions.
   b. Expose the lower conjunctival cul-de-sac.
   c. Wash your hands thoroughly.
   d. Instruct the patient to open the eyes and look up.
   e. Apply light pressure to the lacrimal sac with the index finger.
7. Which of the following actions is most important in ensuring adequate drug delivery of an ophthalmic suspension?
   a. Shake the bottle to distribute the drug thoroughly.
   b. Wash your hands thoroughly.
   c. Gently wipe the tip of the applicator with a sterile cotton ball.
   d. Press the patient's lacrimal sac.
   e. Express a small amount onto a cotton ball.
8. Drugs that paralyze the iris sphincter muscle and dilate the pupil are called
   a. Anesthetics
   b. Short-acting agents
   c. Corticosteroids
   d. Cycloplegics
   e. Miotics
9. Mydriatic agents are used to
   a. Dilate the pupil
   b. Paralyze the iris sphincter muscle
   c. Treat inflammation
   c. Treat accommodation problems
   e. Treat infections
10. Fluorescein and rose bengal aid in
   a. Deadening nerves
   b. Diagnosing certain corneal problems

c. Treating viral infections

d. Inhibiting bacterial growth

e. Treating angle-closure glaucoma

11. Which three kinds of organisms that cause infection do antimicrobials inhibit or kill?

a. Fungi, cysts, and bacteria

b. Bacteria, hormones, and viruses

c. Bacteria, viruses, and osmotics

d. Bacteria, viruses, and fungi

e. Bacteria, microorganisms, and fungi

12. If the doctor's prescription indicates to "apply eyedrops tid," you would advise the patient that this means

a. Use the drops in the morning

b. Use the drops once a day

c. Use the drops three times a day

d. Use the entire prescription of drops before discarding the bottle

e. Use the drops as needed

13. Within a few minutes of applying anesthetic eyedrops, the patient complains of itching around the eye and difficulty breathing. Your best first action to take would be to

a. Loosen the patient's collar

b. Suspect an allergic reaction and call for the doctor immediately

c. Apply corticosteroid drops

d. Begin cardiopulmonary resuscitation (CPR)

e. Have the patient lie down

14. Which of the following best defines *fluoroquinolone*?

a. An antibiotic used to treat bacterial infections

b. An antifungal agent used to treat athlete's foot

c. A sunscreen used for UV protection

d. A medication used to treat migraine headaches

e. A corticosteroid agent used to treat inflammation

SUGGESTED ACTIVITIES

1. Discuss the use and dispensing of ophthalmic drugs with your ophthalmologist. Be thoroughly familiar with any guidelines or procedures for administering medication to patients.
2. Ask your ophthalmologist or a senior technician if you may observe the treatment or testing of patients that requires the instillation of eyedrops or ointments. Take notes and ask questions in a later discussion.
3. With your ophthalmologist or a senior technician supervising, practice instilling eyedrops and applying ointments on coworkers who have agreed to participate. Be sure to ask the doctor to choose a medication that is safe to use for this practice exercise.
4. Review with your ophthalmologist the procedure for the treatment of acute drug reactions. Ask the doctor to outline all the possibilities of what could go wrong and what would be your best immediate response to help the patient.
5. Collect the printed package inserts of the most common medications used in your doctor's practice. Read them thoroughly, paying special attention to the section on side effects or adverse reactions, and discuss any questions you may have with your ophthalmologist or a senior technician.

SUGGESTED RESOURCES

Bradford CA, ed: *Basic Ophthalmology for Medical Students and Primary Care Residents.* 7th ed. San Francisco: American Academy of Ophthalmology; 1999.

Cassin B: *Fundamentals for Ophthalmic Technical Personnel.* Philadelphia: WB Saunders Co; 1995; chap 4.

Physician's Desk Reference for Ophthalmology. Montvale, NJ: Medical Economics Data Production Co; updated annually.

Stein HA, Slatt BJ, Stein RM: *The Ophthalmic Assistant: A Guide for Ophthalmic Medical Personnel.* 7th ed. St Louis: Mosby; 2000.

12 Microorganisms and Infection Control

Microorganisms, or **microbes,** are organisms so small they are visible only with the aid of a microscope. Humans exist harmoniously with many microorganisms, but some can cause disease, including eye disease. Eye disease often starts when harmful microorganisms enter ocular tissues, either through trauma or by means of *contaminated* (microbe-carrying) instruments, hands, solutions, or medications. **Infection** is the invasion and multiplication of harmful microbes in the body tissues.

An important responsibility of the ophthalmic medical assistant is to prevent the transmission of disease-causing microorganisms from one patient to another. This responsibility is part of a program of sanitation and microbial control in the office referred to as **standard precautions.** The purpose of standard precautions is to reduce the opportunity for harmful microbes to flourish and threaten patients and medical personnel, who may be exposed to possibly infectious materials.

This chapter describes the kinds of microbes that can cause eye disease, and their means of transmission and routes of infection. Most important, it covers the techniques, such as standard precautions, disinfection, and sterilization, that are used to control the spread of microorganisms.

TYPES OF MICROORGANISMS

Although microorganisms exist in numerous forms, four groups are most commonly associated with eye disease:

1. Bacteria (singular: bacterium)
2. Viruses (singular: virus)
3. Fungi (singular: fungus), including yeasts
4. Protozoa (singular: protozoan)

Scientists usually classify microorganisms according to their size, structure, method of reproduction, or response to laboratory procedures such as *staining* (dyeing with special coloring agents and procedures). Like all organisms, microorganisms are given names that reflect their classification, with first a *genus* and then a *species* name. The genus name is sometimes abbreviated after the first usage. For example, a common intestinal bacterium with which you may be familiar is named *Escherichia coli* and abbreviated *E coli.*

Bacteria

Bacteria are simple, single-celled microorganisms that reproduce by splitting in two. Although they are widely dispersed in nature, some bacteria cannot live very long when exposed to sunlight and air. Others are relatively resistant and can survive for hours or days on dust particles in the air or on objects. Still other bacteria produce *spores,* a hardy, thick-skinned form that allows them to survive for months and even years until they encounter conditions suitable for growth. Most bacterial infections can be successfully treated with antibiotics.

Bacteria (and certain other microbes) can be classified by their reaction when exposed to dyes in a procedure called **Gram staining.** Knowing an organism's Gram-staining characteristics is useful in determining which antibiotic to select in treating an infection. In the Gram-staining procedure, a glass microscope slide that has been smeared with a microbial specimen is covered with a dye or dyes, which stain the normally colorless microorganisms. Bacteria that stain purple or blue are referred to as *Gram positive*; those that stain pink are referred to as *Gram negative* (Figure 12.1). So that you may familiarize yourself with the names of bacteria that you may see on patient charts and other medical documents, Table 12.1 lists types of bacteria most commonly associated with ocular infections and their Gram-stain characteristics.

For example, the Gram-positive bacterium *Staphylococcus aureus* is a frequent cause of blepharitis, conjunctivitis, and keratitis. Similarly, other *Staphylococcus* species are responsible for infections of the conjunctiva, cornea, lacrimal apparatus, and intraocular fluids. The Gram-negative bacterium *Neisseria gonorrhoeae* can also cause a hyperacute conjunctivitis; this is usually a serious infection (Figure 12.2A) because the bacteria can enter the eye.

Chlamydia trachomatis is responsible for a myriad of ocular infections. These include neonatal conjunctivitis (a conjunctivitis contracted by newborns from

FIGURE 12.1

Photomicrographs of Gram-stained bacteria. (A) Gram-positive *Staphylococcus aureus.* (B) Gram-negative *Neisseria gonorrhoeae.*

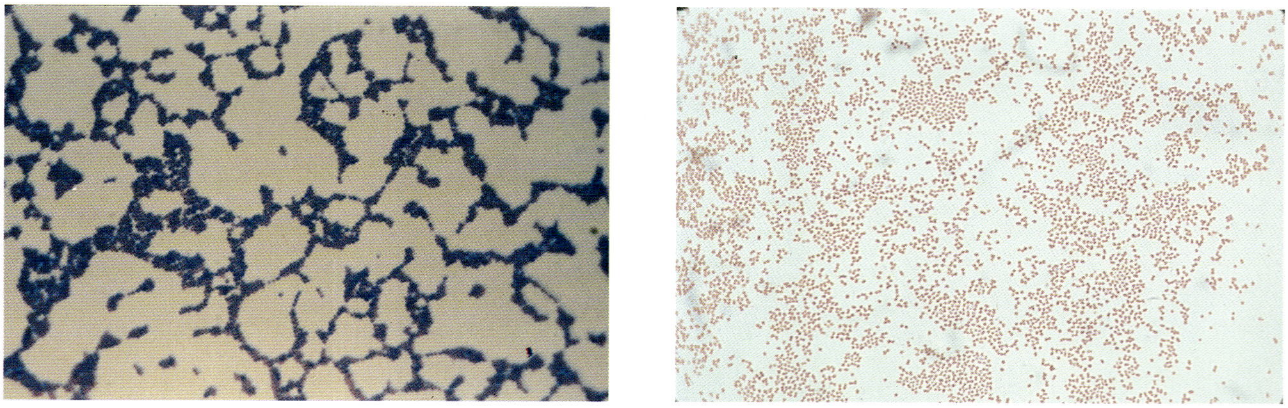

A B

TABLE 12.1 Bacteria Commonly Recovered From Ocular Infections

Gram Positive (G+)	***Gram Negative (G–)***
Actinomyces species	*Haemophilus influenzae*
Bacillus cereus	*Moraxella catarrhalis*
Corynebacterium species	*Moraxella lacunata*
Peptostreptococcus	*Neisseria gonorrhoeae*
Propionibacterium acnes	*Proteus mirabilis*
Staphylococcus aureus	*Pseudomonas aeruginosa*
Staphylococcus epidermidis	*Serratia marcescens*
Streptococcus pneumoniae	
Streptococcus pyogenes	
Streptococcus viridans group	

FIGURE 12.2

Bacterial conjunctivitis. (A) Hyperacute conjunctivitis due to invasion by *Neisseria gonorrhoeae*. (B) Neonatal chlamydial conjunctivitis.

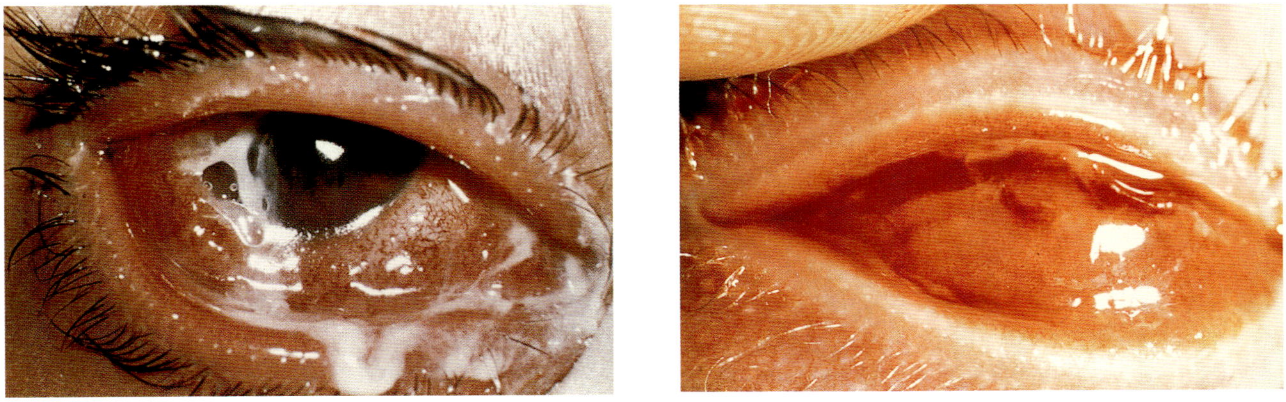

A B

an infected birth canal; Figure 12.2B), inclusion conjunctivitis, lymphogranuloma venereum (LGV), and trachoma, a chronic, scar-producing conjunctivitis. In the United States, trachoma is restricted to the southwestern region, but it remains the leading cause of preventable blindness in the Middle East, North Africa, and Southeast Asia.

Infection caused by *Pseudomonas aeruginosa* can be associated with contact lens overwear. Useful vision may be lost within 48 hours if this infection is not detected or treated properly. This organism is a common contaminant in eyedrops, cosmetics, and hot tubs. Certain other bacteria cause syphilis (*Treponema pallidum*) and Lyme disease (*Borrelia burgdorferi*), both of which can lead to ocular disorders. Infections with these organisms tend to be chronic, cause progressive damage, and involve the nervous system.

Viruses

Among the smallest microorganisms, viruses do not have a cellular structure and so can multiply only in living cells. Because of their unique makeup, viruses are not given genus and species names, but are

FIGURE 12.3

Herpes simplex virus type 1 and one result of its infection of the eye. (A) Photomicrograph of HSV-1. (B) Corneal ulcer resulting from HSV-1 infection. The ulcer has been stained pink with rose bengal dye. (Part A courtesy of John J. Cardamone, Jr/Biological Photo Service.)

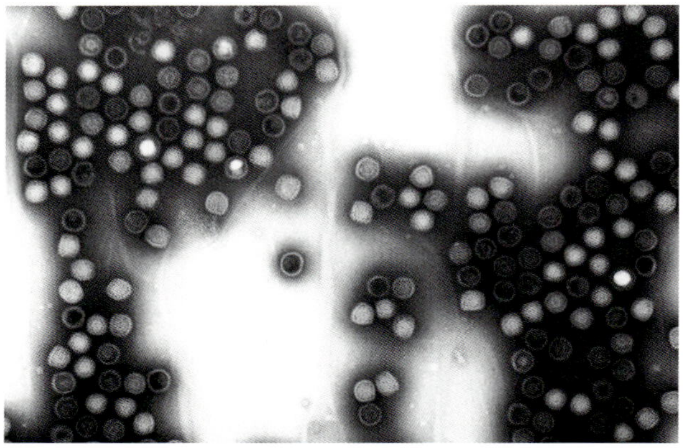

A

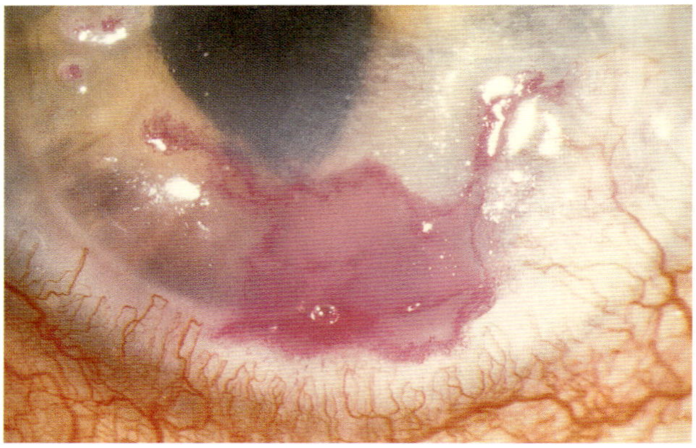

B

instead often named for the diseases they cause or the organisms they infect. Many viral infections are self-limited (this is, the disease they cause runs a definite, limited course), and treatment for these is mainly to alleviate symptoms, not to eradicate the organism. Systemic and topical antiviral drugs can effectively control some viral infections, but they may also be toxic (poisonous) with prolonged use. Viral infections cannot be controlled with antibiotics.

Members of the **herpesvirus** family include herpes simplex virus type 1 (HSV-1), herpes simplex virus type 2 (HSV-2), varicella-zoster virus (VZV), cytomegalovirus (CMV), and Epstein-Barr virus (EBV). These viruses are involved in more than 500,000 cases of ocular disease each year, including blepharoconjunctivitis, keratitis, uveitis, retinitis, and conjunctivitis. **Herpes simplex virus type 1**, which causes commonly seen "fever blisters" on the lips and mouth, is responsible for most of the lesions of the cornea and eyelids (Figure 12.3). **Herpes simplex virus type 2** (HSV-2) more commonly infects the genital region and is transmitted by sexual contact. Newborns exposed to HSV-2 during passage through an infected birth canal are at high risk for ocular infection.

Varicella-zoster virus (VZV) produces the common childhood disease chicken pox. Recovery from chicken pox usually leaves the person immune to recurrence, but VZV may reactivate in certain individuals, producing a painful skin condition called *zoster* or *shingles*. During these outbreaks, the eye can also become involved, resulting in a painful, severe, and sometimes blinding disease called *herpes zoster ophthalmicus* (see Figure B.10 in Appendix B). Oral and topical antiviral drugs are used to minimize inflammation of the eye and orbit. Patients may be treated for many months while the inflammatory reaction to this infection subsides.

CMV retinitis, an ocular infection due to cytomegalovirus, is commonly seen in patients infected with the human immunodeficiency virus (HIV), which causes AIDS (see Figure B.9 in Appendix B). Along with a low white blood cell count, this infection is often the first indication that a patient who has been HIV-positive has made the transition to AIDS.

HIV, which is a type of virus called a *retrovirus*, is indirectly responsible not only for CMV retinitis but also for several other serious infections of the eye. Ocular involvement occurs in 50% to 75% of HIV-infected patients. HIV has been isolated from tears as well as from conjunctival and corneal tissue. HIV may also be isolated from the contact lenses of infected patients. However, the U.S. government agency called the Centers for Disease Control and Prevention (CDC) says that the virus is not in sufficient quantity in these fluids to be considered an infection risk. The route by which HIV reaches the ocular surface tissues and tears remains unknown.

Infections from the *adenovirus* family are responsible for two distinct and common ophthalmic syndromes: epidemic keratoconjunctivitis (EKC) and pharyngoconjunctival fever (PCF), also known as "pink eye." EKC is a highly contagious disease that is spread by direct contact with contaminated medical personnel or instruments. Outbreaks are known to occur in ophthalmic offices and clinics, school locker rooms, and college dormitories. The PCF form of adenoviral conjunctivitis is also contagious, yet it is a milder form that can occur following a respiratory infection.

Fungi

Fungi are multicellular microorganisms with a more complex structure than that of bacteria. Fungi can be divided into two groups: **yeasts,** which produce creamy or pasty colonies, and **molds,** which produce woolly, fluffy, or powdery growth (Figure 12.4). The fuzzy growth seen on old bread is an example of a fungal mold colony.

Ocular fungal infections, especially those involving the cornea, usually are the result of direct trauma, such as a scratch from a tree twig, that introduces plant material or soil into the eye. Intraocular fungal infections can result as an extension of keratitis, from another infected source within the body, or from contaminated instruments or solutions. A common source of fungal eye infections is the *Candida albicans* species of yeast. The fungus called *Histoplasma capsulatum* causes ocular histoplasmosis, an intraocular (inside the eye) infection. Both topical and systemic antifungal medications are available to treat fungal infections.

Protozoa

Protozoa are relatively large and complex single-celled microorganisms found in fresh water, salt water, soil, plants, insects, and animals, including humans. For example, *Acanthamoeba* species flourish in soil, freshwater lakes, hot tubs, swimming pools, and homemade contact lens salt solutions (Figure 12.5). Because this organism can cause a painful infection of the cornea, contact lens wearers must be instructed in special precautions (see Chapter 14). This same type of corneal infection has also been associated with trauma that involves soil or water contaminated with these organisms.

In the eye, infection with the protozoan *Toxoplasma gondii,* called toxoplasmosis, causes inflammation of uveal and retinal structures. Toxoplasmosis is now one of the most common infections seen in patients with AIDS. Oral antibiotics and, occasionally, steroids are used to treat toxoplasmosis.

FIGURE 12.4

Fungi obtained from the cornea of a patient and grown in a laboratory. The left two rows of fluffy streaks are a mold; the right two rows of creamy streaks are a yeast.

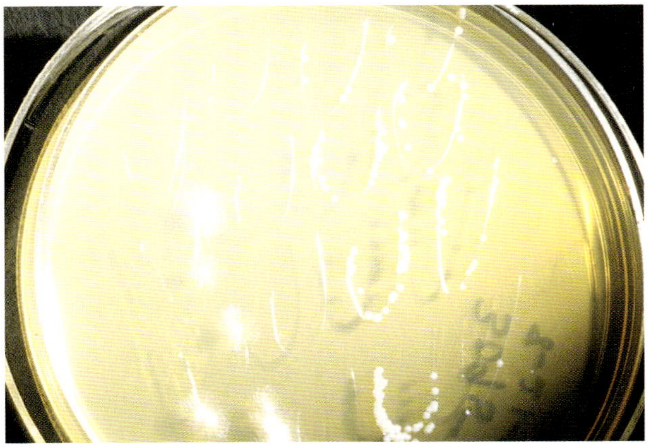

FIGURE 12.5

Photomicrograph of *Acanthamoeba,* the protozoan that causes *Acanthamoeba* keratitis. (Photo courtesy of William Mathers, MD, University of Iowa.)

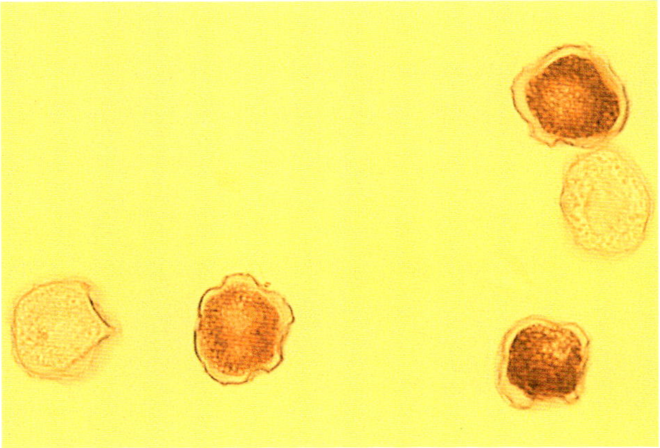

TRANSMISSION OF INFECTIOUS DISEASES

To produce infection, a microorganism must be available, and it must gain access to or cross the protective barriers of the invaded organism. Then it must overcome that organism's natural defense mechanisms and find conditions suitable for reproduction.

Although the external ocular structures, conjunctiva, and cornea are constantly challenged by harmful or potentially harmful microbes, infection rarely results. This is due in part to the eye's natural protective barriers. Protective barriers and mechanisms that help the eye resist infection include intact skin; eyelids and lashes; tears, which contain antibacterial substances; and the mucous layer of the conjunctiva and cornea, which traps and expels invading organisms. As long as the outer layers of the conjunctiva and cornea remain unbroken, they form a barrier against most microbial invasion. However, when the protective layers are broken, such as by trauma, surgery, or debilitating illness, infection can result.

Disease-causing microorganisms are transmitted from a **reservoir** (the animate or inanimate object that provides a microorganism the means for survival and opportunity for transmission) to a **host** (the animal or plant from which a microorganism gains nutrients and conditions necessary for survival and reproduction). The five principal means of infectious transmission are as follows:

1. Airborne droplets and particles containing infectious microbes
2. Direct contact with a contaminated person
3. Indirect contact with a contaminated person or inanimate object
4. Common vehicle, in which microbes are transmitted from a common, inanimate source to several people
5. Vector-borne transmission, which occurs through insects such as mosquitoes and flies (*vectors*).

Except for vector-borne transmission, which is unlikely to be encountered in most ophthalmology offices and clinics in the United States, these forms of transmission are discussed next.

Airborne Droplets and Particles

A person infected with certain disease-causing microbes who coughs or sneezes produces a cloud of water droplets containing millions of infectious organisms. When a susceptible individual inhales these airborne droplets, the microbes are brought directly to cells of the upper respiratory tract and can produce infection in the new host. The varicella-zoster virus that causes chicken pox and the bacterium that causes tuberculosis (*Mycobacterium tuberculosis*) can be spread in this way.

Direct-Contact Transmission

Direct-contact transmission is the direct transfer of an infectious agent from person to person through close physical contact. The fingers are an especially effective means of direct-contact transmission. Physicians or assistants who touch the infected eye of a patient or an infected lesion (such as a cold sore) on themselves can carry infectious microbes on their fingers for minutes, hours, or even longer, depending on the organism. Examining the eyes of another patient without first washing the hands provides the opportunity to transfer the infectious microbes from the fingers to the new patient.

Indirect-Contact Transmission

Indirect-contact transmission involves the transfer of microbes from one host to another via an inanimate object. For example, a tissue or handkerchief used by a person with a cold carries a high concentration of the cold virus, as do objects handled by the infected person shortly after using the handkerchief. Touching these contaminated objects can expose individuals to the virus if they then bring their own hands to their nose or mouth.

An important means of indirect-contact transmission the ophthalmic medical assistant may encounter is contaminated medical instruments, examination equipment, and materials. Door knobs, faucet handles, exam chairs, desk tops, and even paper products are also potential sources for microbial transmission by indirect contact. Indirect-contact transmission can also occur when the skin or eye is penetrated by wood or metal fragments, such as twigs, nails, and knives, which can be contaminated with disease-causing bacteria or fungi. In addition, contaminated eyedrops and other solutions may transmit infection by indirect contact.

Infectious microbes can reside for minutes, hours, or longer on instruments, needles, other sharp implements, swabs, and other reusable or disposable materials that have contacted an infected patient's blood or body fluid. Special care must be taken to decontaminate instruments as well as to clean or dispose of materials in such a way that those who next contact them will not be exposed to infectious or potentially infectious microbes.

Common-Vehicle Transmission

Common-vehicle transmission involves the transfer of infectious microbes from one reservoir to many people. For example, disease-causing organisms can contaminate and multiply in ocular medications, such as eyedrops, that have been improperly stored or handled. Each patient who then has the contaminated eyedrops instilled is exposed and may become infected. Because serious ocular infections can result from the administration of contaminated medications, special precautions for handling them are required in medical offices, clinics, and hospitals (see the box "Administering Eyedrops and Ointments" in Chapter 11, and the section "Aseptic Technique: Handling Sterile Medical Equipment" in this chapter).

INFECTION CONTROL PRECAUTIONS

Ophthalmic medical assistants, as well as ophthalmologists, work in close proximity to patients, some of whom have ocular infections or are carrying disease-causing microorganisms. Many patients have lowered resistance to infection because of systemic disease or age. All medical professionals, including ophthalmic medical assistants, must take the necessary steps to prevent transmission of infectious microbes to the patient, between patients, and to those who may later come in contact with materials contaminated by infectious material from patients. Assistants also have the obligation to protect themselves from infection. A well-designed and scrupulously followed program of microbial control in the medical office can greatly reduce the risk of infection between patients and health care workers.

The Centers for Disease Control and Prevention (CDC) has developed procedures designed to help health care workers protect themselves from various infections. These procedures are of two types, universal precautions and body substance isolation precautions. **Universal precautions** are designed to reduce the risk of transmission of diseases carried in the blood, and were primarily a response to the AIDS epidemic. Universal precautions require medical workers to assume that *all* human blood and body fluids containing visible blood may be infectious for HIV, hepatitis B virus (HBV), and other bloodborne *pathogens* (disease-causing microorganisms). The CDC does *not* consider normal (nonbloody) tears to be subject to bloodborne pathogen precautions. Such precautions include hand washing and the use of appropriate barriers (gloves, masks, goggles, etc) to prevent direct contact with potentially infected body fluids. Also, particular sterilization and disinfection measures and infectious waste disposal procedures are to be followed. See Appendix C, "Universal Precautions," for a complete list of these precautions. The separate standard called *body substance isolation precautions* is designed to reduce the risk of disease transmission by other body fluids and moist areas such as mucous membranes.

The U.S. Department of Labor, Occupational Safety and Health Administration (OSHA) has created a regulation based on universal precautions to help prevent the transmission of potentially life-threatening microbes and diseases to and from workers who come into contact with blood or blood-contaminated fluids. This regulation, called "Occupational Exposure to Bloodborne Pathogens," applies to all medical offices in the U.S. that have at least one worker whose duties may expose him or her to blood or other potentially infectious materials. Ophthalmic medical assistants should consult the physician in their office for detailed information about this standard.

The term **standard precautions** designates the range of procedures used to prevent the spread of infectious microbes to or from patients and personnel in the medical office. Standard precautions combine the earlier universal and body substance isolation precautions and are the precautions commonly followed today in the health care setting. However, only universal precautions ("Occupational Exposure to Bloodborne Pathogens") are mandated by OSHA. (Refer to this publication for complete instructions and precautionary guidelines—see Suggested Resources.) Standard precautions apply to blood, all body fluids, mucous membranes, and nonintact skin.

Six basic activities that make up standard precautions are presented in Table 12.2. However, it is not possible in a physician's office to work with patients in a totally microbe-free environment, nor is it necessary to do so. The following sections discuss specific procedures based on standard precautions to help prevent the spread of infectious microbes. The procedures described here are recommendations and should be confirmed with the physician in charge to ensure that they conform with infection-control practice in your office.

Hand Washing

Hand washing is one of the most important, yet one of the simplest, of the standard precautions. Simply washing with soap and warm water is an effective technique for removing infectious microorganisms from the fingers and hands. Hand washing does not remove *all* organisms, but it substantially reduces the risk of transmitting disease-causing microbes. The hands should be washed immediately before and immediately after contact with each patient, and after any procedure or patient contact that might recontaminate the hands. Keeping fingernails short makes it easier to properly wash the hands.

The box "Washing the Hands Effectively" describes the technique suitable for general purpose and patient testing in the office. If hands-on assistance in surgical procedures is involved, a lengthier "scrub" is required, as described in Chapter 13, "Minor Surgical Assisting in the Office."

TABLE 12.2 Basic Standard Precautions

1. Wash hands between contacts with patients.
2. Wear disposable gloves to avoid contact with body fluids or contaminated objects.
3. Use special receptacles ("sharps containers") for disposal of contaminated needles, blades, and other sharp objects.
4. Properly dispose of, disinfect, or sterilize contaminated objects between uses with patients.
5. Wear a fluid-impermeable gown and mask when splashing of bloody or contaminated body fluids is possible.
6. Dispose of eye patches, gauze, and the like that are saturated with blood (blood that can be wrung or squeezed out) in a special red impermeable isolation bag.

Use of Personal Protective Equipment

Personal protective equipment such as gloves, masks, and gowns minimizes contact between health care workers and patients, and so minimizes the chances of infection. Wear disposable gloves to avoid contact with body fluids or contaminated objects. The gloves should be discarded after use with each patient, and hands should be washed before and after wearing gloves.

Health care workers should wear masks or eye protection whenever there is a possibility of contact with body fluids. Gowns should be worn if soiling of exposed skin or clothing is likely. During resuscitation procedures, pocket masks or mechanical ventilation devices should be used.

Disinfection and Sterilization

Disinfection is the process of inactivating or eliminating most disease-causing microorganisms. Exposure to boiling water for 20 minutes destroys many microorganisms and is a satisfactory method of disinfecting some surgical instruments. However, boiling has disadvantages in that it dulls sharp points and cutting edges and can cause the instruments to rust.

Complex instruments and items made of plastic or certain other substances that can be damaged or destroyed by moist heat can be disinfected by use of a **germicide**, a chemical that kills germs. This germicidal, or chemical, disinfection consists of soaking the item in a solution of the chemical or swabbing those parts that come in contact with the patient's tissues (for example, the prism of the tonometer used to measure intraocular pressure; Appendix A, "Care of Ophthalmic Lenses and Instruments," presents instructions on cleaning tonometers).

Germicides used for chemical disinfection include hydrogen peroxide solution and a number of commercial preparations containing hypochlorite (bleach), formaldehyde, phenol, glutaraldehyde, and other chemicals. The problem with germicides is that few, if any, are effective against spores, and they may leave toxic residues. Nonetheless, for certain purposes (such as cleaning the tonometer), they are very useful. Consult manufacturers' recommendations for specifics regarding disinfection of ophthalmic equipment.

Sterilization is the destruction of *all* microorganisms. Different sterilization methods can be selected, depending on the object or substance to be sterilized. If the sterilized item is to contact sensitive tissues such as those of the eye, the sterilization method chosen must allow no residue of the sterilizing agent to remain that might irritate or damage the tissues. Commonly used methods of sterilization include moist heat and ethylene oxide gas.

Moist Heat

An **autoclave** is a metal chamber equipped to use steam under high pressure to destroy microorganisms (Figure 12.6). In principle, it operates much like a kitchen pressure cooker; the increased pressure permits steam to reach temperatures of at least 250° F for 30 minutes or 272° for 15 minutes (the temperatures and times usually required for sterilization). The time and temperature used for autoclaving can be varied, depending on the materials to be sterilized.

Autoclaving is commonly used to sterilize glass and stainless steel objects, some solutions, and materials such as towels and sponges. Items other than solutions are wrapped in paper and tied or taped closed. After sterilization, they are permitted to dry in the autoclave and stored. If the paper cover is unopened, the items will remain sterile for several months or longer.

Ethylene Oxide Gas

Ethylene oxide is a gas that can effectively sterilize instruments and various materials with little damaging effect on the articles themselves. It is often used for items made of plastic, rubber, and other substances that would be destroyed by heat or exposure to chemical agents. The disadvantages of ethylene oxide sterilization are that it is slow and costly and the gas is highly flammable and toxic. Still, it is widely used commercially for the production of sterile disposable (single-use) articles such as hypodermic syringes and needles, scalpels and blades, rubber gloves, bandages, sutures, and plastic equipment.

Aseptic Technique: Handling Sterile Medical Equipment

After an instrument or container has been sterilized, it is *sterile*, and that sterility needs to be maintained until it is used. Even when the hands and fingers are properly washed and gloved, they may still contami-

WASHING THE HANDS EFFECTIVELY

1. Turn on the faucets and adjust the water to the warmest comfortable temperature.
2. Wet your hands, wrists, and about 4 inches of your forearms.
3. Apply antiseptic soap from a dispenser and wash your hands with circular strokes for at least 15 seconds.
4. Rinse your hands and forearms.
5. Hold dry paper towels to close the faucets, and discard them when finished.
6. Dry your hands with clean paper towels.

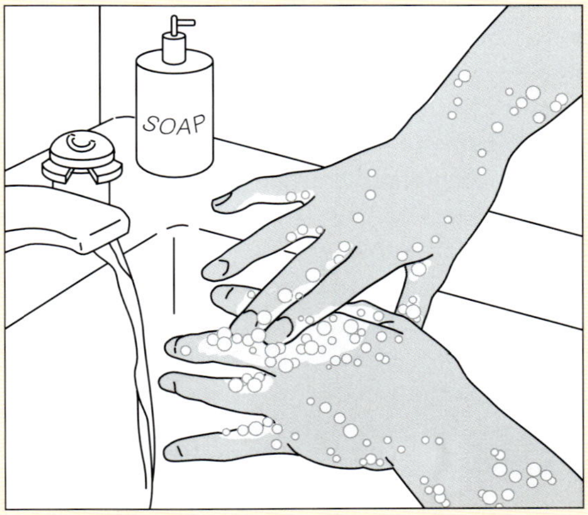

FIGURE 12.6

An autoclave, used to sterilize materials with moist heat.

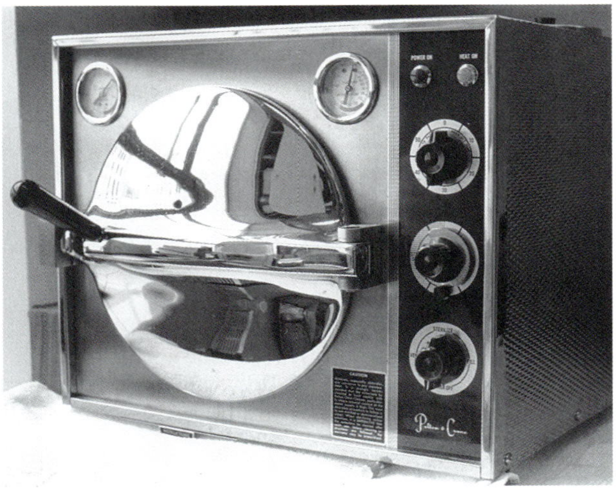

nate a sterile instrument, bottle, or other item; this contamination is a transmission risk, especially if it occurs at the *functional surface* of the article. The assistant and physician must therefore use **aseptic technique** to protect an article's sterility before and during its intended use. (See Chapter 13 for a discussion of aseptic technique in minor surgical assisting.) In practice, this means handling the item only on a part that will not come in contact with the patient or with other sterile materials.

Proper aseptic technique requires that instruments that have been disinfected or sterilized be picked up by their handles or a nonfunctional part. With sterile gauze pads, adhesive bandages, and similar materials, avoid touching the portions that will contact the wound they are intended to cover.

Relatively inexpensive items such as eyedroppers, rubber gloves, hypodermic syringes, and scalpels are available in single-use, disposable form. These articles are individually paper-wrapped and are sterile. When an item is to be used, carefully open the wrapper and grasp the article by a part that will not be in contact with the patient or with other sterile materials. Disposable eyedroppers, gloves, syringes, and other items are intended to be used once and discarded. They should never be stored and reused. Once used, they must be considered not only nonsterile, but contaminated.

Occasionally, when handling a sterile article, you may accidentally touch the sterile functional surface. If this occurs or if you are unsure whether the sterility of the article has been compromised, discard or resterilize the item as appropriate. The cost of the disposable item or of resterilization is less than the damage that can result from contamination.

The rules for handling sterile items apply equally to containers of eyedrops, other liquids, and ointments. Remove the cap without allowing your fingers to touch the lip or tip of the bottle or the inner surface of the lid. Finger contact compromises the sterility of the fluid in the container. Similarly, when instilling topical drops or applying topical ointments, never allow the tip of an eyedropper, dropper bottle, or ointment tube to contact the patient's lashes, lids, or eye. If this occurs, consider the container of medication to be contaminated and discard it.

Sterile eyedrops, fluids for washing contact lenses, and other solutions intended for use more than once are packaged in small bottles and contain a chemical preservative to help prevent bacterial or fungal contamination. Always inspect bottles before use for cloudiness or particulate matter in the liquid, indicating possible contamination. If either is present, do not use the fluid, and discard the container. Single-dose bottles of fluids are also available and are intended to be discarded after a single use. Never store or reuse such items once opened; the fluids contain no preservatives and must be considered contaminated.

Handling and Decontaminating Contaminated Materials

Any instrument, needle, swab, bandage, or other item that has come in contact with a patient's eye must be considered contaminated with potentially infectious microorganisms. Contaminated reusable objects must be decontaminated before they are used again; disposable items must be discarded. According to standard precautions, assistants should assume that fingers that have contacted a patient's eyes or face are contaminated and treat them accordingly. This means proper washing of the hands, even if contact occurred while wearing gloves.

Medical instruments and other reusable items are always first decontaminated by washing with soap and water to remove grease or protein matter, then stored and packed for later sterilization and reuse. Some offices require that these items be soaked in a chemical disinfectant before cleaning and sterilization. Check the preferred procedure in your office. Tonometers and some other reusable ophthalmic instruments with complex or delicate parts cannot be fully immersed or safely washed in this manner. Parts of such complex instruments that have touched a patient's eye should be disinfected with alcohol, bleach, or hydrogen peroxide after each patient contact. Follow the manufacturers' instructions (or check with the manufacturers) for proper disinfecting of such instruments. Be certain that the disinfectant has been rinsed off completely with sterile water or normal saline before it comes in contact with a patient's eye, to prevent eye irritation or damage to the ocular tissues.

Avoiding sticks with contaminated needles, sharp medical implements, and similar objects is an important office safety measure, especially in preventing the spread of HIV and hepatitis B. Take particular care in handling and disposing of scalpel blades, syringe needles, broken glass, and other sharp objects. Place these items, after using them, in a rigid, puncture-proof biohazard container (called a *sharps container*). When the container is full, close and dispose of it as biohazardous waste, according to the procedures used in your office.

Hygienic Practices in Potentially Infectious Situations

The ophthalmic assistant who has a common cold has the potential for transmitting the infection to a patient, particularly if the assistant is sneezing or coughing or has a runny nose. In these cases, the assistant should discuss with the physician the advisability of temporarily performing duties other than working directly with patients.

All medical professionals, including medical assistants, must take special precautions to prevent their own cuts and abrasions, even inapparent ones, from contacting the blood or body fluids of an infected patient, and vice versa. If the assistant has cuts, abrasions, or lesions on the hands, clean or sterile rubber gloves should be worn after washing the hands, to protect both the assistant and the patient. Health care professionals who have open lesions, dermatitis, or other skin irritations should avoid direct patient care activities or handling of contaminated equipment.

If a patient has a fever blister, ophthalmic medical assistants should avoid touching the patient's face near the mouth with fingers or instruments. To protect themselves and other patients, assistants should wear gloves, carefully wash their hands after completing any tests, and be certain that any instruments used with the infected patient are properly sterilized, or disinfected when sterilizing is not possible.

COLLECTING SPECIMENS FOR THE IDENTIFICATION OF MICROORGANISMS

In many cases, the appearance of an infected eye helps the physician determine the type of infecting microbe. For example, bacterial conjunctivitis often produces a white or yellow creamy discharge, while conjunctivitis caused by a virus generally produces a clear or yellowish watery discharge. If bacterial infection is suspected, rather than wait for the results of laboratory tests to identify the particular organism, the physician may begin **empiric treatment**, that is, immediately prescribe an antibiotic capable of destroying a range of bacteria.

At the same time, the physician may have a specimen of the discharge taken from the infection site and order laboratory tests to isolate and identify the causative microorganism and to determine its specific antibiotic susceptibility. This is done through microscopic observation of the microbes in specimen materials that have been stained or *cultured* (grown on specially prepared substances that promote recovery of the organism). In some viral, chlamydial, or protozoan diseases, stains may be the only method of confirming the presence of an infectious agent. Specimens should be collected for testing before empiric treatment is initiated, because the treatment might interfere with the ability to obtain a sample of the true disease-causing organism. If empiric treatment fails, results from microbiologic testing will be available and will enable effective treatment to be initiated.

Although ophthalmic medical assistants usually do not perform microbiologic testing, taking such specimens and forwarding them to a microbiologic laboratory are the ophthalmic medical assistant's responsibility in some offices. The sample of infectious material from the patient is obtained by swabbing or scraping the infected site, such as the conjunctiva or cornea, with a sterile swab or spatula (Figure 12.7). Materials taken this way from the site of infection are then transferred directly onto glass microscope slides (for staining) or onto a culture dish. The sample may also be transferred into a tube filled with a substance that preserves the sample until it can be used for testing. Assistants who are required to obtain and handle microbiologic specimens receive instructions from the physicians or technicians in their office; a more detailed discussion is beyond the scope of this book.

FIGURE 12.7

A sterile swab can be used to collect materials from the conjunctiva and lid margins for culture.

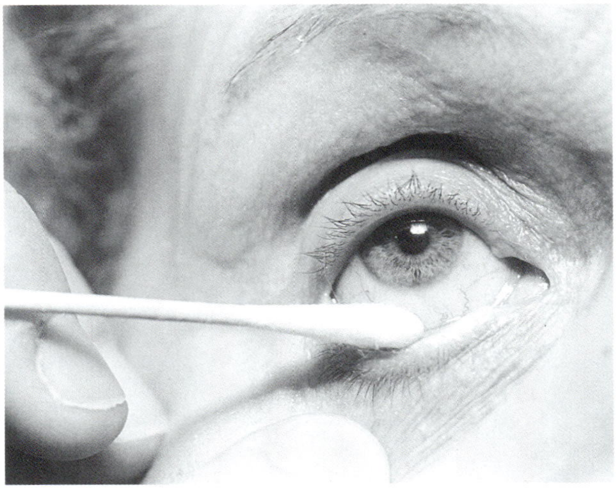

REVIEW QUESTIONS

1. Name the four groups of microorganisms that commonly cause eye disease.
2. List the five principal means of transmitting disease-causing organisms from a reservoir to a host.
3. What is the practical purpose of microbial control (aseptic technique) in the medical office?
4. State at least three of the six basic infection control activities known as standard precautions.
5. Describe the special precautions to be taken to prevent infection when (1) the assistant has a herpes simplex lesion ("fever blister") and (2) the patient has a herpes simplex lesion.
6. Describe the basic hand-washing technique.
7. Distinguish between disinfection and sterilization.
8. Name the two principal methods of sterilization.
9. Describe the method of handling sterile items to maintain sterility.
10. List at least two aseptic precautions in the use of multidose containers of sterile eyedrops.
11. Describe the procedure for the handling and disposing of contaminated sharp objects such as scalpel blades, syringe needles, and broken glass

SUGGESTED ACTIVITIES

1. Ask an experienced office staff member to show you the hand-washing technique and materials that are used in your office.
2. Ask a senior staff member to demonstrate the procedures for disinfecting office diagnostic and examination equipment.
3. Ask a senior office staff member to demonstrate the procedures for decontaminating instruments and disposing of contaminated waste materials.
4. Ask a senior staff member in your office to demonstrate the various procedures used to sterilize medical instruments, equipment, and other items in the office. Ask for a demonstration of how to handle sterile instruments and how to unwrap and handle disposable sterile items and bottles.
5. Ask to observe office procedures used to obtain microbial specimens from patients and to send them to the microbiology laboratory.

SUGGESTED RESOURCES

Forbes BA, Sahm DF, Weissfeld AS, eds: *Bailey and Scott's Diagnostic Microbiology*. 10th ed. St Louis: Mosby; 1998.

Garner JS, Hospital Infection Control Practices Advisory Committee: Guideline for isolation precautions in hospitals. *Infect Control Hosp Epidemiol* 1996;17:53–80.

Hill JE, ed: *Ophthalmic Procedures: A Nursing Perspective—Office and Clinic*. Rev ed. San Francisco: American Society of Ophthalmic Registered Nurses; 2001.

Murray R, ed: *Manual of Clinical Microbiology*. 7th ed. Washington, DC: American Society of Microbiology Press; 1999.

Stein HA, Slatt BJ, Stein RM: *The Ophthalmic Assistant: A Guide for Ophthalmic Medical Personnel*. 7th ed. St Louis: Mosby; 2000.

Tabbara KF, Hyndiuk RA, eds: *Infections of the Eye*. 2nd ed. Boston: Little, Brown and Co; 1996.

Tortora GJ, Funke BR, Case CL: *Microbiology: An Introduction*. 7th ed. San Francisco: Benjamin Cummings; 2001.

US Department of Labor, Occupational Safety and Health Administration. *Occupational Exposure to Bloodborne Pathogens*. (OSHA 3127). Washington, DC: OSHA; 1992.

13 Minor Surgical Assisting in the Office

Ocular surgery is not performed exclusively in an operating room. A number of minor ophthalmologic health problems requiring some type of surgical procedure can be treated in the ophthalmologist's office. Such procedures are known as minor surgery or office surgery. Ophthalmic medical assistants serve as invaluable team members in the care of patients undergoing minor office surgery. They can help to answer patients' questions, provide printed informational materials, and prepare patients for surgery. In addition, the ophthalmic medical assistant may sterilize and prepare surgical instruments and materials for the doctor's use, assist the doctor during the operation, and attend to cleanup and patient care afterward.

This chapter presents information about patient preparation, surgical materials and instruments, and practical skills that make the ophthalmic medical assistant an important aide to the ophthalmologist before, during, and after minor surgery. It discusses the types, principles, and requirements of office surgery and surgical procedures.

PATIENT PREPARATION BEFORE SURGERY

Patients must be prepared for surgery not only physically but also intellectually and emotionally. The ophthalmic medical assistant plays a vital role in this patient preparation.

Informed Consent

Before any surgery can be performed, the physician discusses with the patient not only the details of the operation itself but also the risks and benefits of the proposed surgical procedure, so that the patient can decide whether or not to have the operation based on a full understanding of all the facts. This process, known as obtaining **informed consent**, helps protect both the doctor and the patient. It ensures that everyone involved knows the reasons for and possible results of the surgery and, because of this understanding, all parties agree that the procedure should take place.

The discussions of informed consent usually start during the office visit when the physician describes and diagnoses the condition of the patient's eye. Generally, the doctor outlines the **complications**, or problems that might occur as the result of a proposed surgical treatment; the doctor might provide statistical information about the chance that the surgery may cause a problem.

Finally, the ophthalmologist judges whether the patient comprehends the risks and benefits of the surgery. This discussion of informed consent is recorded on the patient's chart, and a written operative permit may be obtained for the file as well. Often, a standardized informed consent form, to be signed by the patient, is used by the ophthalmologist as documentation. Ophthalmic medical assistants should become familiar with the routine of their ophthalmologist's practice for recording informed consent and filing documentation.

Patient Assistance

Because ophthalmic medical assistants often meet and prepare patients for their surgical office visit, they have the opportunity to put patients at ease and make their visit as comfortable as possible. A reassuring, calm manner helps reduce the patients' anxiety. Informing patients about what to expect throughout the visit by describing the preparatory steps as you perform them also aids in lowering their anxiety and increases their cooperation as well. Care should be taken to avoid comments about the nature or extent of the condition being treated, which can make a patient anxious and apprehensive. It may reassure patients to be told that the doctor is experienced in treating conditions like theirs (if that is the case).

For most minor surgical procedures, the preparation of the patient is similar. The patient is escorted to the office surgery room and asked to lie down on the operating table or to sit in the examining chair, depending on the instructions of the ophthalmologist. The ophthalmic medical assistant should offer to help patients onto the table or into the chair and steady them as they become more comfortable in their position. The patient's head should be positioned in a way that is comfortable for the patient and appropriately placed for the ophthalmologist/surgeon performing the procedure (Figure 13.1). According to office policy, assist the patient in removing or loosening clothing, shoes, and the like.

Patient Questions

Because ophthalmic medical assistants spend time with the patient prior to the surgery, they often will be asked questions about the upcoming operation. You may answer questions regarding how the patient will feel during and after the procedure if you are comfortable answering them. Refer the patient's questions about the surgical procedure itself or the outcome to the doctor. Bring up these questions when the surgeon enters the room to ensure that the inquiries are satisfactorily addressed before surgery begins.

ADMINISTRATION OF ANESTHETICS

Most minor office surgical procedures require that the patient receive an anesthetic. The most common methods of delivering anesthesia are by topical eyedrops and by injection. Ophthalmic medical assistants are often required to instill topical anesthetic drops, but the doctor gives injections.

Either proparacaine or tetracaine, anesthetics formulated in a topical solution, is usually instilled in both eyes before the presurgical cleansing routines known as **prepping** (short for *preparing*). Proparacaine and tetracaine anesthetize the ocular surface and decrease the patient's blink rate, making it easier to perform minor surgery around the eye. These

FIGURE 13.1

Helping to position the patient in the operating chair.

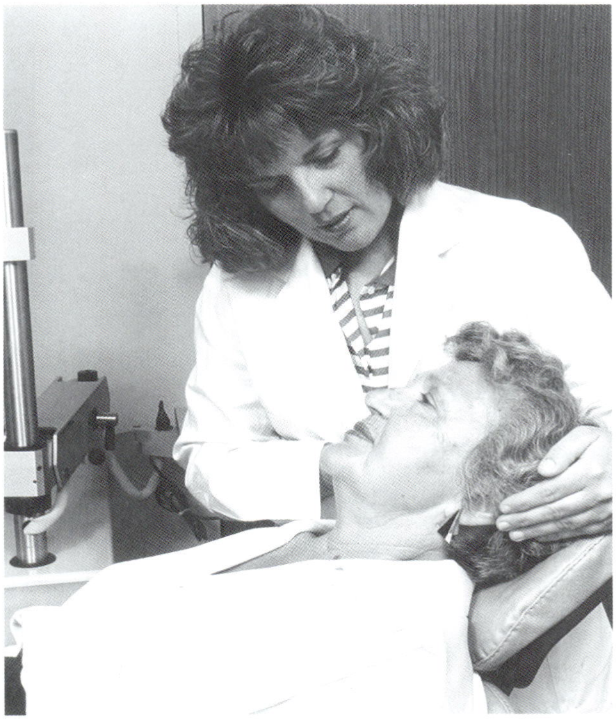

FIGURE 13.2

Applying an anesthetic-soaked pledget.

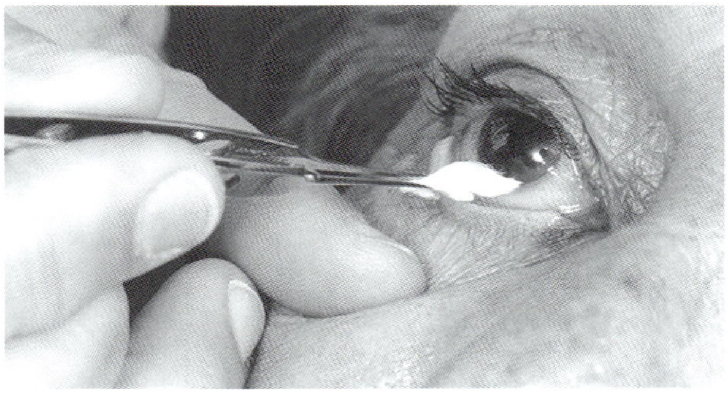

drugs also prevent the sting that can result if any of the germicidal cleansing solutions used to prepare the patient's eye area accidentally contacts the eye. Topical lidocaine 4% may be used to numb the conjunctiva and punctum. A **pledget**—a small tuft of cotton soaked in anesthetic solution—is often applied directly to these areas (Figure 13.2).

Lidocaine, injected with a hypodermic syringe, is frequently used to anesthetize the lids before prepping begins for several minor surgical procedures. Lidocaine immediately numbs the area. The initial needle stick can be painful and the medication may burn as it infiltrates under the skin. Patients should be advised of these possible reactions so that they can control the response to the pain. The ophthalmic medical assistant can help the ophthalmic surgeon by steadying the patient's head, holding the patient's hand, and asking the patient to gaze in a direction indicated by the doctor. Even though an allergic or sensitivity reaction to injected or topical anesthetics is rare, the patient should not be left alone for more than a few moments at a time for 15 to 20 minutes after such drugs have been administered. Actions to take in the case of a drug reaction are described in Chapter 9, "Patient Interaction, Screening, and Emergencies."

SURGICAL MATERIALS AND INSTRUMENTS

The ophthalmic surgeon employs a variety of specialized instruments and materials before, during, and after minor surgery. Principal materials include sutures and needles, while major surgical instruments are forceps, scissors, needle holders, clamps and curettes, scalpels and blades, lacrimal instruments, and cannulas. Within each instrument category, many different types with various specific purposes are available to the surgeon. The choice of instruments is quite individualized, however. Each surgeon has a favorite tool for performing a given task. It is important to realize that a variety of ways exist for performing the same procedure, and the best way is the one that allows a particular surgeon to accomplish the task with minimal trauma to the tissues.

Ophthalmic medical assistants perform a valuable service by preparing materials and instruments for use and caring for them before and after the surgical procedures. In many cases, ophthalmic medical assistants participate during surgery by passing materials and instruments to the doctor as requested. Therefore, ophthalmic medical assistants must become familiar with the names and appearances of common instruments and materials used in office minor surgery.

Sutures and Needles

The term **suture** describes the action of stitching a wound closed, the pattern of the stitch itself, and the thread-like material used to make the stitch. As in embroidery or sewing, suturing requires specialized threads and needles. And, just as many different

FIGURE 13.3

Suture materials.

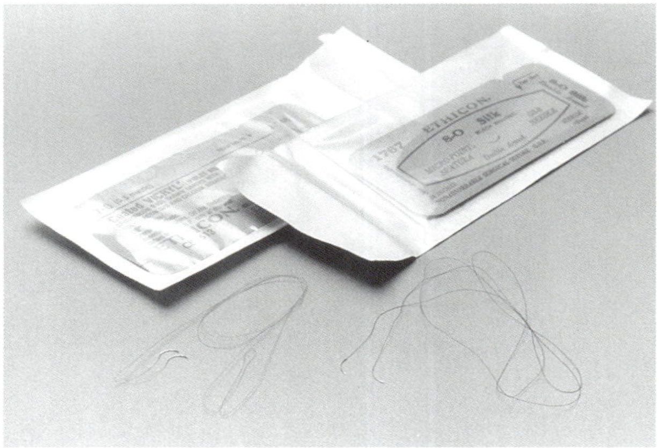

FIGURE 13.4

Four basic shapes of needle points used in ocular surgery. (A) Taper point. (B) Cutting. (C) Reverse cutting. (D) Spatula.

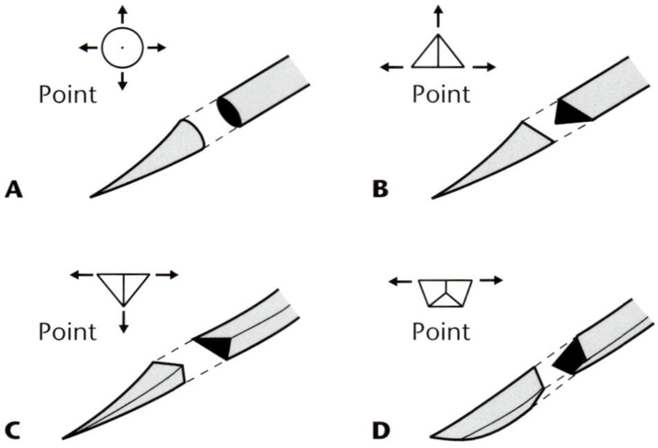

forms of embroidery stitches exist, so do many diverse forms of suture stitches. The particular suture stitch used depends on the type of surgical closure needed, the requirements of the patient, the kind of suture material used, and the type of needle attached.

Sutures are classified by the type of needle, kind of material from which they are made, and their diameter (Figure 13.3). Some suture materials are absorbed by the body; others are not.

- Absorbable sutures are degraded by the body over time and do not need to be removed. Examples of absorbable natural suture materials include surgical gut and collagen. An example of an absorbable synthetic suture material is polyglactin 910 (brand name: Vicryl).
- Nonabsorbable suture materials are not degraded by the body but remain at the surgical site until or unless they are removed. The nonabsorbable sutures are made of silk, nylon, polypropylene, or polyester fibers, such as Dacron and Mersilene.

In addition to the materials from which they are made, sutures are also defined by their diameter, which may range from thread-like to almost microscopically thin. The larger the suture, the smaller the number that is assigned to it. The finest diameter for a suture is 11-0 (pronounced *eleven-oh*). Generally, for use around the eye, the largest diameter of suture is 4-0 silk. In intraocular surgery, a finer 10-0 nylon suture is often used to close the eye. For procedures involving the eyelid, 5-0 to 8-0 suture size is employed.

Suture needles used in ophthalmic minor surgery are classified by two characteristics: the curvature and the point.

- Needle curvature is measured in degrees of extent: one-quarter of a circle equals 90°, one-half of a circle equals 180°, and five-eighths of a circle equals 225°.
- Needle points are available in four basic shapes (Figure 13.4):
  1. Taper point: a cone-shaped single point on a round shaft; used for delicate tissues
  2. Cutting: a triangular point with two-sided cutting edges and an upper cutting edge; largely replaced by the reverse-cutting needle
  3. Reverse cutting: a triangular point with two-sided cutting edges and a lower cutting edge; used for resistant tissue
  4. Spatula: a rhomboid-shaped point with two-sided cutting edges; used in the cornea and the sclera where the plane of penetration must be precise

Needles also come in different diameters, usually to match the diameter of the suture material to which they are attached.

FIGURE 13.5

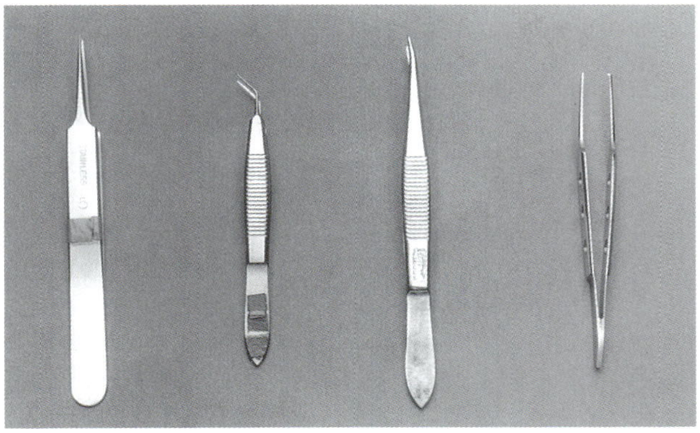

Forceps.

FIGURE 13.6

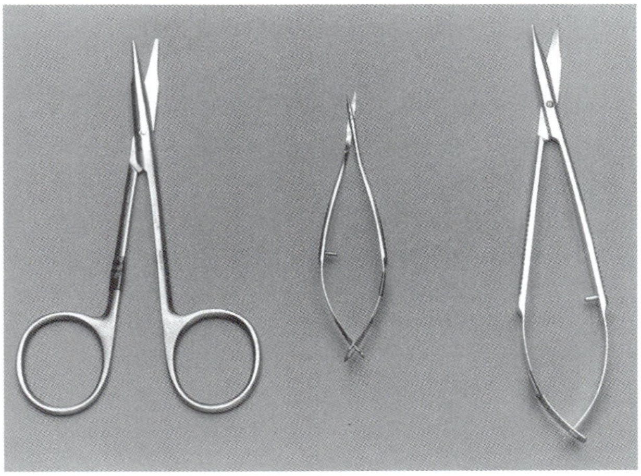

Ophthalmic surgical scissors.

Forceps

In general shape and manner of operation, forceps resemble tweezers with very delicate and fine points (Figure 13.5). Forceps are used to grasp or move body tissues, sutures, or other materials. Each has a handle and a set of jaws. The inner surface of the jaws may be rounded, flat, serrated, or toothed. The instrument itself may be curved, angled, or straight and may contain a locking device on its handle.

The two basic categories of forceps—toothed tissue forceps and nontoothed tying forceps—reflect the different purpose of each. Tissue forceps usually have teeth or serrations and are used to grasp ocular tissues to allow suturing, fixation, or dissection. Tying forceps aid the surgeon in tying sutures and usually have a broad, flat, nontoothed tip to permit grasping suture materials without tearing them. Nontoothed forceps are available for other surgical uses as well.

FIGURE 13.7

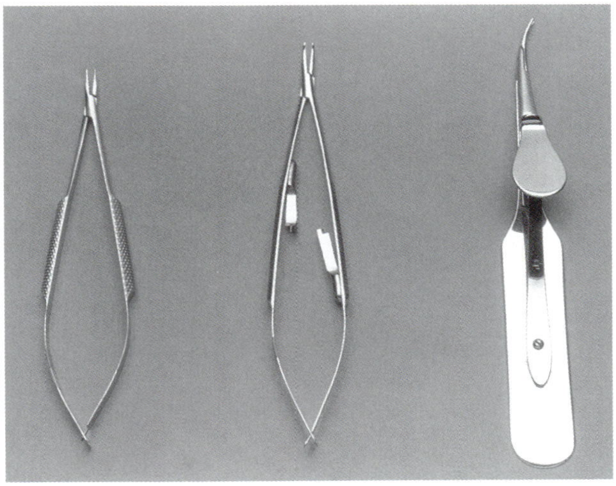

Needle holders.

Scissors

A variety of scissors serve ocular surgery (Figure 13.6). The type of scissors used during an operation depends on the tissue that the scissors must cut. Depending on the surgical purpose, scissors may be blunt or sharp, curved or straight, and may feature either spring action or direct action.

Needle Holders

Needle holders are used to hold the suture needle, which provides more control of the suturing process for the surgeon (Figure 13.7). In shape, needle holders resemble a combination of tweezers and scissors. These instruments may be nonlocking or have a locking device. The handle may or may not be spring-loaded, and the tip may be curved or straight, wide or narrow, serrated or nonserrated, or any combination of these features. Some are cradled like a pencil; others have finger loops like ordinary scissors.

Clamps and Curettes

Clamps (Figure 13.8 left) are used in ophthalmic surgery to hold or fasten onto an area of tissue to help

FIGURE 13.8

Clamp (left) and curette.

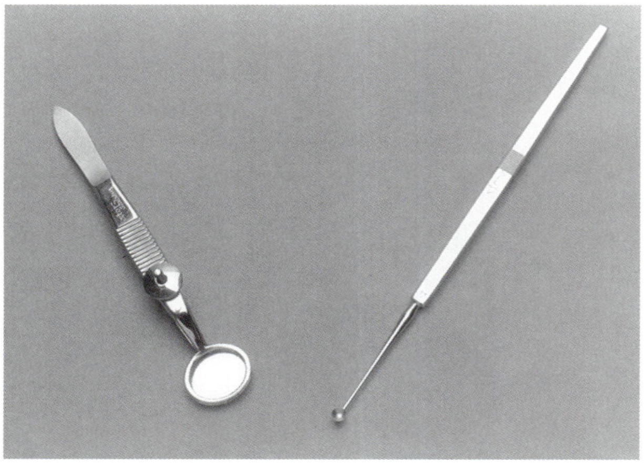

FIGURE 13.9

Blade (top) and scalpel.

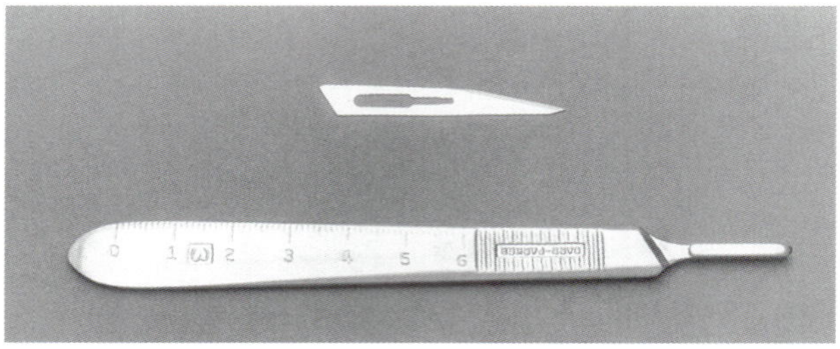

FIGURE 13.10

Lacrimal set. (Left to right) Punctum dilator. Medicine glass. Syringe. Lacrimal needle. Set of four lacrimal probes.

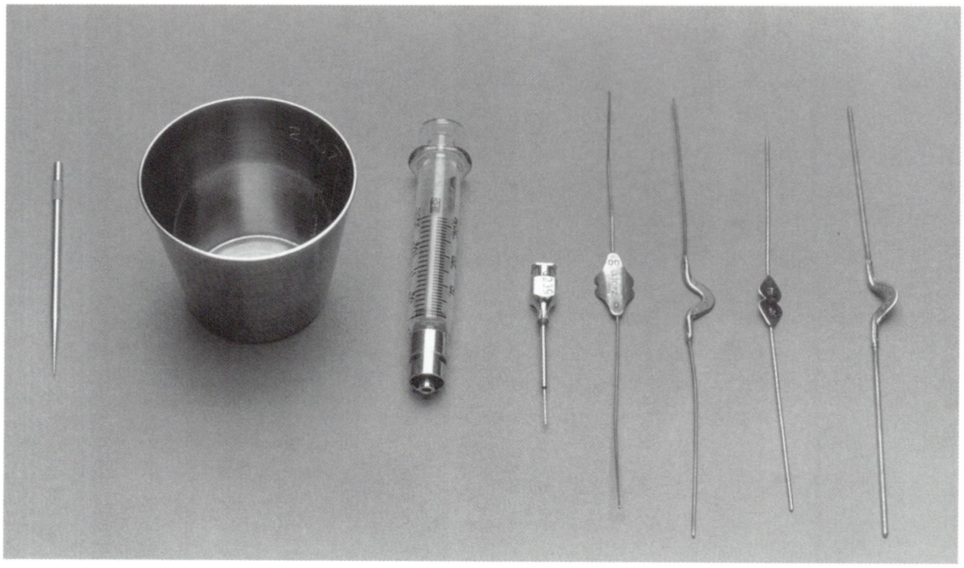

expose it for the procedure or for **hemostasis** (control of bleeding). The surgeon employs curettes in the scooping actions required to remove unwanted tissue. Curettes (Figure 13.8 right) consist of a slim handle with a small bowl-shaped end, which can be either rounded or serrated.

Scalpels and Blades

A variety of scalpels and blades may be used by the ophthalmic surgeon during minor office surgery (Figure 13.9). The types of scalpels employed by the physician for a procedure depend mainly on the preference of the surgeon.

Lacrimal Instruments

Special instruments are used to locate and clear obstructions of the tear duct. Sometimes called a **lacrimal set** (Figure 13.10), this group of instruments includes a **punctum dilator**, to enlarge the punctum; a sterile medicine glass, to hold sterile saline solution or an antibiotic solution; a **syringe** and a blunt **lacrimal needle** (cannula), to introduce the

FIGURE 13.11

Cannulas.

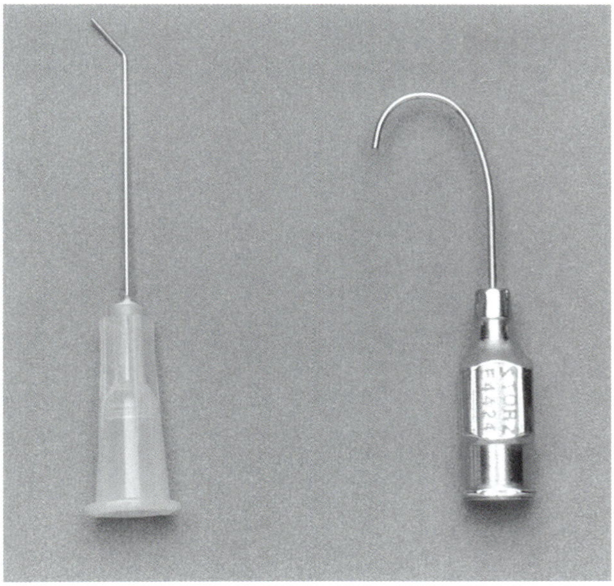

TABLE 13.1 Principal Instruments and Materials Used in Three Types of Minor Surgery

Instrument	***Chalazion***	***Other Lid Lesions***	***Lacrimal Probing***
Forceps	■	■	■
Scissors	■	■	■
Needle holder		■	
Clamp	■*	■	
Curette	■		
Probe			■
Scalpel	■	■	
Cautery	■*	■	
Material			
Suture/needle		■	
Eye pad	■	■	

*Instrument choice often depends on surgeon preference.

solution into the duct; and **lacrimal probes**, to clear the duct.

Cannulas

A **cannula** is a surgical device that resembles a small, thin tube. Cannulas are frequently used in ophthalmic surgery to inject or extract fluid or air (Figure 13.11).

COMMON MINOR SURGICAL PROCEDURES

The most common minor surgical procedures are chalazion surgery, removal of other eyelid lesions, and lacrimal-system probing. Each of these procedures requires specialized protocols and instrumentation. Table 13.1 lists the principal instruments and materials used in each type of surgery.

Chalazion Surgery

The type of lid lesion called a *chalazion* results when a meibomian gland fails to drain because of a blockage. Inflammation occurs within the lid, and the gland becomes distended and nodular. The purpose of chalazion surgery is to incise (cut open) and drain this pocket of chronic inflammation.

After the eyelid is injected with anesthetic and sterile preparation is completed, a special chalazion clamp is placed on the lid to expose the conjunctiva and to maintain hemostasis (Figure 13.12). The clamp generally is screwed down to a firm tightness, which collapses all the blood vessels surrounding the chalazion and prevents excessive bleeding from occurring when the incision is made. After the clamp is set, the doctor makes a vertical incision with a scalpel through the tarsal conjunctiva of the lid and removes the granulomatous material with a curette. As the clamp is released, bleeding may be observed and controlled. Either the doctor or the surgical assistant then applies an antibiotic ointment to the incision site and secures a special form of eyepad called an *occlusive dressing* or a *pressure patch* over the eye.

Other Lid-Lesion Surgery

Many small lid lesions occurring around the eyelid and ocular adnexa can be safely removed in the office. Xanthomas, papillomas, and benign epithelial cysts represent the most common eyelid lesions other than chalazion.

FIGURE 13.12

Chalazion clamp in place on lid.

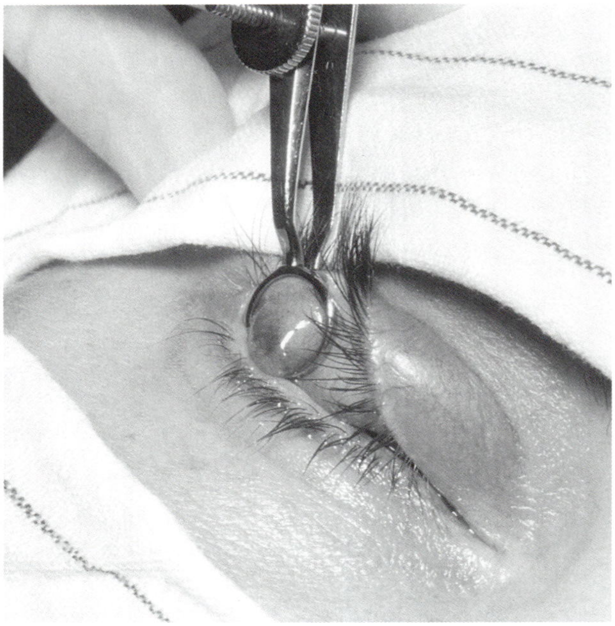

FIGURE 13.13

Cauteries.

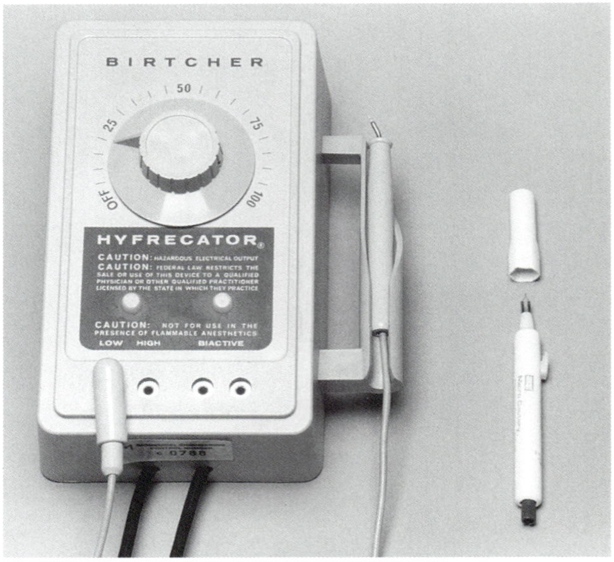

In lid-lesion surgery, the area of the eyelid lesion is anesthetized with a local infiltration of lidocaine. The doctor then removes a portion of the lesion for biopsy or excises the lesion completely with a scalpel and/or scissors. Depending on the size of the lesion, suturing may be required. If the base of the lesion is not extensive, a local **cautery** (the application of an electric current by means of a specialized instrument) may be used to destroy the lesion and prevent bleeding (Figure 13.13). Usually, if cautery is used, no suturing is necessary.

In addition to the instruments required for basic eyelid surgery, a specimen bottle, which usually contains the preservative formaldehyde, should be available for the surgeon to preserve the lesion tissue if desired for basic pathologic examination.

Lacrimal-System Probing

Minor surgery of the lacrimal apparatus occurs often in the office. When the lacrimal drainage system is blocked, **epiphora** (excessive tearing) results.

At the start of the lacrimal probing procedure, a pledget of lidocaine is often used to instill the anesthetic at the punctal area. This action is sometimes followed by a local infiltration of anesthetic. The surgeon may use a punctum dilator to enlarge the small punctal opening sufficiently to admit a needle or probe. Then, to determine the location of blockage within the lacrimal duct system, the surgeon may irrigate the tear duct by injecting a saline solution or other fluid through the punctum with a syringe and lacrimal cannula. The doctor then inserts a slim probing device through the punctum to clear the blockage and reirrigates the duct to verify that it is no longer blocked.

A congenital nasal lacrimal obstruction commonly occurs in children under the age of 1 year. Some ophthalmologists prefer to perform this probing with the infant restrained in a large blanket or on a papoose board. The ophthalmic medical assistant may therefore be required to help hold the infant. The infant may or may not receive anesthetic, depending on the surgeon's decision. Most other ophthalmologists conduct the lacrimal probe procedure in young children under general anesthesia in a hospital or formal operating room. In adults, however, almost all probing of the tear duct is done under local anesthesia in the office.

During the actual probing, the patient's head must not move while the probe passes through the canaliculus. If the patient can't keep the head still, the assistant may be asked to hold it.

Patients should be informed that when the irrigation of the lacrimal area occurs, they may taste the irrigant in back of the throat and may feel like cough-

APPLYING PRESSURE PATCHES AND SHIELDS

1. Set out two sterile eye pads and adhesive surgical tape. Tear the tape into 5- to 6-inch lengths to facilitate the patching process.
2. Instruct the patient to close both eyes tightly.
3. Clean the forehead and the area around the cheekbone and toward the ear with an alcohol pad to remove the skin oils. This helps the tape stick to the skin.
4. Fold one pad in half, place it over the closed eye, and hold it in place with one hand.
5. Apply an unfolded eye pad over the folded one.
6. Tape the unfolded pad firmly to the forehead and cheekbone (Figure A). To prevent blinking, further bleeding, or swelling, the patch must exert some pressure on the lids. The patient should not be able to open the eyelid beneath the patch. The tape should not extend to the jawbone because jaw movement could loosen the patch.
7. If the patient has any contusion or laceration of the globe or its adnexal structures, apply and tape a fenestrated aluminum (Fox) shield, instead of a pressure patch, over the globe, to protect these tissues from further damage until healing occurs or definitive repair is performed. Rest the shield on the bony eyebrow and cheekbone (Figure B). Do not patch an open globe tightly.

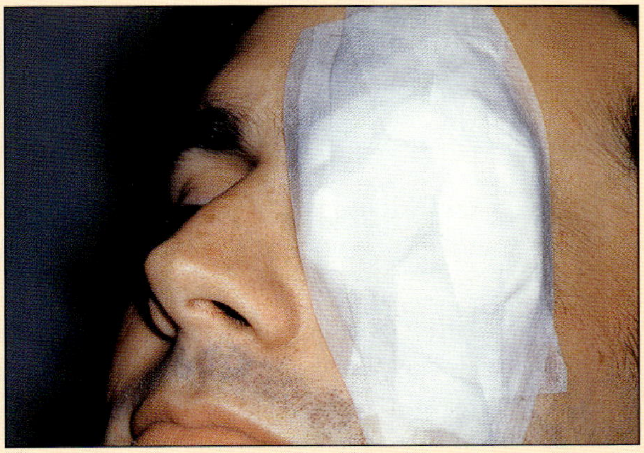

Figure A

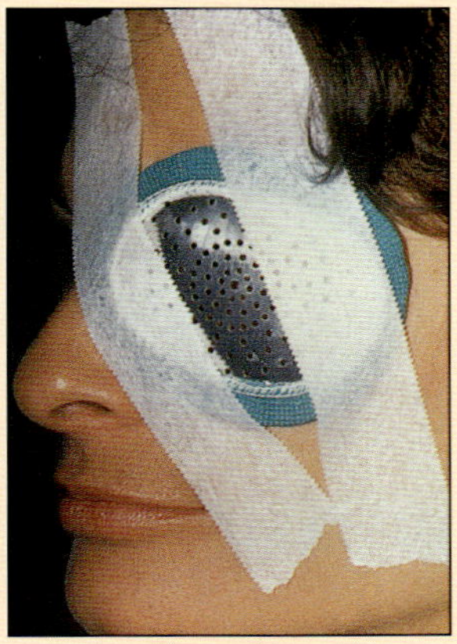

Figure B

ing. Alerting patients to this possible event before irrigation helps to prepare them, so they will not be startled by the irrigant and possibly swallow the solution or move unnecessarily. After the probe and irrigation, the ophthalmologist may instill an antibiotic solution into the punctum to avoid possible infection.

POSTSURGICAL DRESSING AND PATCHING

Dressings, usually in the form of antibiotic ointments, are applied after some kinds of minor surgery to promote healing and avoid infection. A pressure patch, made of gauze, soft cotton, or multiple eye pads, may also be applied over the eye to minimize postsurgical bleeding and immobilize the eyelid. Generally, no dressing or patch is used after nasal lacrimal probing.

The procedure for patching is described in the box "Applying Pressure Patches and Shields." A patch may not be indicated with some minor eyelid procedures. Rather, the incision site will be covered with ophthalmic ointment and a sterile adhesive strip (for example, Steri-strip) applied to it. This option depends on the size and location of the surgical incision.

FIRST SURGICAL EXPERIENCE

It is not unusual for ophthalmic medical assistants to develop faintness when observing surgery for the first time or two. If you feel faint, excuse yourself, sit down, and place your head between your knees. It is important to recognize and deal with faintness before you actually collapse, since you could injure yourself and others if you fall.

Some patients, too, may develop faintness when surgery is performed around their eyes. It is usually wise to ask the patient to stay seated for at least a few minutes after any procedure. After minor surgery, when the patient is asked to sit up, the ophthalmic medical assistant should be alert to any signs that the patient feels weak or dizzy. If the patient complains of feeling hot, dizzy, or weak, the ophthalmic medical assistant should help the patient lie down again. No patient should be dismissed until the ophthalmologist thinks the patient is steady enough to leave the office. A drink of water or a snack may help the patient who feels faint.

SURGICAL ASSISTING SKILLS

When assisting in minor surgery, the ophthalmic medical assistant's main responsibilities are to

- Ensure asepsis (strict cleanliness) of the surgical area and materials
- Prepare the instrument tray
- Prepare the patient for surgery
- Assist the doctor during the procedure
- Clean and dispose of instruments and materials after surgery

Aseptic Technique and Office Surgery

As described in Chapter 12, *aseptic technique* is the term given to the procedures followed in the medical environment that minimize the chance of infection. Four main components of aseptic technique are applied in the context of office surgery to help reduce the number of microorganisms that come into contact with the surgical wound:

1. Sterilizing all instruments
2. Preparing the patient's operative site with germicidal (organism-killing) solutions (an activity called *prepping*)
3. Scrubbing of the surgeon's and the surgical assistants' hands and donning of sterile gloves (on occasion, donning gowns and face masks as well)
4. Handling instruments, solutions, and protective drapes in such a way that prevents contamination with microorganisms

Aseptic technique is critical during any surgical procedure because it greatly reduces the incidence of postoperative infection. In the formal or hospital operating room, strict protocol is followed for scrubbing and for preparing the instruments. In minor surgery performed in the office, the same principle applies but, in reality, true asepsis—the complete absence of microbes—cannot usually be totally maintained.

Areas and the materials within these areas that have undergone sterilization are considered to be the **sterile operating field**, or simply *sterile field*. The area designated as the sterile field includes

- Sterile table and trays containing instruments and supplies and any accessory instruments that have been sterilized or covered with a sterile drape
- Portions of the patient's body that have been cleansed (prepped) and covered with sterile drapes
- Portions of the body of the personnel (doctor, nurse, and ophthalmic medical assistant) that have been cleansed and gloved

Only the front portion of a sterile gown between the waist and just below the neck is considered part of the sterile field. Masks are not sterile because they are in contact with the nose and mouth.

Scrubbing, Gloving, Prepping, and Draping

When assisting the ophthalmologist during minor surgery and before the procedure begins, ophthalmic medical assistants must scrub their hands and forearms and then put on gloves. For the majority of office surgery, most surgeons will require their assistants to scrub with warm water and germicidal soap for 3 to 5 minutes, using the standard hand-washing technique (described in Chapter 12, "Microorganisms and Infection Control"). The forearms are usually included in the scrub. Because scrubbing procedures as well as surgeon preference may vary, you should request specific scrubbing instructions from the surgeon in your office. After the washing, sterile packaged gloves may be put on without assistance while

FIGURE 13.14

Prepping procedure.

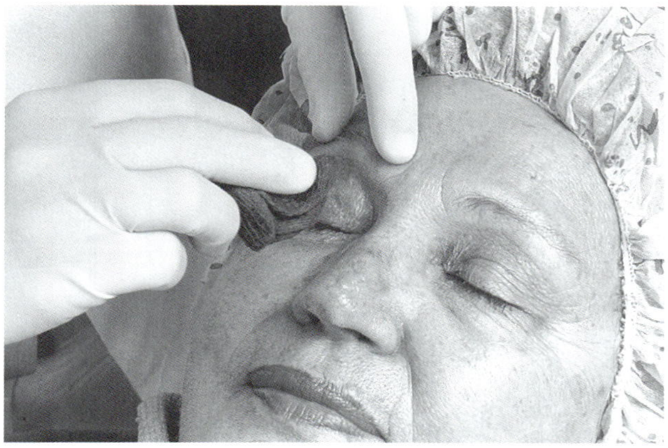

FIGURE 13.15

Standard instrument tray set up for minor surgery.

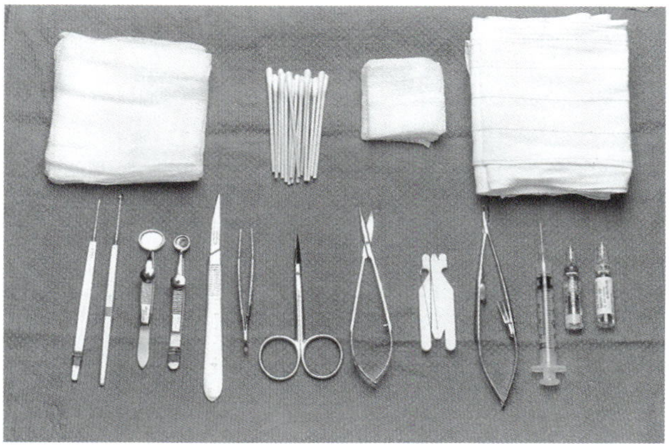

maintaining sterility to their outside working surfaces. Your doctor or another trained assistant can show you this relatively simple technique. Masks, if required, are donned before scrubbing and before gloving. Gowns, if required, are donned after scrubbing and before gloving. After these procedures, do not touch anything outside of the sterile field. If gloves or gowns become contaminated before surgery begins, remove them and put on new ones.

For minor office surgery, prepping consists of washing the external area of the eye to be operated on with a cotton ball, swab, or gauze pad soaked with a germicidal solution, which usually contains iodine, hexachlorophene, or chlorhexidine (Figure 13.14). Precautions should be taken to avoid dropping or splashing any of the solution into the patient's eye because it may cause irritation later in the day. Prepping is usually performed while wearing sterile gloves and precedes final scrubbing and donning a fresh pair of sterile gloves.

After the patient has been prepped with the germicidal solution, **sterile drapes** (large, sterilized protective sheets or cloths) may be placed around the patient's eye to provide a clean operating field. The draping also provides a sterile area on which the doctor and assistant may rest their hands and instruments during the procedure.

Preparation of the Instrument Tray

The tray containing the array of instruments and materials the surgeon will need is generally set up within the sterile field. The ophthalmic medical assistant prepares the instrument tray after scrubbing and putting on gloves.

The instrument tray itself must be covered with a sterile cloth or paper to provide a sterile surface onto which the sterile instruments can be placed. The cloth and instruments are usually wrapped in a sterile package, previously prepared by the ophthalmic medical assistant or other office personnel depending on the office practice. The outer sterilization wrappers, if present, are removed before scrubbing and gloving. The sterilized packages are opened, and the sterilized instruments and materials are handled only with sterile gloves on. The instruments are placed on the sterile tray in the order in which they are to be used (Figure 13.15). The ophthalmologist or the ophthalmic medical assistant thus knows where each instrument is for the next step in the procedure.

All sharp-pointed instruments (also called *sharps*), such as suture needles, hypodermic needles, and disposable blades, must be counted when the tray is prepared. These sharp instruments are then recounted after surgery to ensure that no sharp objects have been left near the patient.

In addition to the wrapped or packaged instruments on the sterile tray, cotton-tipped applicators are often included. Cotton-tipped applicators are available in 3-inch or 6-inch sizes in sterile packages and are used to absorb fluids, hold back certain tissues, and apply solutions or ointments. Cellulose sponges or spears are sometimes preferred to cotton-tipped

FIGURE 13.16

Cotton-tipped applicators and cellulose spears.

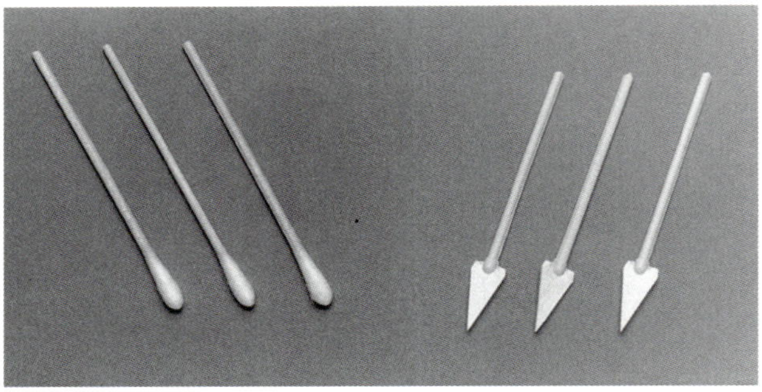

FIGURE 13.17

Correct technique for passing instruments.

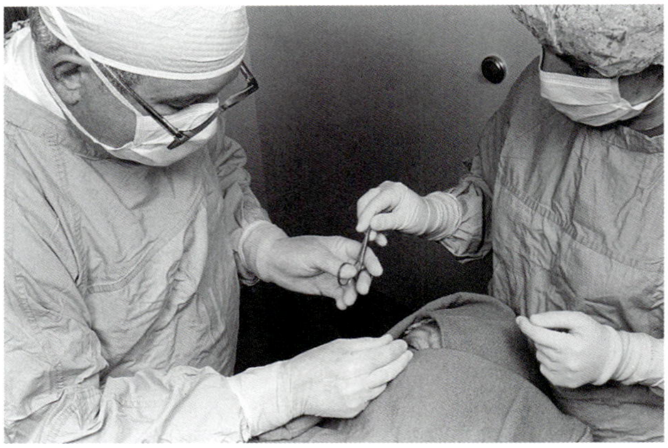

applicators because they do not shed cotton fibers and tend to be more absorbent (Figure 13.16). Suture materials may also be needed on the tray, as well as sterile syringes, needles, and solutions. Every surgeon has personal preferences as to the exact kinds and numbers of items that must be included on the tray.

Tasks During Surgery

During most minor surgical procedures, the ophthalmic medical assistant can best help the ophthalmic surgeon by anticipating the next step of each procedure. This requires a good understanding of a particular surgical procedure and a working knowledge of the physician's preference for instruments. By anticipating the surgeon's needs, the ophthalmic medical assistant helps expedite the operation and minimize the chance for complications. Knowing which instrument the surgeon will call for next comes with practical experience in assisting your doctor over time.

During the actual surgical procedure, the duties of the ophthalmic medical assistant center on providing better operative exposure for the surgeon. In chalazion surgery, for example, this might be accomplished by holding the chalazion clamp during the incision and curettage. In addition, the ophthalmic medical assistant may be asked to use a cotton-tipped applicator or a cellulose sponge to blot any blood or maintain hemostasis so the surgeon can see an incision site.

The ophthalmic medical assistant can also help the operation go smoothly by passing the surgeon the necessary instruments when requested. It is very important during this passing that the instruments are not brought over the eye or face of the patient—especially sharp instruments such as scalpels or needles. Instruments should be passed to the surgeon around and off the operative field, and in a way that minimizes an inadvertent wound with the sharp end of any instrument (Figure 13.17).

Many of the instruments used in ophthalmic surgery are quite delicate and expensive. They should always be treated gently and carefully. Avoid touching the tips of instruments with any hard object, such as other instruments or the instrument tray, as the tips can often be easily damaged.

Disposition of Instruments and Materials

At the conclusion of the surgical procedure, the ophthalmic medical assistant removes the instruments from the field. The assistant re-counts sharps, such as suture and hypodermic needles and disposable blades, to ensure that no sharp objects are left anywhere near the patient. Disposable sharps are placed in safety containers so that they will not injure office personnel or waste collectors. Other disposable supplies, including drapes, are discarded into appropriate safety containers. Nondisposable drapes and gowns are placed in the office linen hamper for laundering and resterilization.

The instruments used during the surgery are taken to a sink to be washed, rinsed, and prepared for sterilization. Surgical gloves should be worn while cleaning the instruments. Ophthalmic medical assistants must be careful not to expose their skin to any of the patient's body fluids. Protective eyewear may also be useful to prevent the splashing of body fluids or other solutions into the eyes.

Each instrument should be separated from the others and cleaned individually, either by rinsing in water or by using a commercial instrument cleansing solution. All blood, tissue, and solution must be removed from the instruments before sterilization. Jointed instruments must be cleaned thoroughly and carefully. Scissors must be open to their fullest position and all blood removed, especially from the joints. Tissue should be removed from the jaws of such instruments. After complete cleaning and drying, the sharp and delicate tips of the instruments should be covered with an instrument guard to protect the points, teeth, or cutting edges as well as to protect office personnel. This step is important because many instruments used in ophthalmic minor surgery are delicate and easily damaged. Mishandling or rough handling of these instruments can cause the jaws to become misaligned or the points to become dull. After cleaning, instruments are rewrapped for sterilization.

REVIEW QUESTIONS

1. Name the process by which the physician and patient discuss the risks and benefits of a proposed surgical procedure.
2. A patient asks you a specific question about the outcome of surgery just before the operation. Which is the best action to take?
   a. Answer the question as best you can, based on your experience with similar surgical situations.
   b. Excuse yourself, leave the room to ask the doctor, and report the answer to the patient.
   c. Reassure the patient that there is nothing to worry about.
   d. Suggest that the patient ask the doctor, and bring up the question as soon as the doctor arrives.
   e. Record the question in the patient's medical record.
3. Name the two principal methods used to deliver anesthetizing drugs to the eye for minor surgery.
4. Identify from left to right the instruments shown in the photograph.

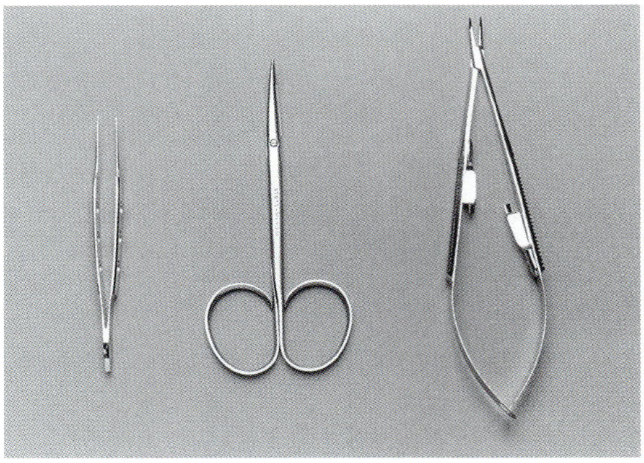

5. What are the four types of suture needle points?
6. Name the two classifications of suture materials, and identify at least two materials used for each kind.

7. List the three principal types of minor office surgery.
8. What are the main purposes of a pressure patch?
9. State the principal purpose for aseptic technique in the office surgical environment.
10. List the four components of aseptic technique that apply to minor office surgery.
11. What does *prepping* the patient for minor surgery mean?
12. Name the elements of the sterile field.
13. Why is a drape used in ophthalmic minor surgery?
14. Describe the special actions taken with sharps after surgery and explain why they are necessary.

SUGGESTED ACTIVITIES

1. Discuss your responsibilities related to minor surgery with the ophthalmologist for whom you work. Be sure to ask any questions now, rather than during the surgery itself.
2. With the ophthalmologist in your office supervising, role-play with a fellow employee the following minor surgery activities:
   a. Assist the patient onto the operating table, position the patient's head, and give instructions for fixation of gaze to prepare the patient for an anesthetic injection.
   b. Handle some typical patient questions.
   c. Using an inert fluid suggested by the doctor, practice administering anesthetic by the topical drop and the pledget methods.
   d. Prepare (prep) the patient's operative area with germicidal solution, using sterile inert liquid.
3. With the senior technician or ophthalmologist supervising, practice scrubbing, gloving, and postsurgical instrument removal and cleaning.
4. Under supervision, lay out an instrument tray for
   a. Chalazion surgery
   b. Other lid-lesion removal
   c. Lacrimal-system probing
5. Discuss with the ophthalmologist the correct procedure to follow when you or the patient feels faint.
6. With the ophthalmologist's permission, observe several different minor surgical procedures. Take notes and ask questions in a discussion with the surgeon and assistant afterward.
7. Practice applying a pressure patch on either a dummy head or a coworker. Have an experienced person critique your technique.

SUGGESTED RESOURCES

Atkinson LJ: *Berry & Kohn's Introduction to Operating Room Technique*. 8th ed. St. Louis: Mosby-Year Book; 1996.

Boess-Lott R, Stecik S: *The Ophthalmic Surgical Assistant*. Thorofare, NJ: Slack; 1999.

Cassin B: *Fundamentals for Ophthalmic Technical Personnel*. Philadelphia: WB Saunders Co; 1995; chap 25.

Jackson-Williams B: *Ophthalmic Surgical Assisting*. 2nd ed. Thorofare, NJ: Slack; 1993.

Stein HA, Slatt BJ, Stein RM: *The Ophthalmic Assistant: A Guide for Ophthalmic Medical Personnel*. 7th ed. St Louis: Mosby; 2000.

14 Principles and Problems of Contact Lenses

Prescribing and fitting contact lenses have become an integral part of today's comprehensive ophthalmology practice. More than 30 million people in the United States wear contact lenses, with the majority using them for cosmetic purposes. Other reasons for wearing contact lenses include occupational preferences, sports, and therapeutic uses.

Beginning ophthalmic medical assistants may function in a contact lens practice by taking a patient history, obtaining basic preliminary refractive measurements, and performing lensometry and keratometry. With experience, responsibilities may include assistance in the fitting of the lenses, confirming lens parameters, and suggesting lens modifications. Because assistants often are required to help educate patients in the proper use and care of their contact lenses and to help assess patients' related problems, a basic understanding of contact lens principles, types, appropriate use, and problems is necessary.

This chapter describes how contact lenses work to correct vision, how they differ from eyeglasses, and the types of lenses available and their uses. Lens care is emphasized because improper care can lead to problems. Procedures for inserting and removing lenses are presented, as well as a discussion of commonly encountered problems and of the types of patients who may be unable to wear contact lenses successfully.

Although you can read extensively on the subject of contact lenses, the most productive and practical knowledge will come from observing contact lens fitting, talking to patients who have worn contact lenses, and actually trying on contact lenses yourself. When in doubt about your role in the ophthalmologist's office, exercise caution, never assume diagnostic responsibility, and always readily and appropriately discuss a patient's symptoms and signs with the ophthalmologist.

FIGURE 14.1

Physiology and refractive result of contact lens. Dotted line: focal point/plane without contact lens; solid line: focal point/plane with contact lens.

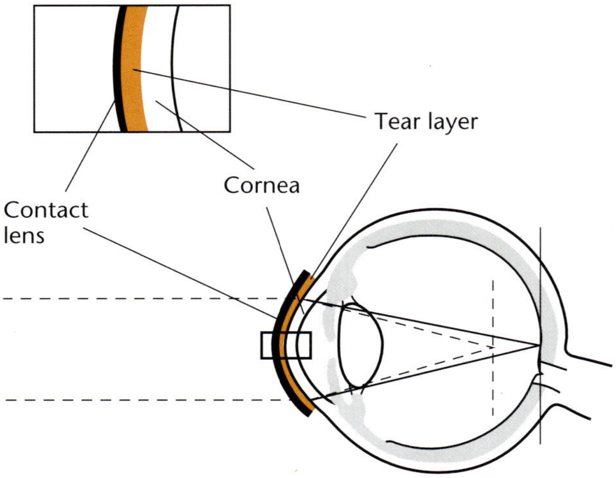

FIGURE 14.2

A typical responsibility of the ophthalmic medical assistant is to help educate patients in the proper wear and care of their contact lenses.

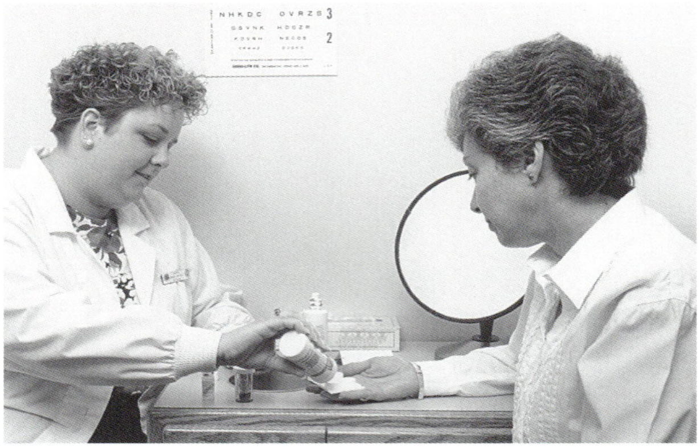

BASIC PRINCIPLES

The contact lens places a new refractive surface (the contact lens) over the surface of the cornea. The contact lens itself rests on a thin liquid cushion, the tear layer, and not on the eye. This fluid lying between the back surface of the contact lens and the front surface of the cornea fills out corneal irregularities, converting the interface between the contact lens and the cornea into a smooth, spherical surface. In principle, the contact lens then alters the refractive power of the eye by providing a radius of curvature (the front of the contact lens) different from that of the cornea. This new front curvature is selected to correct the optical error of the eye and allow light to focus on the retina, thereby correcting the patient's spherical and astigmatic refractive error to the extent possible by a given lens material (Figure 14.1).

The following procedures are used to arrive at a contact lens prescription:

- Determination of the refractive error (refraction/refractometry)
- Definition of the curvature of the cornea, using the keratometer to determine the flattest and steepest corneal meridians and the axis (in degrees) in the central visual axis of the eye (keratometry)
- Use of both refraction and keratometry measurements to provide a starting point from which to choose the appropriate lens material, lens, base and peripheral curve, diameter, and power

According to their experience and office policy, ophthalmic medical assistants may perform some of these procedures as well as take a contact lens patient's history and instruct patients in lens care and wear (Figure 14.2).

The contact lens must allow normal corneal metabolism by enabling adequate oxygen to reach all of the cornea and by promoting the flushing of metabolic waste products from underneath the lens itself. Depending on the type of lens material used, oxygen can reach the cornea either directly through the contact lens or indirectly by the *tear pump*. The tear pump results from blinking; the movement of fresh tears under the lens carries oxygen to the cornea and pushes out the old tears with their metabolic wastes. In addition to maintaining corneal metabolism and promoting waste removal, the contact lens must also sustain the integrity of corneal epithelium and normal corneal temperature. These objectives are met by the following kinds of contact lenses:

- **Soft lenses**, which provide oxygen and carbon dioxide diffusion through the lens material itself with a minimal tear pump (the movement of tears under the contact lens)

- **Rigid gas-permeable (RGP) lenses**, which provide oxygen and carbon dioxide diffusion through the lens material and a tear pump
- **Polymethylmethacrylate (PMMA) lenses**, which provide oxygen by means of a tear pump only and no diffusion of oxygen and carbon dioxide through the lens

Contact Lenses vs Eyeglasses for Vision Correction

Contact lenses are useful for cosmetic purposes, such as avoiding thick and heavy or unsightly eyeglasses, concealing a disfigured eye, or achieving a fashionable or different eye color. Contact lenses can be a real boon for patients whose eyeglasses irritate or actually inflame their ears or nose. Some advantages of contact lenses over eyeglasses are that they

- Do not impair or distort peripheral vision
- Do not fog or become easily dislodged during work or sports or under adverse environmental conditions
- Permit better correction of the types of refractive errors that occur with keratoconus, nystagmus, congenital albinism, or irregular astigmatism caused by corneal scars
- Provide a normal retinal image size, especially in those who have large refractive errors or who have had cataract surgery without an intraocular lens implant
- Can provide 24-hour vision (with extended-wear lenses)

Some disadvantages of contact lenses are that they

- Require fastidious, continuous, careful maintenance
- Carry the risk of infection and other adverse physiologic effects on the cornea
- Are inappropriate in some environments, such as in the presence of dust, smoke, or caustic agents
- Cost more than eyeglasses, particularly because lenses can be lost or damaged more easily than eyeglasses and require replacement more frequently

Contact Lens Specification vs Eyeglass Prescription

The specification for a patient's contact lenses differs from a prescription for eyeglasses. A prescription for eyeglasses includes such information as the refractive error expressed as sphere and cylinder (either plus or minus), with bifocal or prism included if required and vertex and pupillary distance as appropriate. In contrast, a contact lens prescription (specification) requires the following information:

- Spherical equivalent of refractive error (power)
- Keratometry readings (corneal curvature), determining the flattest and steepest corneal meridians in the visual axis
- Diameter of lens required
- Base curve
- Lens thickness
- Material of the lens
- Water content (soft lens)
- Specific brand or type of lens to be dispensed
- Edge blends or peripheral curves (if any)
- Lens tint (if any)
- Wearing instructions

The ophthalmic medical assistant helps gather some of this information and takes some of the measurements, such as refractometry and keratometry.

TYPES AND MATERIALS OF CONTACT LENSES

After determining the preliminary specifications for a patient's contact lenses, the ophthalmologist chooses the lens type and material that will provide the best vision and fit and meet the physiologic and comfort needs of the patient. Ophthalmic medical assistants may be called upon to educate patients in the advantages and disadvantages of the different types and help instruct patients in the insertion and removal of contact lenses, in wearing schedules, and in lens care.

More than 85% of those wearing contact lenses today use soft contact lenses. Also called **hydrophilic** lenses because they do not repel water, soft contact

FIGURE 14.3

(A) Soft contact lenses are made of flexible, gel-like materials. (B) Hard contact lenses comprise RGP and PMMA lenses.

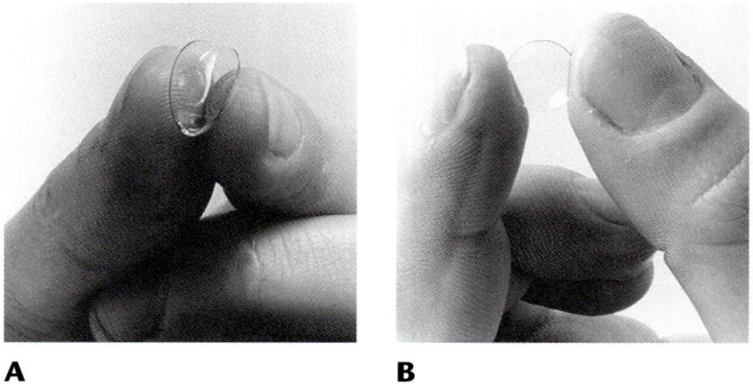

FIGURE 14.4

RGP contact lenses permit oxygen and carbon dioxide to diffuse through their semiflexible plastic structure.

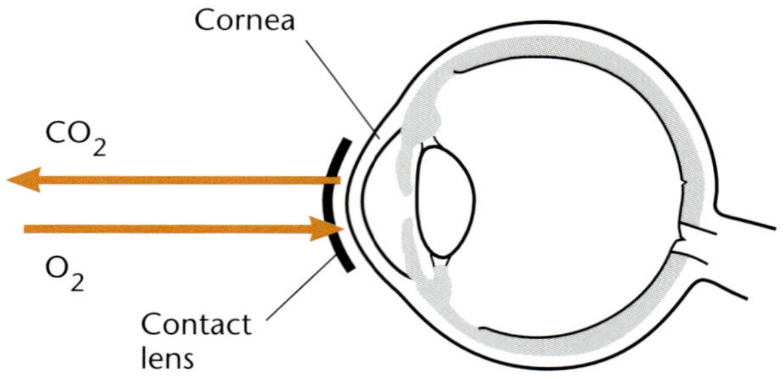

lenses are made of flexible, gel-like materials that contain more than 10% water or silicone (Figure 14.3A). Approximately 12% to 15% of contact lens users wear rigid gas-permeable (RGP) lenses, a hard lens made of materials that bend or flex only slightly (Figure 14.3B). The RGP lenses allow direct passage of oxygen and carbon dioxide through the lens materials. Some 4.5 million individuals use soft or RGP lenses for extended wear; of these extended-wear lenses, a significant number are disposable soft lenses. A small number of contact lens wearers use the older, original polymethylmethacrylate (PMMA) "hard" lenses. The following sections describe the various types of lenses in detail.

PMMA and RGP Hard Lenses

Polymethylmethacrylate (PMMA) was the plastic material used in the original hard contact lenses, but it is infrequently used today. The non–gas-permeable PMMA material allows oxygen to reach the cornea only by the pumping of oxygenated tears around and under the lens. Today's rigid gas-permeable (RGP) contact lenses, however, are made from materials that permit oxygen and carbon dioxide to diffuse through their semiflexible plastic structure (Figure 14.4). These kinds of hard contact lens materials include cellulose acetate butyrate (CAB), silicone acrylates, silicone resins, styrene, fluorosilicone acrylates, and fluorine and silicone materials. These newer RGP contact lens materials offer several advantages in that they

- Are easier to adapt to than PMMA lenses
- Provide better comfort than PMMA
- Maintain corneal physiology because of their oxygen and carbon dioxide permeability
- Have applications for difficult visual problems, such as in keratoconus, large amounts of astigmatism, or irregular corneas, compared to soft lenses
- Offer good vision potential from larger optical zones
- Minimize **spectacle blur** (temporary blurred vision upon switching from contact lenses to eyeglasses), compared to PMMA
- May be modified after manufacture to alter fit, size, or power

The disadvantages of the RGP contact lens materials are that they

- Are more fragile, compared to PMMA
- May warp (especially thinner or higher–oxygen-permeable RGP lenses)
- May scratch easily or craze (silicone acrylate)
- May require special solutions or have other increased requirements for cleaning
- Are more susceptible than PMMA lenses to protein deposits that can blur vision or irritate the eye
- May cost more than either PMMA or soft lenses

Soft Lenses

Soft, or hydrophilic, contact lenses are made of gel-like hydrogel materials and owe their softness to the hydrogel's ability to absorb and bind water. The advantages of this type of material are that the lenses

- Are comfortable, and thus easy to adapt to and wear
- Rarely cause spectacle blur (the patient can easily switch from contact lenses to eyeglasses), and so can be worn intermittently
- Rarely become "lost" in or dislodged from the eye
- Rarely lead to overwear symptoms
- Are a useful alternative for patients who were unsuccessful in wearing rigid contact lenses
- Can in some cases be inexpensively and accurately mass-produced
- Are available as disposable lenses

The major disadvantages of soft contact lenses are that they

- Can cause variable vision due to dehydration of the lenses, uncorrected astigmatism, or lenses becoming dirty because of improper care
- Are less durable than rigid lenses
- Have increased deposit formation
- Cannot be modified after manufacture, as RGP and PMMA lenses can
- Require meticulous and somewhat expensive care, cleaning, and disinfection
- Have limited use for some patients with astigmatism

Extended-Wear Lenses

Extended-wear lenses include soft contact lenses that have increased oxygen permeability and certain RGP lenses of high oxygen permeability that have been approved by the United States Food and Drug Administration (FDA) for overnight wear for up to 7 days. Some patients choose to wear their extended-wear lenses on a flexible schedule of just 1 or 2 nights of extended wear, while others opt for wearing their lenses for the FDA-recommended maximum wear of 7 days without lens removal. Certain disposable lenses are also approved for extended wear.

Extended-wear lenses are associated with increased incidence of adverse corneal effects and corneal ulcers, and it is especially important that patients receive and follow instructions in the care and wearing schedules of their lenses. Further information may be obtained from the American Academy of Ophthalmology Information Statement *Extended Wear of Contact Lenses.*

Daily-Wear Lenses

Daily-wear lenses comprise both rigid and soft contact lenses that are intended to be worn for fewer than 24 consecutive hours, while the wearer is awake. Significant corneal problems can occur if a lens approved only for daily wear is worn overnight. Such corneal injury results from the deprivation of oxygen to the cornea under the closed eye and/or from mechanical trauma.

Disposable Lenses

Disposable lenses include those soft contact lenses that are predominantly made by a molding process or by spin-casting and are designed for either daily or extended wear and disposal after 1 day to 2 weeks of use. Disposability serves as a way to categorize these lenses rather than as an indication of a specific lens material. Because they are worn for only a short time and then discarded, disposable lenses usually require minimal or no cleaning, but they must be disinfected after removal and before reinsertion. Many contact lens wearers feel that the time and money they save in maintenance offsets the cost of frequent replacement of disposable lenses.

Planned-Replacement Lenses

Planned-replacement lenses, also referred to as programmed-replacement lenses or frequent-replacement lenses, are soft contact lenses that are replaced at intervals of 1, 2, 3, or 6 months. In planned replacement, lenses are replaced before the contact lens material is significantly degraded. The frequency of replacement is determined by the ophthalmologist, based on the response of both the contact lenses and the patient's eyes to the patient's wearing conditions. Planned-replacement lenses require lens care, including cleaning and disinfection after each removal and before reinsertion. Enzyme cleaning may be required, depending on how long the lenses are used and how the patient's eyes respond to wearing lenses.

FIGURE 14.5

This patient is wearing a cosmetic opaque fashion lens in the right eye that is tinted to alter her normal iris color from brown to blue.

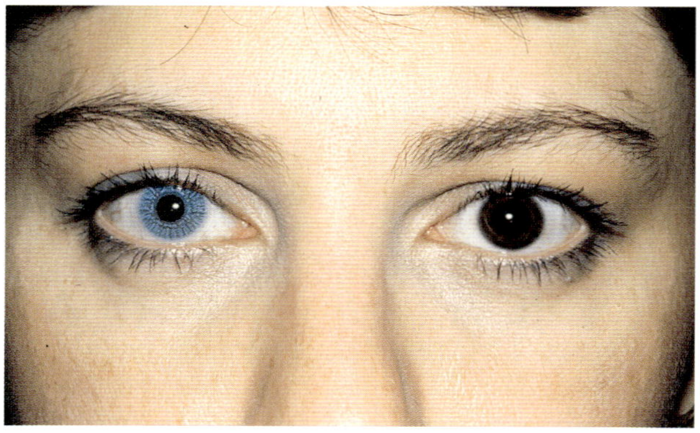

FIGURE 14.6

A patient with hyperpigmentation of the iris and sclera of the left eye (A) can wear an opaque soft contact lens as a cosmetic restorative lens on the right eye to equalize iris color (B).

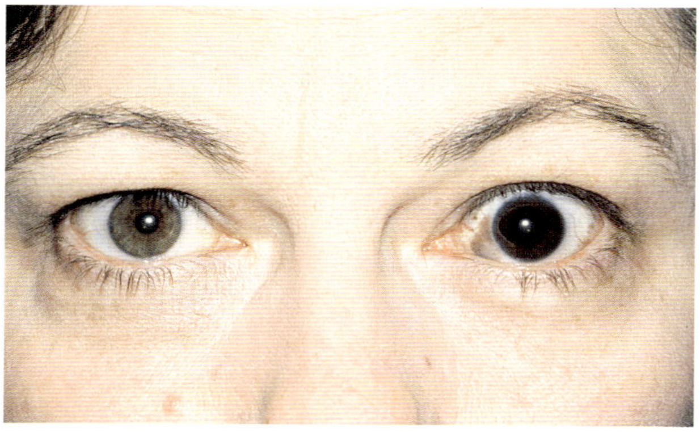

A

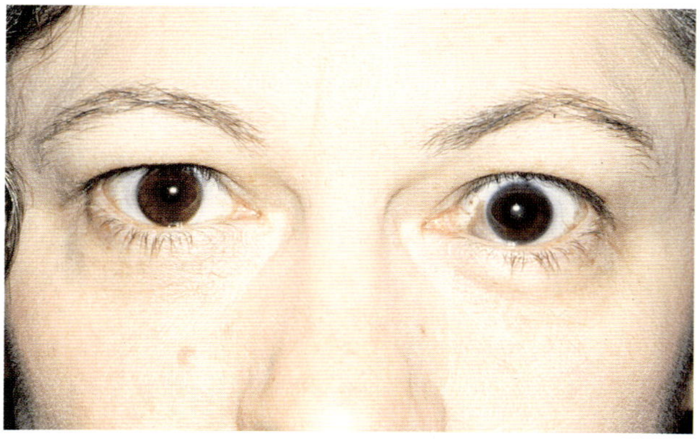

B

LENS DESIGNS FOR SPECIAL PURPOSES

Contact lenses can meet the special needs of individuals who require a prosthetic device to conceal ocular disfigurement or treatment for certain ophthalmic disorders. Some of the possible uses for unique contact lens designs are described below.

Cosmetic Fashion Lenses

Conventional lenses can be tinted to enhance or change the color of a person's iris (Figure 14.5). Although changing the color of the eyes usually serves no therapeutic purpose, tinted contact lenses may offer some relief from photophobia in glare-sensitive individuals. In addition, contact lenses with a handling, or visibility, tint may help patients, especially those with hyperopia or presbyopia, to find their lenses more easily than they could colorless lenses. The light handling tint does not affect the eye color, however. Cosmetic tinted lenses can have a clear pupillary area or a total overall color. The tint itself may eventually fade ("weather") over time. Some cleaning solutions promote this fading process.

Cosmetic Restorative Lenses

Contact lenses can serve a cosmetic restoring function, such as being used as a prosthetic device for eyes disfigured by trauma, infection, or other condition (Figure 14.6). These contact lenses can have a sclera, iris, or pupil painted, printed, or laminated onto them. Such lenses can be used with eyes that have no visual potential or functional vision.

Toric Lenses

Toric contact lenses have two different radii of curvature on their anterior and/or posterior surfaces. This type of contact lens corrects the vision of patients whose astigmatism cannot be adequately corrected by other types of contact lenses. Toric contact lenses correct for astigmatic errors in the same way eyeglasses do. In special cases, a toric design may help center the lens on the cornea. These lenses are available as both soft and rigid lenses.

Bifocal Lenses

Bifocal contact lens design attempts to provide individuals with correction for both near and distance vision. These lens designs are based on alternating

FIGURE 14.7

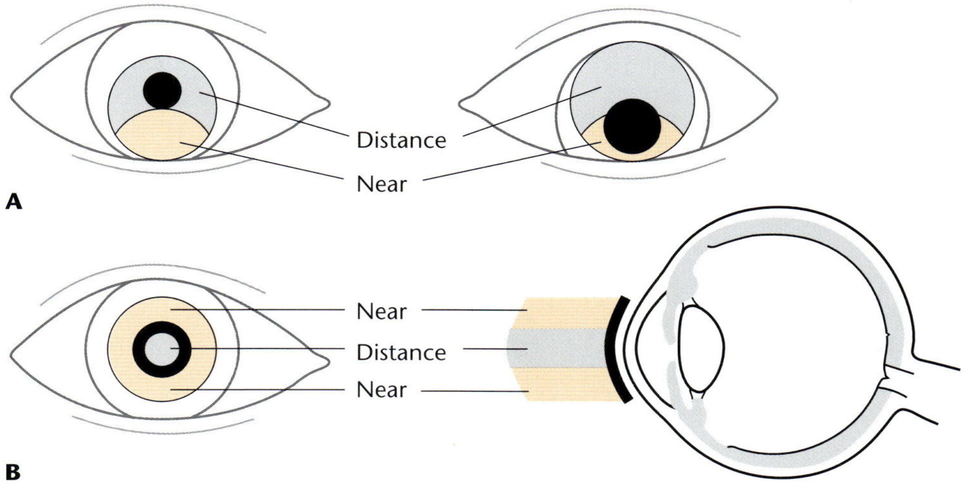

Bifocal contact lens. (A) For alternating vision, the distance segment is positioned over the pupil (left); as the patient looks down toward the reading position, the lower lid pushes up the contact lens so that the near segment covers the pupil for reading (right). (B) For simultaneous vision, the distance (or near) optical portion of the lens is made smaller than the pupil so that light rays from both distance and near pass through the pupil simultaneously. The lens wearer chooses either the central portion of the contact lens for distance vision or the peripheral portion for near vision.

vision or simultaneous vision in which the wearer "chooses" either distance or near (Figure 14.7). Bifocal contact lenses have numerous drawbacks, such as poor vision at distance or near, ghosting of images, and halos or flaring around headlights at night. Such drawbacks have led to these lenses' limited use. The most successful presbyopic contact lens correction occurs using monovision, in which one eye (usually the dominant eye) is focused at distance and the other eye at near.

Keratoconus Lenses

Keratoconus is a progressive thinning and cone-like protrusion of the cornea. How and why keratoconus occurs remain unknown. This condition most often affects both eyes, but one eye can have a more advanced cone than the other eye. Most patients with keratoconus are fitted with specially designed RGP lenses for the irregular astigmatism associated with the condition and for the stable refractive surface this type of lens provides.

Therapeutic Lenses

Soft contact lenses can serve as therapy for various ocular problems. Soft contact lenses can be used as "bandage lenses" to cover damaged or painful corneas. They provide therapeutic covers for abrasions or recurrent corneal epithelial breakdowns and protect exposed nerve endings present in corneal bullous edema. Soft contact lenses can also operate as a vehicle to deliver high concentrations of drugs to the cornea. Both rigid and soft contact lenses have been used for occlusion and patching to treat amblyopia or to eliminate diplopia.

CARE OF CONTACT LENSES

The most important aspect of contact lens care is to minimize bacterial contamination. To ensure that patients achieve clear vision and wear their lenses safely and comfortably, all contact lenses require cleaning so that the lens surface remains free of mucus and other debris. Contact lenses also require disinfection to remove contaminants and, in some cases, the use of lubricating ("wetting") and soaking solutions. Patients must understand that the lenses should feel comfortable when placed in the eye after a suitable period of adjustment. Discomfort may signal a poor lens fit or may be caused by a lens that needs cleaning or lubrication, or that is torn, chipped, or spoiled beyond repair. Numerous cleaning, disinfecting, and lubricating solutions exist for lens care. Contact lens wearers should be instructed in appropriate lens care and urged to read their lens manufacturer's printed recommendations and the labels of lens care solutions carefully to ensure that the solutions they use are compatible with the type of lens they wear.

FIGURE 14.8

Surface deposits that collect on a contact lens surface may not be visible to the patient but show up when the ophthalmologist views the lens in place by the light of a slit lamp.

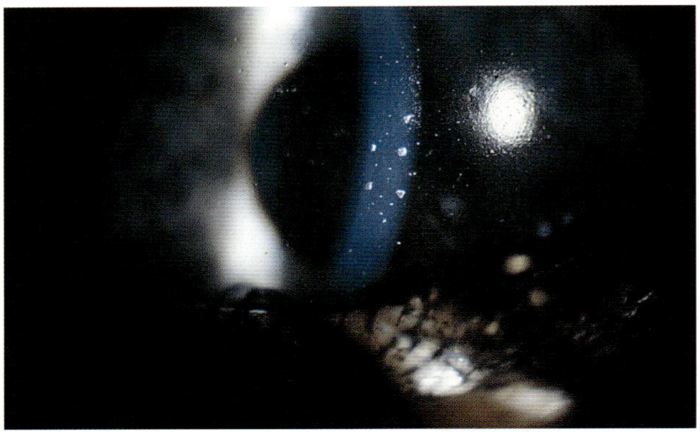

Cleaning

Contact lens wearers must understand that deposits of protein and other debris can form on their lenses, although this matter may be invisible to the patient (Figure 14.8). If not removed by cleaning, the deposits can become thick, blur vision, and/or irritate the eye when the lenses are worn and can serve as a reservoir for microorganisms. Some people develop deposits on their contact lenses rapidly; others rarely do.

Lens cleaning requires using **surfactant cleaners** (specially designed detergents) and rubbing the lens with clean fingers. Surfactant cleaners are designed to help remove surface deposits, thereby increasing clarity of vision and reducing irritation caused by coated lenses. Because foreign deposits can interfere with the disinfecting step of lens care, **enzyme cleaners** have been specifically developed to remove accumulated protein deposits.

Disinfection

Disinfection is a critical step in contact lens care because it prevents organisms such as bacteria, viruses, and fungi from growing. Any of these organisms may cause a potentially blinding infection of the cornea. Two methods are commonly used for disinfecting contact lenses:

- Chemicals with antimicrobial action, such as hydrogen peroxide, thimerosal, chlorhexidine, quaternary ammonium compounds, BAK (benzalkonium chloride; not for soft lenses), and PAPB (para-aminopolybiguanide)
- Heat, which is less popular but more effective (for soft lenses only, although heat can damage certain hydrophilic lenses that have a high water content)

Some patients have sensitivity reactions to at least one, but usually not all, of the preservatives or disinfectants used in contact lens solutions. These problems are discussed later in this chapter. Both PMMA and RGP lenses are less susceptible than soft lenses to contamination and are easier to clean and disinfect.

Ophthalmic medical assistants who handle trial contact lenses in the office should keep abreast of current procedures for the care of contact lenses with reference to persons infected with the human immunodeficiency virus (HIV), which causes acquired immunodeficiency syndrome (AIDS).

Lubrication

Lubricants, or wetting/cushioning solutions, are used by contact lens wearers to keep the lens surface hydrophilic. These solutions act like a cushion between the contact lens and the cornea and between the lens and the eyelid. Patients may wish to use lubricants when they insert their contact lenses, but usually their own tears perform the cushioning function. It is important to note that patient's saliva should never be used to wet contact lenses because of the possibility of infection.

Storage

The ophthalmic medical assistant should make certain the contact lenses stored in the office remain in a clean, ready-to-wear condition. Contact lenses that have been tried on but not dispensed should be cleaned, disinfected appropriately, and returned to the fitting sets. Rigid contact lenses should be stored in individual containers with the proper storage solutions or in a dry state, according to the ophthalmologist's instructions. Soft contact lenses should be cleaned with surfactant cleaners, disinfected with heat or chemical solutions, and kept in individual sealed containers. Be sure that patients understand appropriate similar storage methods for their lenses at home. Patients should store their lenses in the contact lens case that is recommended by the ophthalmologist and should be instructed to clean and dry the case daily and replace it at intervals recommended by the doctor.

INSERTION AND REMOVAL OF CONTACT LENSES

An important part of the dispensing of both soft and rigid contact lenses is the instruction to the patient, by the ophthalmic medical assistant, on how to insert and remove the lenses. The insertion and removal of soft and rigid lenses require different techniques. These methods are best learned by experience, but the basic principles for insertion and removal apply. Clean hands, appropriate solutions, near-sterile techniques, and clean containers are prerequisites for both lens types.

Soft Lenses

Although there are variations in technique, in general the soft contact lens is placed below the cornea on the lower white of the eye (sclera) and gently positioned onto the cornea by massaging through the

INSERTING SOFT LENSES

Instruct the patient to insert a soft contact lens as follows:

1. Wash your hands and dry them with a lint-free towel. Be sure all traces of soap are rinsed off.
2. Remove the clean lens for the right eye from the case with your clean finger or pour the contents of the contact lens vial into the palm of your hand, allowing the solution to drain between your fingers into the sink.
3. Rinse the lens with an FDA-approved saline solution. If you do this over a sink, placing a stopper or drain plug perforated with small holes over the drain opening can prevent the lens from being accidentally washed down the drain.
4. Place the lens on the tip of a dry index finger or middle finger of your dominant hand. You may allow the lens to dry for 10 to 20 seconds in the air until it "rounds up"; thicker lenses require little or no drying. Check the lens contour to be sure it is not inside out.
5. With small lenses, look up, pull down the lower lid with the middle or third finger of the hand holding the lens, and, while looking upward, place the lens onto the lower sclera (see the figure). Larger lenses are best placed directly on the central cornea by holding the upper lid up with the opposite hand.
6. Express any air under the lens by pressing gently, remove your index finger, and gently release the lower lid.
7. Carefully close your eyes and center the lens by lightly massaging the lower eyelid of the eye that is closed over the contact lens.
8. Repeat steps 1 through 7 for the left lens.

When inserting or removing a soft lens from a patient's eye, the ophthalmic medical assistant should follow all steps outlined above while the patient performs the ocular movement; that is, the patient looks up and closes the eye, and the ophthalmic medical assistant holds the lens, places it on the sclera, compresses the lens between the thumb and index finger, and removes it. At all times, both patient and assistant should conduct these procedures only with thoroughly washed and dried hands. In addition, ophthalmic medical assistants should keep their fingernails short and their hands free of lotions, oils, and soap residues.

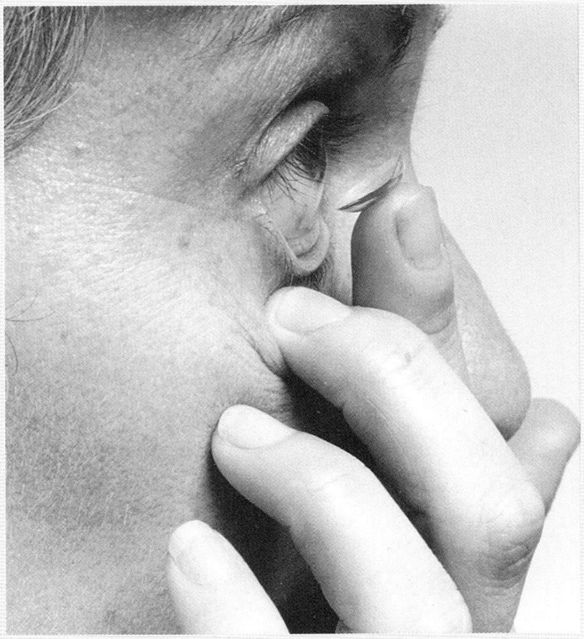

REMOVING SOFT LENSES

Instruct the patient to remove a soft lens as follows:

1. Wash your hands and dry them with a lint-free towel. Be sure all traces of soap are rinsed off.
2. To make certain the lens is in place on the cornea, check that the eye's vision is clear by gazing at a distant object with the opposite eye covered.
3. Begin with your right eye. Look up, then pull down the lower lid with your middle or third finger and place your index finger on the lower edge of the lens.
4. Move the lens down to the sclera.
5. Compress the lens between your thumb and index or middle finger to break the suction (see the figure).
6. Remove the lens from your eye.
7. Clean the lens appropriately and place it in the case for disinfection. Be sure to place the right contact lens in the compartment of the lens case marked "right."
8. Repeat steps 1 through 7 for the left lens.

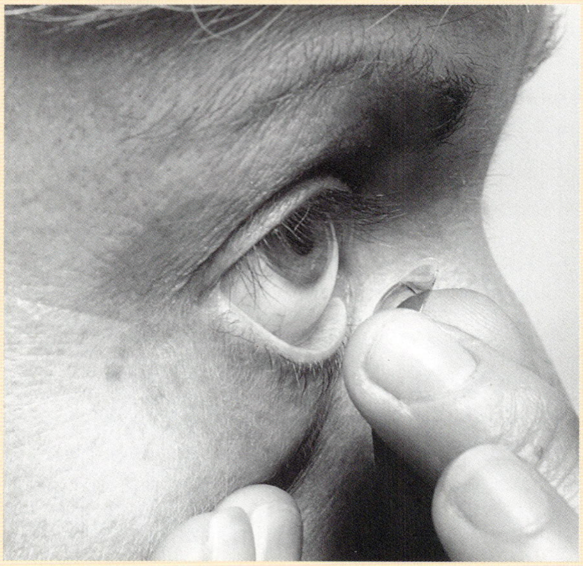

lower eyelid. To remove the soft contact lens, the lens is first decentered by sliding it with the index finger to the lower sclera and is then pinched off the eye. The boxes "Inserting Soft Lenses" (page 225) and "Removing Soft Lenses" (above) describe these actions in detail. Many equally effective techniques appear in contact lens booklets accompanying solution kits.

Rigid Lenses

As opposed to most soft lenses, which are placed on the sclera and massaged into place, rigid lenses must be placed directly on the cornea. Because they are not flexible, rigid lenses are removed by pulling aside an eyelid and blinking, which makes them pop out. Details of these procedures are presented in the boxes "Inserting Rigid Lenses" (right) and "Removing Rigid Lenses" (page 228).

An alternative method for inserting and removing a rigid contact lens uses a special suction cup. This procedure is best performed by the ophthalmic medical assistant rather than by the patient, because the patient could accidentally apply the suction cup to the cornea and cause an abrasion. An ophthalmologist or a senior technician in your office can demonstrate the use of the suction cup to you. The ophthalmic medical assistant should at all times conduct these procedures with thoroughly washed and dried hands, keep fingernails trimmed, and be sure hands are free of hand lotions, oils, and soap residues.

PROBLEMS WITH CONTACT LENSES

Because the ophthalmologist treats problems that can occur with the use of contact lenses, the ophthalmic medical assistant should recognize and understand the symptoms and causes of the difficulties that are typically seen in contact lens wearers in order to assist the ophthalmologist. Ophthalmic medical assistants play an important role in educating patients in the prevention of these problems, in alerting patients to the danger signals of potential problems, and in encouraging patients to comply with appropriate lens care and wear.

The ophthalmic medical assistant should instruct all patients to remove their contact lenses and call

INSERTING RIGID LENSES

Instruct the patient to insert a rigid contact lens as follows:

1. Wash your hands and dry them with a lint-free towel. Be sure all traces of soap are rinsed off.
2. Begin with the right eye. Using an approved sterile solution, rinse off the storage solution from the clean rigid lens and wet it with the appropriate wetting solution.
3. Use your right hand for inserting the right contact lens and your left hand for the left lens, or, if more comfortable and natural, use your dominant hand for both eyes.
4. Position the lens concave side up on the tip of your index or middle finger.
5. Look straight down, place your chin on your chest, and keep both eyes open.
6. Hold your upper lid at the eyelash margin with the finger of the opposite hand, pressing up against the brow. Hold the lower lid at the eyelash margin with the third or fourth finger of the hand that is holding the lens and press down against the cheek (see the figure).
7. Bring the finger holding the lens directly up to the eye until the lens comes in contact with the cornea of the eye (see the figure). This is facilitated by staring with the other eye at a convenient straight-ahead target and keeping the eye open.
8. Immediately release the lower lid and then slowly release the upper lid.
9. Cover the opposite eye and check vision to be certain the lens has been inserted.
10. Repeat steps 1 through 9 for the left lens.

As with soft lenses, when the ophthalmic medical assistant inserts or removes a rigid contact lens from the patient's eye, all steps of each procedure should be conducted with the patient performing the ocular movements and the ophthalmic medical assistant's fingers placing the contact lens on the cornea or, in the case of contact lens removal, moving the eyelid and retrieving the lens into the cupped hand as the patient blinks.

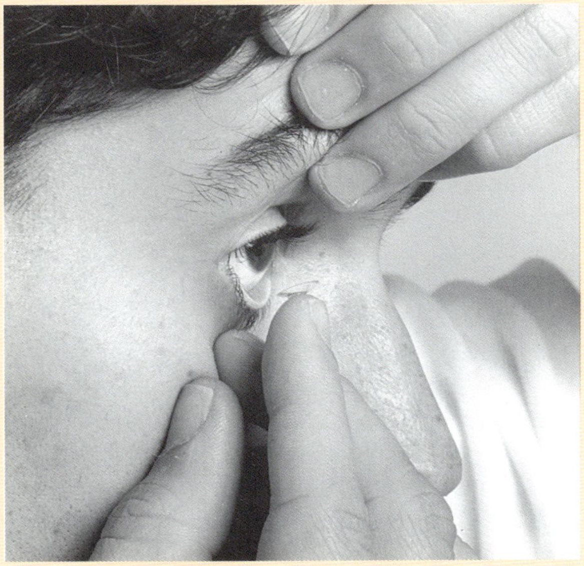

the ophthalmologist's office whenever they experience the following symptoms:

- Redness in the eye
- Increased light sensitivity
- Watery or tearing eye
- Discharge from the eye
- Blurred or decreased vision
- Pain or burning

Allergy

About 10% to 20% of contact lens wearers have sensitivity reactions to at least one (but usually not all) of the preservative or disinfectant chemicals used in contact lens solutions. Such allergic reactions occur more often among soft lens wearers. In a hypersensitivity reaction, the patient may complain of irritation, fogging, redness, tearing, and decreased wearing time within days to months after using the solution containing the offending chemical. The preservative

REMOVING RIGID LENSES

Instruct the patient to remove a rigid contact lens as follows:

1. Wash your hands and dry them with a lint-free towel. Be sure all traces of soap are removed.
2. Begin with your right eye.
3. To be sure the lens is centered on the eye, check for clear vision by gazing at a distant object. If not centered, manipulate the lens gently through the lid to center it on the cornea.
4. Look down and cup your left hand under your right eye to catch the lens (see the figure).
5. Place your right forefinger on the outer corner of the eyelid and pull the upper lid aside toward the upper ear as you blink. The lens will pop out (see the figure). If it slides off the cornea, slide it back before again attempting removal.
6. Clean the lens and place it in an appropriate disinfectant solution in the case or store it clean and dry in a cleaned case. Be sure to place the right lens in the compartment of the contact lens case marked "right."
7. Repeat steps 1 through 6 for the left eye.

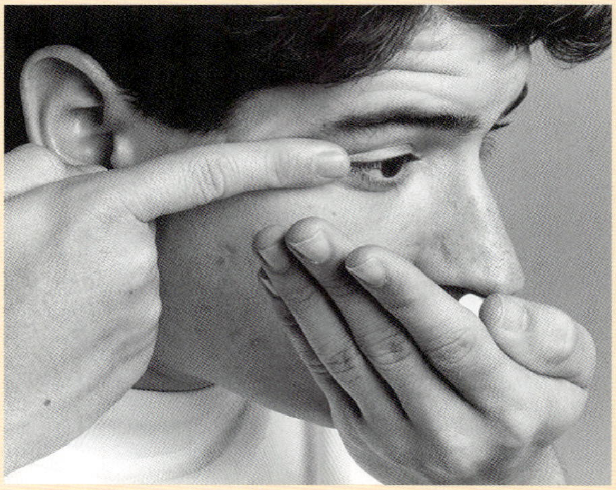

thimerosal most commonly causes this type of allergic reaction. Other preservatives implicated in solution sensitivities include sorbic acid, chlorhexidine, and ethylenediaminetetraacetic acid (EDTA). The diagnosis of a sensitivity reaction to a preservative agent is confirmed when the signs and symptoms disappear after the patient uses a solution free of the offending chemical. Currently, most soft lens saline solutions are sold as "preservative-free," but these should be used as rinses since they are not "disinfecting."

Overwearing Syndrome

Overwearing syndrome, as its name suggests, usually results from wearing a PMMA contact lens longer than recommended and is caused by inadequate amounts of oxygen reaching the cornea. Symptoms and signs of the overwearing syndrome include moderate to severe eye pain, lid swelling, tearing, and marked light sensitivity. The pain can be very intense, usually occurring 2 to 3 hours after removal of the lens. Upon examination with fluorescein, the cornea of the affected eye shows diffuse fluorescein staining over its central area. Topical anesthetic drops instilled by the ophthalmologist into the eye immediately stop the pain but are never given to patients to use on their own, because patients may unknowingly allow severe injury or even permanent damage to occur to the anesthetized eye.

Overwearing syndrome usually responds within about 24 hours to an analgesic for pain, and a short-acting cycloplegic to relieve ciliary spasm. The eye is usually not patched. Occasionally, non-preserved lubricating drops are necessary to treat the keratitis. Although symptoms can resolve overnight or within a day, the actual healing can take up to several days. Overwearing syndrome can be largely avoided by ensuring that patients are properly instructed in their contact lens wearing schedule.

Improper Lens Fit

A contact lens that fits improperly can produce discomfort and blurred vision. It may even lead to corneal abrasions and/or corneal edema, both of which can promote corneal infections.

A loose-fitting lens may cause variable visual acuity because the lens moves too much and thus the optical portion of the contact lens may not always cover the visual axis. A loose fit can be corrected by providing the patient with a lens that is larger, has a steeper curvature, or both. Excessive movement of a loose hard lens can also result in a corneal abrasion.

Alternatively, a tight-fitting contact lens causes a stagnation of tears because of lack of movement of the lens. This can lead to corneal edema from oxygen deprivation. A tight lens should be replaced with a lens that is smaller, flatter in curvature, or both. With a steeply curved contact lens, vision is usually clear right after a blink and then fades. The examiner may see an indentation on the white of the eye in a patient wearing a tightly fitting soft contact lens. The lens does not move easily and the eye becomes irritated as the patient continues to wear the lens.

An improperly fit rigid contact lens can result in a semipermanent change in the corneal curvature, called *warping*. This problem can be treated by refitting the contact lens correctly.

Irritation and Tearing

Irritation, often described by the patient as "the eye doesn't feel right," may be due to early lens deposits or tiny particles trapped by the lens. A contact lens patient reporting occasional mild eye irritation or tearing can often safely be instructed to remove and clean the contact lens, then reinsert it. If the irritation was due to dust, particles, or something temporary, the symptoms probably will not recur. If the symptoms persist, an examination by the doctor may be warranted.

Corneal Problems

Wearing lenses too long, wearing lenses that have been improperly cleaned and disinfected, wearing damaged lenses, wearing spoiled lenses, and wearing lenses that do not fit properly are the principal causes of the majority of contact lens problems. Acting singly or together, these factors and certain others can lead to a variety of corneal problems.

Corneal edema, or swelling, occurs because of a lack of oxygen to the cornea (Figure 14.9). In addition to overwear and improper lens hygiene and fit, the use of a lens material that does not allow sufficient corneal oxygenation will cause edema. Improving tear exchange or oxygen penetration can help reduce or overcome this problem. With rigid contact lenses, flattening the lens curve can allow better tear exchange; when soft lenses are being used, they may be exchanged for a type that is flatter, smaller, thinner, or of higher water content. Corneal edema needs to be remedied promptly before it leads to permanent corneal injury. Corneal edema is usually visible with slit-lamp examination, but early cases may require pachymetry for diagnosis.

Corneal vascularization, an ingrowth of superficial or deep blood vessels into the cornea, is another serious sign of corneal oxygen deprivation (Figure 14.10). It requires prompt adjustment of the causative factor, whether lens fit, improper hygiene, or wearing schedule.

FIGURE 14.9

Corneal edema (swelling) occurs from poor oxygenation under the contact lens. Compare the swollen cornea (A) with the appearance of a normal cornea (B). (Part A courtesy of Thomas D. Lindquist, MD, PhD.)

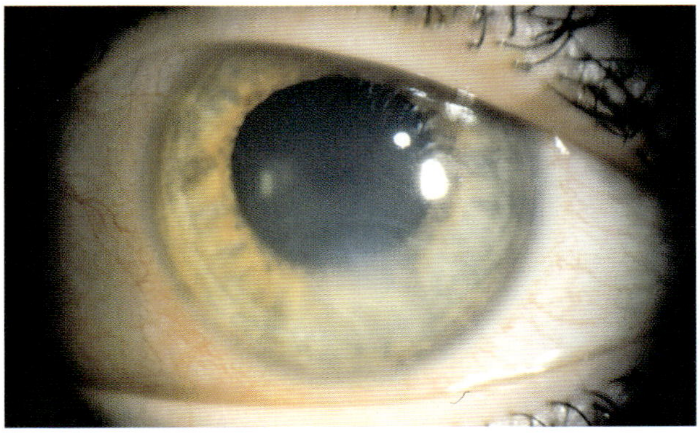

A

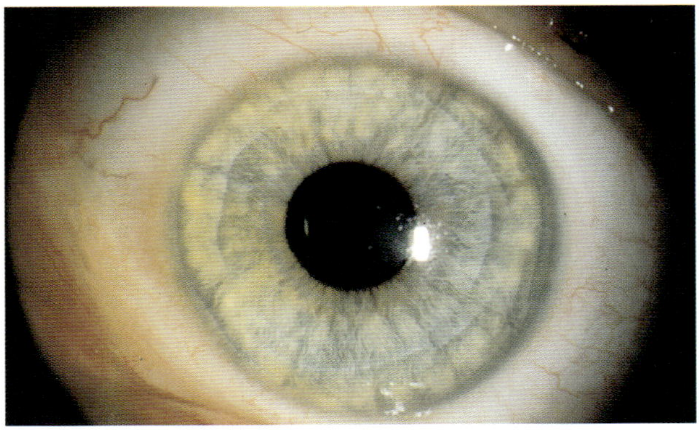

B

FIGURE 14.10

Slit-lamp view of corneal vascularization occurring from oxygen deprivation due to a poor-fitting soft contact lens. (Photo courtesy of Thomas D. Lindquist, MD, PhD.)

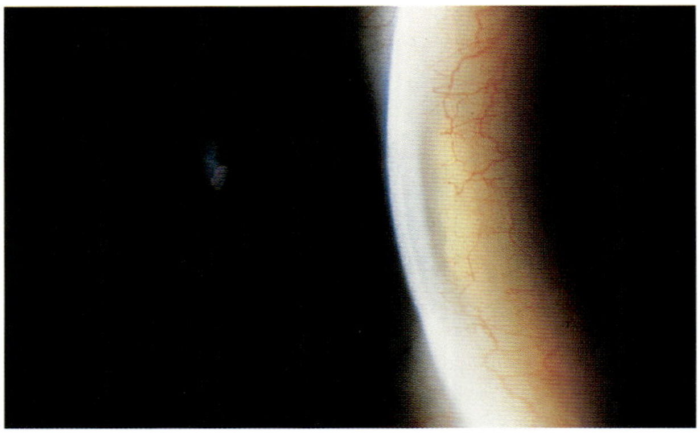

The most serious complication of improper lens wear or care is corneal ulcer, a defect in the corneal tissue usually accompanied by infection. Symptoms may include pain, redness, irritation, tearing, and diminished vision. The ophthalmologist may order laboratory smears or cultures made from corneal scrapings for diagnosis. Antimicrobial medications are used to treat corneal ulcers.

A corneal abrasion may occur not only from overwear or improper hygiene or fit but also from foreign material lodged between the contact lens and the cornea. This condition is extremely painful for rigid lens wearers, but the effects of the abrasion can be masked in soft lens wearers by the "bandage" effect of the soft lens itself. A corneal abrasion has the potential to become infected. Because reports have appeared in the ophthalmic literature of *Pseudomonas* corneal ulcers developing after a patch for what seemed to be a simple corneal abrasion in a contact lens wearer, today ophthalmologists consider all contact lens abrasions to be potentially infected and treat them with frequent topical antibiotics and cycloplegic agents, and do not patch the eye.

Corneal infections are severe complications of improper use of contact lenses, but they can be avoided by ensuring that patients are properly instructed in careful lens handling and maintenance and that scrupulous lens hygiene is also followed in the office. Because therapy for infections is sometimes limited, with resulting corneal scarring and decreased vision, prevention is most important. Preventing contact lens infections is the responsibility not only of the patient but also of the ophthalmologist and the ophthalmic medical assistant.

Pseudomonas aeruginosa is a serious pathogen in bacterial corneal ulcers in patients who wear either daily-wear or extended-wear contact lenses. Because these infections can progress rapidly, early recognition, diagnosis, and appropriate antibiotic treatment are imperative. *Acanthamoeba*, a microorganism found abundantly in soil and water, can produce serious, severely painful corneal infections. Corneal infections caused by this organism have been associated with the use of salt tablets and tap water or improperly sterilized distilled water for making a saline solution at home. Therefore, contact lens wearers must understand that they should never use homemade saline solutions, tap water, or distilled water to care for their soft lenses. In addition, they should avoid wearing their lenses in hot tubs or swimming pools, where this organism is found.

Giant Papillary Conjunctivitis

Giant papillary conjunctivitis (GPC) is characterized by large raised bumps called *papules* on the tarsal conjunctiva. Associated mainly with soft contact lenses, GPC can occasionally occur with rigid lenses. This condition can develop months to years after seemingly successful contact lens wear. Symptoms include ocular itching, foreign-body sensation, redness and mucus, and decreased lens wearing time. Considered an autoimmune response to the patient's own proteins on the contact lens or to the "trauma" of lens wear, GPC is treated by aggressive lens cleaning, change of lens materials, use of disposable lenses, and/or use of cromolyn 4% or lodoxamide 0.1% ocular drops.

Solution–Lens Interaction

Not all contact lens solutions are compatible with all materials used in contact lenses. The ophthalmic medical assistant must help ensure that each patient uses the proper and compatible solutions for the particular contact lens being dispensed. In addition, heat and certain chemical disinfectants may not work well together for a specific kind of lens. Chemical incompatibility can result in binding of the chemical to the lens materials, changes in lens parameters or oxygen permeability, discoloration, and other deleterious effects. Improper combinations of lenses and solutions can lead to ocular irritation, itching, tearing, hazy vision, redness, and a gritty feeling. The package inserts that come with the contact lenses and contact lens solutions explain in detail which lenses and which solutions are compatible. Always consult the lens and solution manufacturers' instructions before giving the patient information.

Inability to Insert or Remove Lenses

Patients may have difficulty inserting or removing their contact lenses, especially during the initial trial period of lens wear. Sometimes patients become panicky if their first attempts fail, making the situation worse. The ophthalmic medical assistant can best assist the patient by providing calming advice. For most individuals, taking a few minutes to rest and relax before retrying leads to success. When teaching patients proper lens insertion and removal techniques, remind them to remain relaxed and not to panic. If patients are truly unable to remove the contact lens, they should immediately see the ophthalmologist or seek emergency room care.

Lens "Lost" in Eye

It is impossible for a contact lens to be truly lost in the eye because the conjunctiva, which lines both the globe and the inner lid, prevents the lens from disappearing behind the eye. On rare occasions, a patient may displace a lens into the cul-de-sac or to the side of the eye. In the office, fluorescein drops may aid in locating a "lost" soft contact lens. If the "lost" lens is a rigid type, careful office examination and double eversion of the upper lid will assist in finding the lens. Rigid lenses can often be located and removed by the patient, but soft lenses may fold or tear in the eye and become lodged in the superior cul-de-sac, requiring in-office removal.

CONTRAINDICATIONS FOR CONTACT LENSES

The term **contraindication** describes any condition that renders a particular treatment, medication, or medical device inadvisable because complications or adverse effects may result. Patient-related complications from contact lens wear can be overcome by considering the possible complications and taking steps to prevent them before fitting the patient with a contact lens. A thorough ocular history and a total ocular examination by the ophthalmologist must be completed, with special emphasis on the lids, conjunctiva, cornea, and tears, as well as inquiries into the possible history of allergies and the success or failure of previous contact lens wear. Emphasis should be placed on inquiring about the patient's commitment to compliance and dedication to proper contact lens wear and care.

Even with care to avoid complications, some patients who desire contact lenses may be poor candidates for their use. The ophthalmologist may choose to discourage these patients from wearing contact lenses in order to avert potentially serious eye problems. The following list of contact lens contraindications names conditions and characteristics of patients who are likely to have a lower rate of success in contact lens wear.

- Individuals with certain ocular pathologic conditions (for example, severe allergies, chronic blepharoconjunctivitis, pterygium, seventh-nerve paresis, or anesthetic cornea)
- Those who have inappropriate nervous and emotional temperaments
- People who have poor or no blink reflexes
- Those with dry eyes (because all contact lenses require adequate tear production)
- Persons with disability conditions such as parkinsonism (tremor) or arthritis (deformed hands), which make insertion and removal of contact lenses difficult
- Those in certain occupations that expose workers to dusty, dirty, or particulate environments or to caustic chemicals in the air

REVIEW QUESTIONS

1. Briefly describe how a contact lens provides a new refractive surface for the cornea and corrects refractive error.
2. Name the four objectives that a contact lens must meet to maintain the health of the cornea.
3. Name at least five elements that may be required in determining the specification of a contact lens.
4. Match the type of contact lens with the most appropriate possible use.

    ____ cosmetic restorative

    ____ cosmetic fashion

    ____ therapeutic

    ____ toric

    a. Corrects astigmatic error
    b. Acts as a prosthetic device for a disfigured eye
    c. Enhances or changes iris color
    d. Corrects irregular astigmatism associated with keratoconus
    e. Corrects both near and distance vision
    f. "Bandages" a damaged or painful cornea
5. Briefly describe the different methods by which soft lenses, PMMA hard lenses, and RGP hard lenses provide oxygenation to the cornea.
6. Briefly compare the purpose of contact lens cleaning with the purpose of contact lens disinfection.
7. Name the two most common methods of disinfecting contact lenses.
8. What are the purposes of a contact lens lubricant, or wetting solution?
9. What is the first step to take in inserting a contact lens?
10. Name five symptoms that may indicate an allergic or sensitivity reaction to a contact lens solution.
11. Define and state the cause of warping caused by contact lenses.
12. Name the five principal types of corneal problems that may occur in contact lens wearers.
13. Why is it impossible for a contact lens to become "lost" behind the eye?
14. Name at least three possible contraindications for contact lens use.

SUGGESTED ACTIVITIES

1. Ask permission to observe several contact lens fittings for a variety of types of patients. Take notes and ask questions in a later meeting with the ophthalmologist or the technician overseeing the fitting.
2. Talk to friends, family, or patients who wear or have worn contact lenses to understand the advantages and disadvantages of their use.
3. With your ophthalmologist's permission and under supervision, try on a set of contact lenses yourself to appreciate your patients' reactions. Follow the steps for insertion and removal outlined in this chapter.

4. On your next trip to a pharmacy, visit the contact lens solutions section. Discuss the many choices of contact lens solutions with the pharmacist or your ophthalmologist so that you can better advise patients.
5. Under supervision of the ophthalmologist or an experienced technician in your office, practice cleaning and disinfecting the trial lenses used in your ophthalmologist's practice.

SUGGESTED RESOURCES

Cassin B: *Fundamentals for Ophthalmic Technical Personnel.* Philadelphia: WB Saunders Co; 1995; chap 23.

Extended Wear of Contact Lenses. Information Statement. Revised. San Francisco: American Academy of Ophthalmology; 1997.

Freeman MI: Selecting rigid versus soft contact lenses. *Ophthalmol Clin North Am* 1989;2:229–234.

Freeman MI, Rakow PL, Campbell RC: *Basic Principles of Contact Lens Fitting.* Clinical Skills videotape. San Francisco: American Academy of Ophthalmology; 1993. Reviewed for currency: 1999.

Kastl PR, ed: *Contact Lenses: The CLAO Guide to Basic Science and Clinical Practice.* 3rd ed. Dubuque, IA: Kendall/Hunt Publishing Co; 1995.

Key JE, ed: *The CLAO Pocket Guide to Contact Lens Fitting.* New Orleans: Contact Lens Association of Ophthalmologists; 1994.

Mackie IA: *Medical Contact Lens Practice.* Boston: Butterworth-Heinemann; 1993.

Stein HA, ed: *CLAO Home Study Course for Contact Lens Technicians.* 3rd ed. New York: CLAO Home Study Course Corp; 2001.

Stein HA, Freeman MI, Stein RM, Maund LD: *Contact Lenses: Fundamentals and Clinical Use.* Thorofare, NJ: Slack; 1997.

Stein HA, Slatt BJ, Stein RM: *Fitting Guide for Rigid and Soft Contact Lenses: A Practical Approach.* 4th ed. St Louis: Mosby; 2002.

Stein HA, Slatt BJ, Stein RM: *The Ophthalmic Assistant: A Guide for Ophthalmic Medical Personnel.* 7th ed. St Louis: Mosby; 2000.

Appendix A: Care of Ophthalmic Lenses and Instruments

Ophthalmic medical practice today employs a large variety of instruments and equipment, both hand-held and freestanding, to diagnose and treat patients with eye disorders. Whether ophthalmic medical assistants use such equipment themselves or not, they often have the responsibility of caring for, maintaining, and performing minor servicing of ophthalmic equipment in the office. These duties may include cleaning lenses and equipment, protecting instruments from dust and damage, replacing light bulbs and fuses, and performing minor adjustments and selective calibration.

Many of the lenses and instruments used in the modern ophthalmology practice are delicate and costly. In addition, these items must remain clean and in good condition to best perform their diagnostic or other medical function. It is important to observe certain precautions in keeping them clean and in proper working order, not only to protect the instruments themselves but also to protect patients from infection caused by microorganisms left on unclean equipment. This appendix presents general guidelines for the care of lenses and selected instruments, including special cautions to observe and techniques to employ for their handling, cleaning, and maintenance.

CARE OF LENSES

Lenses, whether hand-held or incorporated into instruments, whether contact or noncontact, comprise a significant portion of the diagnostic equipment in an ophthalmology office. All optical lenses used in the ophthalmic practice must be free of dust, dirt, fingerprints, and oils to perform correctly. However, careless cleaning can mar the anti-reflective coating on ocular instrument lenses or even ruin a precision optical lens. In addition, not all lenses and mirrored optical surfaces can be cleaned safely.

The general guidelines below apply to the care of all types of diagnostic lenses in the ophthalmology office. They are followed by more specific information pertaining to contact and noncontact diagnostic lenses and their care.

Standard Care Guidelines

- To ensure that a given lens can be cleaned safely, always consult the lens manufacturer's instructions or your office policy before attempting a cleaning procedure.
- Never rub a dry lens; dragging abrasive dust or dirt across a lens surface can scratch it. Always use wet friction or, if liquid cleaners cannot be used, remove dust by blowing or brushing it off.
- Use only those cleaning fluids that are approved by the lens manufacturer or by your office policy. Inappropriate cleaning fluids can scratch and permanently damage a lens.
- Use only special lens-cleaning paper, cotton balls, or soft lint-free ophthalmic cloths. Avoid using ordinary tissue papers, paper towels, cloths with high lint content, nylon, and handkerchiefs, which can be abrasive enough to scratch the lens surface; plastic lenses are particularly easy to scratch in this way.

Lenses That Do Not Contact the Eye

Examples of lenses that do not contact the eye are the Hruby lens, condensing lenses, and hand-held fundus lenses used in conjunction with a slit lamp.

The **Hruby lens** is a –55 diopter lens attached to the slit lamp (Figure A.1). It allows careful magnified binocular study and examination of the vitreous and central fundus. To avoid accidental damage, always return the Hruby lens to its storage position on the side of the slit lamp after use.

FIGURE A.1

Hruby lens in use.

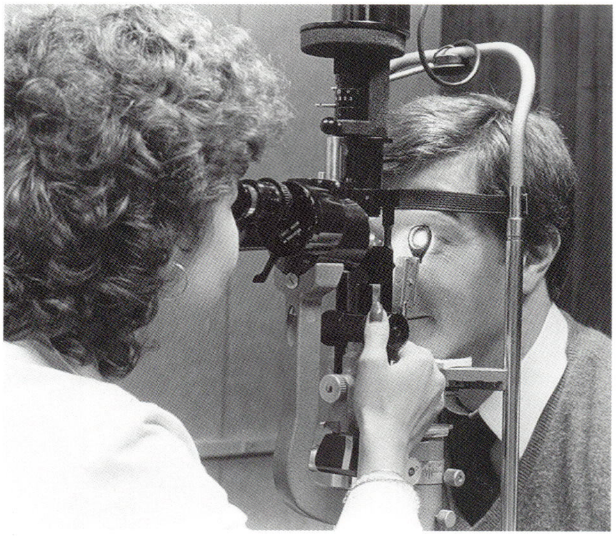

FIGURE A.2

Condensing lens.

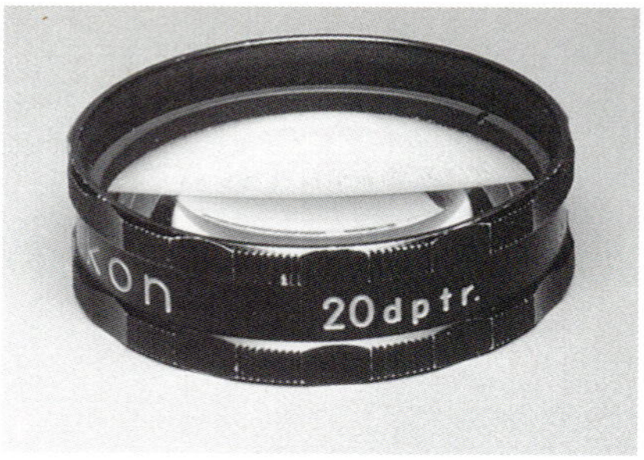

Condensing lenses, also known as *aspheric* or *panretinal viewing lenses*, are hand-held, noncontact biconvex lenses available in powers of +14 to +40 diopters (Figure A.2). Condensing lenses are used to view the ocular fundus as a real, inverted image in conjunction with the indirect ophthalmoscope.

Hand-held, noncontact **funduscopic lenses** of +60, +78, and +90 diopters are used in conjunction with the slit lamp for stereoscopic observation of the fundus within various fields of vision and under magnification.

Although individual types of lenses require specialized care, the standard care guidelines presented above may be applied to most hand-held and instrument lenses, optical filters, and other highly polished glass surfaces (including coated lenses) that do not come into contact with the patient's eye. The box

CLEANING LENSES THAT DO NOT CONTACT THE EYE

1. Remove dust from lenses or mirrors that cannot be cleaned with a liquid by blowing it off with a dry, empty bulb syringe or with a blast of air from a can of commercial compressed air or by brushing it off gently with a photographic lens brush or a loosely wadded lens-cleaning paper.
2. Remove fingerprints or oils from cleanable glass and polymethylmethacrylate (PMMA) plastic lenses by moistening a cleaning paper, cotton ball, or lint-free cloth with a special photographic liquid lens cleaner and rubbing the lens surface gently, using a circular motion.
3. Be sure that all cleaning agents are completely removed from the lens surface. Leaving a residue on the lens can diminish its clarity and effectiveness.
4. Dry lenses with clean lens paper or a lint-free cloth.

Additional Tips

- Clean only the exposed front and back surfaces of a complex lens system. Never disassemble such a lens system; that procedure is reserved only for the instrument specialist or manufacturer's representative.
- Generally, thorough cleaning of optical mirrors in ophthalmic instruments is best left to professionals. For routine cleaning, a blast of air from a dry bulb syringe or from a can of commercial compressed air will usually suffice.
- Clean the trial lens set lenses, diagnostic lenses, and easily accessible phoropter lenses regularly. Do not wait until the ophthalmologist or other user becomes aware of a dirty lens.

"Cleaning Lenses That Do Not Contact the Eye" presents more detailed instructions for this procedure, as well as additional care tips.

Lenses That Contact the Eye

Examples of lenses that contact the eye include diagnostic contact lenses, such as the fundus lens, the goniolens, and the Koeppe lens (Figure A.3). They are used to examine the inner aspects of the eye with greater magnification, often in conjunction with the slit lamp or other magnification and illumination source.

Any lenses that come in contact with the patient's eye may become clouded with diagnostic solutions, smeared with eye make-up, or contaminated with ocular secretions that could become a source for the spread of infection. These lenses must be cleaned immediately after contact with the eye, generally by rinsing thoroughly with water to remove the contaminants. Lenses that contact the eye may also be either disinfected or sterilized. The appropriate procedure depends on the purpose of the lens (such as diagnostic or surgical), the type of lens, and the materials used in its manufacture. The boxes "Cleaning Lenses That Contact the Eye" and "Disinfecting Lenses That Contact the Eye" on page 238 present general instructions for these procedures. Guidelines for lens sterilization follow.

Lens Sterilization

Lenses usually do not need sterilization unless they have been grossly contaminated or will be used during surgery or on a recently operated eye. Generally,

FIGURE A.3

(Left to right) Fundus contact lens. Goniolens. Koeppe lens.

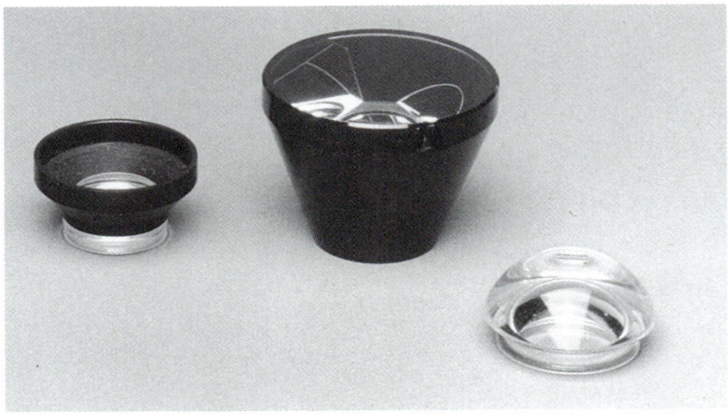

CLEANING LENSES THAT CONTACT THE EYE

1. Using a rotary motion, carefully wash the lens in lukewarm water with a moistened cotton ball that contains a few drops of clear dishwashing liquid.
2. Rinse the lens completely with lukewarm water.
3. Blot the lens dry using a lint-free lens-cleaning paper or a soft lint-free absorbent lens cloth.
4. Store the lens in a dry state in its original case.

DISINFECTING LENSES THAT CONTACT THE EYE

1. Soak the lens for either
   a. 10 minutes in a disinfecting solution such as 2% aqueous solution of glutaraldehyde, or
   b. 5 minutes in fresh 1:10 dilution of household bleach, or
   c. the length of time indicated on a prepackaged commercial disinfectant solution

   Note: To be sure the solution will not damage the lens, consult the lens and solution manufacturers' directions.
2. Remove the lens from the disinfecting solution and rinse thoroughly with cool running water to remove all residual disinfectant solution.
3. Blot the lens dry, using a lint-free lens-cleaning paper or a soft lint-free absorbent lens cloth.
4. Store the lens in a dry state in its original case.

lenses cannot be sterilized in an autoclave, but some made specifically for use in an operating room can be.

Some general guidelines concerning lens sterilization are as follows:

- Use ethylene oxide gas and nonheat aeration that does not exceed 125°F.
- Use the appropriate gas-sterilization container bags with safety markers to ensure complete sterilization, according to the operations manual of the sterilizer, and write on the sterilization bag the date that the sterilization will expire.
- Use the standard unit cycle and aeration time specified in the operations manual of the sterilizer.
- Do not use wood storage cases in the gas-sterilization process because wood will not be sterilized by the gas.
- For *glass* surgical lenses with stainless-steel components:
  a. Before sterilization, clean with soap and water to remove ocular secretions and debris.
  b. Sterilize the components with ethylene oxide or autoclave for 5 minutes at 270°F.
- For glass surgical lenses used during fluid–gas exchange procedures (such as intravitreal surgery):
  a. First make certain that any oil on the lens surface is removed by careful cleaning with soap and water.
  b. Next, fully rinse the lens, blot dry with lint-free lens-cleaning paper, and wipe with alcohol before placing the lens in the receptacle for sterilization.
- For ocular instrument lenses made of polymethylmethacrylate (PMMA):
  a. Never autoclave or boil.
  b. Never use cleaning agents such as acetone, alcohol, or peroxide.

TROUBLESHOOTING INSTRUMENT FAILURE

If an electrical instrument fails to work, check the following:

1. Is the instrument plugged into an electrical outlet?
2. Are all plugs and connections on the instrument securely in place?
3. Is the bulb burned out or darkened?
4. Is the instrument fuse burned out?
5. Are the central wall outlet and electrical fuse for the circuit functioning?

If a battery-powered instrument fails to work, check the following:

1. Is the battery fresh or recharged?
2. Is the bulb burned out or darkened?

CARE OF INSTRUMENTS

Ophthalmic medical assistants often clean electrical and battery-powered office instruments and perform simple maintenance, such as bulb replacement or minor calibration. The general guidelines below apply to the care and maintenance of all instruments in the ophthalmology office. The box "Troubleshooting Instrument Failure" provides a simple checklist to follow when an ophthalmic instrument fails to operate.

Standard Care Guidelines

- Read the operations manuals or the use and care guidelines for each piece of equipment you are responsible for, and keep the manuals in one place in the office. If some instruction manuals or user guides are missing, ask the optical company supplier or distributor or the instrument manufacturer directly to provide replacements.
- Check each instrument's user manual for instructions on the proper cleaning solutions and methods and follow the recommended procedures given.
- To prevent instrument optics or other delicate components from becoming dusty, dirty, or accidentally damaged, ensure that each instrument is in its storage or carrying case or protected with an individual dust cover when it is not in use.
- To avoid electrical shock, always disconnect an instrument from its power source before any servicing, even changing light bulbs or fuses.
- Bulbs and batteries and their replacement techniques vary by instrument. Always check the instrument user's manual for the correct bulb type, battery type, and replacement procedure.
- Because oil from fingers can etch an instrument bulb once it heats up, diminishing its effectiveness and life, always handle instrument bulbs with lens tissue paper. If you or someone else has handled an instrument bulb without using tissue paper, remove fingerprints from the bulb with photographic-lens cleaning fluid and lens tissue or a soft lint-free lens cloth.
- To avoid burning your fingers when servicing an instrument or replacing a bulb, make certain the instrument is turned off and the housing is cool. A recently burned-out bulb can be very hot; you may need to use a cloth to remove it.
- To maintain an adequate reserve of bulbs, batteries, and fuses for all instruments used in the office, check the office inventory of these and other supplies frequently and reorder as necessary. Keep these supplies handy and be sure their whereabouts are known so that replacement can be immediate.
- Turn off all instruments when they are not in use to prolong the life of bulbs and batteries. (This does not apply to instrument rechargers, which should be plugged in and/or turned on whenever the instrument needs charging.)

FIGURE A.4

Retinoscope.

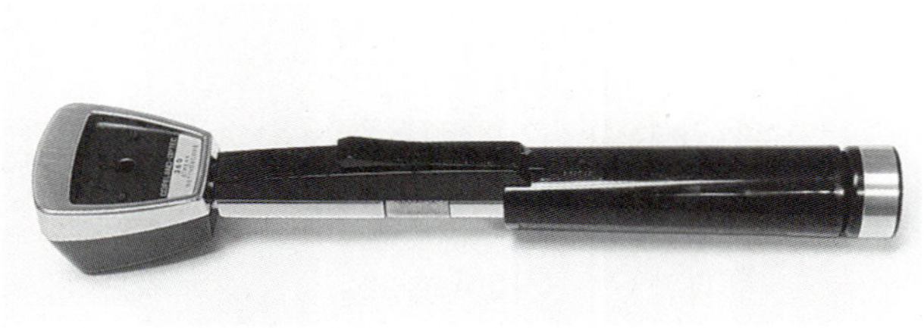

FIGURE A.5

Phoroptor.

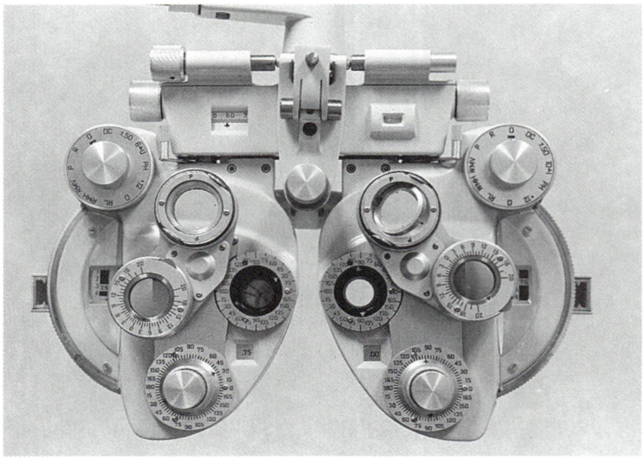

SELECTED OFFICE INSTRUMENTS

For protecting instruments from dust and damage, avoiding shock, and handling bulbs or batteries, follow the instructions given in the section "Standard Care Guidelines" earlier in this appendix. In addition, consult the manufacturer's guidelines for any special instructions concerning the cleaning and care of a specific instrument. This section briefly describes the major ophthalmic instruments, followed by any additional instructions or precautions for safe, effective operation that apply to the instrument.

Retinoscope

The retinoscope is a hand-held instrument used with either trial lens set lenses or the phoropter to define a patient's objective refractive error before beginning subjective tests. The instrument contains a light source in the handle and a mirrored light-projection and viewing system (Figure A.4). Most retinoscopes today are powered with batteries and rechargeable power packs.

Special Care and Cautions

- Clean the front surface of the mirror by blowing off dust with a dry, clean, empty bulb syringe.
- Always maintain an adequate supply of spare bulbs in the examining room.

Phoroptor

The Phoroptor, or manual refractor, is used in performing refraction/refractometry. A Phoroptor consists of a unit that holds a series of trial lenses, both spheres and cylinders, mounted on a wheel used to select lenses to place before the patient's eye (Figure A.5). The instrument includes built-in accessory lenses such as a pinhole, retinoscope lens, Maddox rod, Risley prism, polarizing lens, cross cylinder, and others to aid in measuring the refractive error of the eye.

Special Care and Cautions

- If your office has an American Optical (Reichert) Phoroptor, periodically wash the reusable nylon face shields with soap and water. The shields also may be disinfected by soaking for a few minutes in alcohol or disinfectant solution or boiling in water, then rinsed and allowed to air-dry. Other brands of manual refractors have disposable shields, which should be discarded after each patient use.
- Never put your finger into the lens aperture because you can get fingerprints on the Phoroptor's enclosed lenses.
- Clean the enclosed trial lenses by blowing off dust with a clean, dry, empty bulb syringe.
- Clean the accessory lenses located on the outside of the Phoroptor casing with a photographic-lens cleaner and lens tissue.
  a. If your office has an American Optical (Reichert) Phoroptor, clean only the back lenses (that is, the retinoscopic and polarizing

FIGURE A.6

Lensmeter.

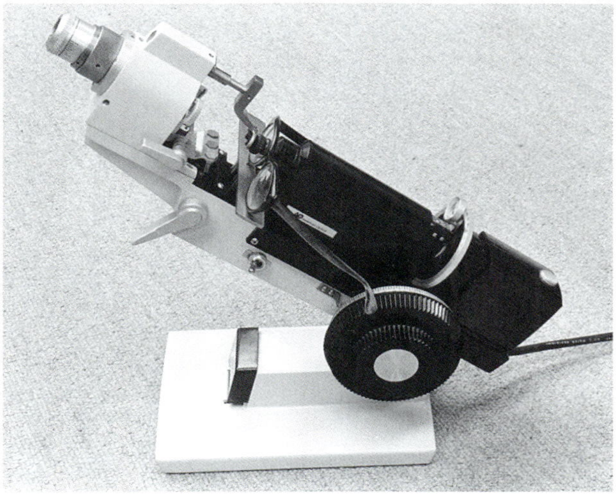

FIGURE A.7

Keratometer.

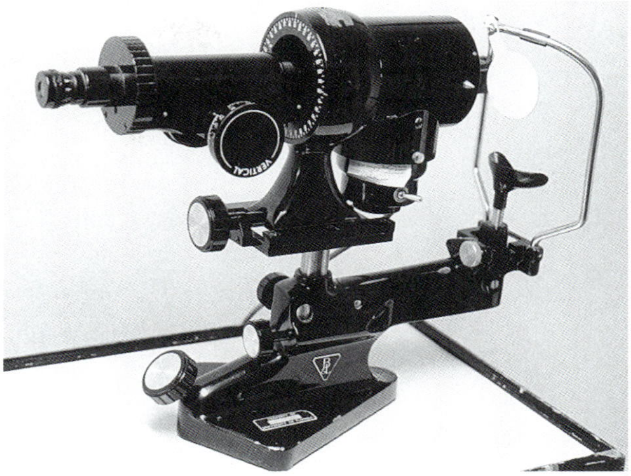

lenses) with photographic-lens cleaner and cotton-tipped swabs.

b. If your office has a Green's manual refractor, clean only the retinoscopic and +0.25-diopter lenses with photographic-lens cleaner and cot ton swabs. These lenses become soiled easily because they come in contact with the patient's eyelashes.

c. If your office has another brand of manual refractor, review the instruction manual to find out which accessory lenses you should clean.

- Schedule authorized maintenance service every 2 years to clean the internal trial lenses and to prevent any major malfunctions.
- Never use alcohol on any part of a Phoroptor.
- Never use cleaning solutions on the lens power numbers; clean only with a dry soft cloth.

Lensmeter

The lensmeter is used to determine the prescription of an eyeglass or contact lens. The lensmeter measures the spherical and cylindrical powers in diopters and can define the optical center of a lens, the axis of a cylindrical lens, the presence and direction of a lens prism, and the power of a bifocal or trifocal lens. The lensmeter unit includes a focusable eyepiece, lens holder, light source, and adjustment knobs (Figure A.6).

Special Care and Cautions

- If dust falls onto the surface of the lenses of the lensmeter, blow it off with a clean, dry rubber bulb syringe or compressed air.
- Wipe the instrument's enamel finish with a soft cloth occasionally to prevent dust from collecting.
- Do not attempt to lubricate the instrument. If it feels tight to the operator, call a qualified service technician.

Keratometer

The keratometer, or ophthalmometer, is used to measure corneal curvature objectively and to fit contact lenses (Figure A.7). It uses the mirror effect of the cornea's surface to measure the curvature of the central 3.3 mm of the anterior corneal surface in its two meridians.

Special Care and Cautions

- Check the lamp bulb for sooty carbon deposits, which can obscure the mirror image. Replace the bulb with a new bulb if these are present.
- Do not attempt to adjust the instrument if it seems out of alignment. Call an optical service technician to repair it.

FIGURE A.8

Slit lamp (biomicroscope).

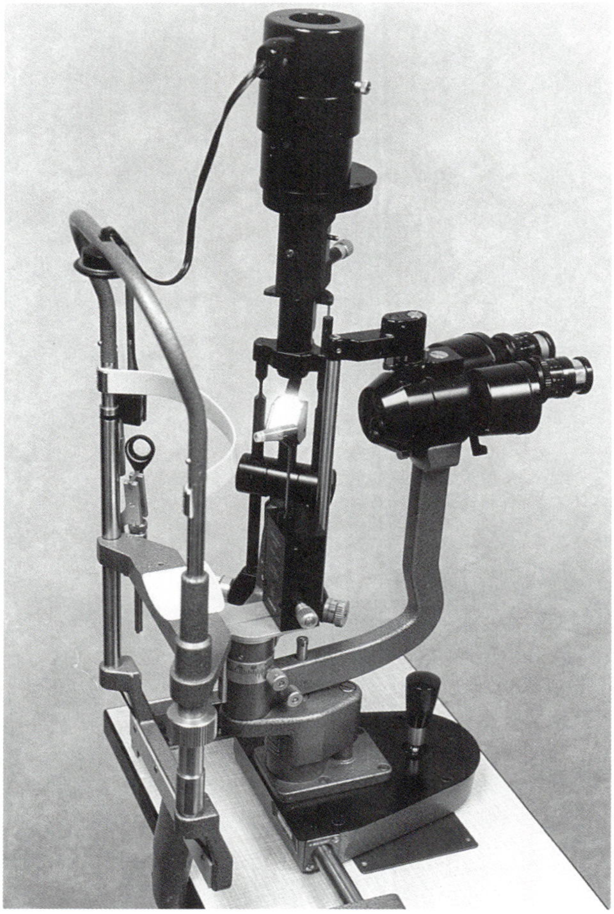

Slit Lamp

The slit lamp, or biomicroscope, combines a microscope and specialized illumination system that delivers a freely movable slit beam of light (Figure A.8). It provides a binocular, stereoscopic view of the cornea, sclera, and anterior segment of the eye (lens, iris, anterior chamber, and anterior vitreous) at magnification levels ranging from 10× to 40×. The instrument can also be used with additional lenses to examine more closely the chamber angle of the eye and the vitreous as well as the central and peripheral fundus. In addition, the slit lamp can function with a special instrument attachment to perform applanation tonometry.

Special Care and Cautions

- A blast of air or a lens brush is usually sufficient for routine maintenance of the mirror on a Haag-Streit type of slit lamp. If that doesn't work, try dusting and then wiping carefully with a soft lint-free cloth or chamois that will not scratch the mirror surface. If dirt remains, carefully spray the mirror with a photographic-glass cleaner. Wipe the surface dry with cotton balls, using downward strokes only. Be careful not to scratch the mirror surface. Repeat wiping with fresh cotton balls until dry.
- If the operating handle becomes difficult to move, clean the pad with a standard household cleaning solution. Then apply a thin coat of sewing-machine oil to the pad in the area of the ball joint.
- Always check any electrical connections, making sure that all wires are plugged into the transformer after each cleaning and maintenance procedure.
- If the slit-lamp light does not operate after you have checked all electrical connections, replace the bulb even if it seems to be in good condition, using the standard guidelines for bulb replacement given earlier.
- Special instructions for cleaning the tonometer used with the slit lamp appear later in this appendix.

Projector

The projector—with accompanying slides, mirrors, and screens—is used to conduct the Snellen or other visual acuity tests. The projector unit consists of a housing for the bulb, a tube containing a lens system for focusing, and an opening between the bulb and the lens system for glass target slides (Figure A.9). The projector directs images from the glass slides onto a projection screen located 20 feet away or employs multiple mirrors to create the visual effect of 20 feet.

Special Care and Cautions

- Blow or brush superficial grit off the projector.
- Wipe the glass slides and external lens surfaces of the focusing tubes with a soft clean lint-free cloth or photographic-lens paper at appropriate intervals to prevent dust from accumulating.
- Clean the projector slides only with a dry photographic- or optical-lens tissue. Do not use water or other cleaning agents.

FIGURE A.9

(A) Projector. (B) Glass slides.

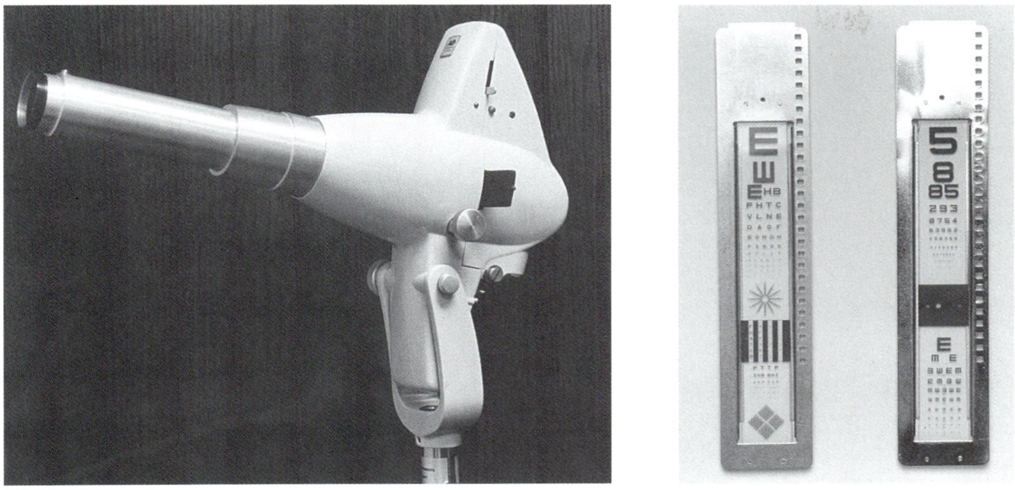

A B

- Clean the patient viewing mirrors (plate glass with silvering on the back surface) and projecting mirrors (silvering on the front surface) with a blast of canned air or with a lint-free photographic cloth. To remove stubborn dirt, use a small amount of household glass cleaner and dry with cotton balls, using downward strokes only, not back-and-forth rubbing motions. Repeat with fresh cotton balls until the surface is dry.
- Never take apart the lamp reflectors, which are assembled and positioned at the factory. The reflector behind the bulb can be cleaned as above.
- Check to determine whether your office's projector screen can be cleaned (some cannot). If it can, clean the projector screen carefully because it is easily scratched or smeared with fingerprints and scratches can never be removed. To remove fingerprints, use a mild household detergent solution and damp cotton balls or a damp lint-free cloth to wipe the screen surface gently.
- Never operate the projector with the lamp compartment open. The lamp operates under pressure and at a high temperature and must be protected at all times from abrasion and contact to avoid shattering.
- Do not attempt to remove lenses from the projector barrel.
- You may observe that the projected image becomes dim, particularly in one half of the screen, shortly before the bulb fails. You may wish to replace the bulb at this point to ensure that acuity testing remains accurate.

Applanation Tonometer

The Goldmann-type applanation tonometer consists of a biprism in an eyepiece, attached by a rod to a housing that delivers measured pressure by use of an adjustment knob (Figure A.10). The Goldmann applanation tonometer, mainly used attached to a slit lamp, measures intraocular pressure by flattening a small area (3.06 mm) of the cornea with the biprism by a known pressure or force. The intraocular pressure is given directly (in 10× units) from a calibrated dial on the adjustment knob.

Because the tip of the Goldmann tonometer contacts the patient's eye during use, it must be carefully cleaned after each use to avoid the possibility of spreading infection. Although ophthalmic medical assistants should consult the ophthalmologist for the preferred cleaning method in their office, either of the two methods below is generally acceptable.

Special Care and Cautions

- To clean the tonometer, wipe the entire tonometer tip carefully and thoroughly with an alcohol sponge and allow it to air-dry for 1 to 2 minutes

FIGURE A.10

(A) Goldmann applanation tonometer.
(B) Slit-lamp–mounted Goldmann applanation tonometer in use.

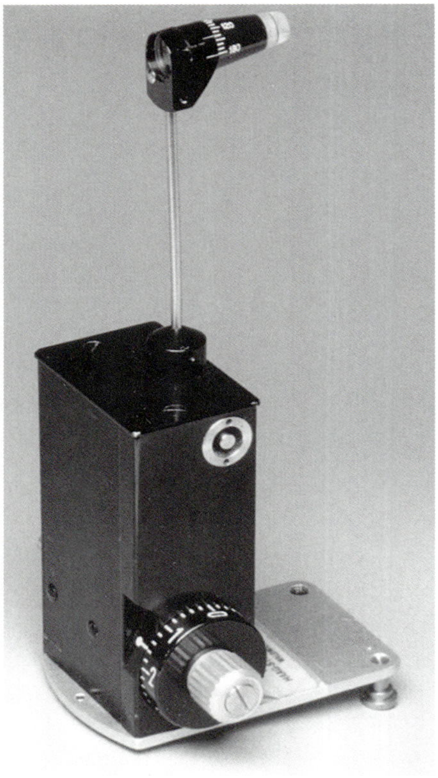

A

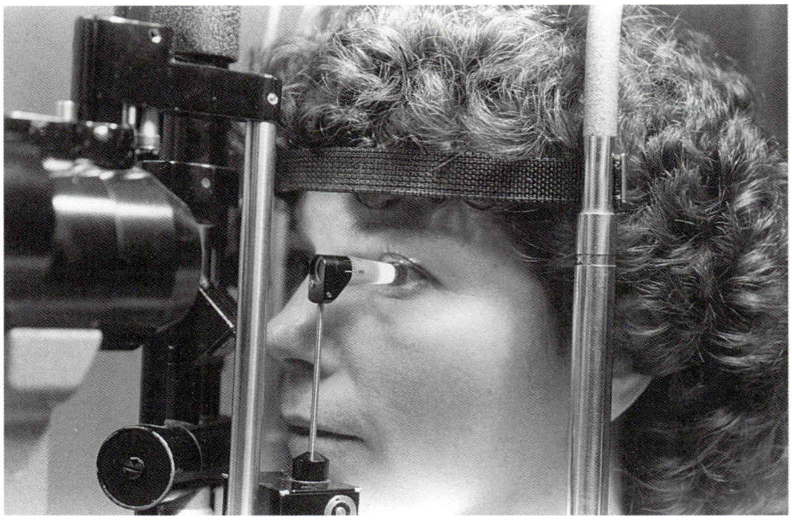

B

before reuse. Alternatively, remove the entire prism from the tonometer and soak it for 5 minutes in 3% hydrogen peroxide or a 1:10 dilution of household bleach. Then rinse the tip under running tap water and allow it to dry before reuse. The bleach solution should be changed at least once a day, and the peroxide solution twice a day.

- Be sure to rinse off the disinfectant and allow for thorough air-drying; if the patient's eye comes in contact with a disinfectant solution, corneal damage, pain, and discomfort could result.
- Calibrate the tonometer at the intervals determined by the ophthalmologist, using the controlled weight supplied with the instrument by the manufacturer.

Indentation Tonometer

The indentation, or Schiøtz, tonometer consists of a plunger in a barrel, attached to a footplate assembly that includes a pressure scale (Figure A.11). The plunger is fitted with one of several available weights, and intraocular pressure is measured by indenting the cornea with the plunger. The intraocular pressure reading shown on the pressure scale is interpreted by using a printed conversion table.

Like the Goldmann applanation tonometer, the Schiøtz indentation tonometer contacts the patient's eye directly. Therefore, to prevent contamination and the spread of infectious diseases, the tonometer and its barrel and plunger must be cleaned and disinfected after use with each patient.

Special Care and Cautions

- To clean the tonometer, disassemble it and clean the barrel first with a pipe cleaner soaked in alcohol, then with a dry pipe cleaner. Clean the footplate with an alcohol-soaked cotton swab. Do not touch the plunger directly with your fingers after cleaning. Allow all tonometer surfaces to dry before reassembling.

FIGURE A.11

Indentation (Schiøtz) tonometer.

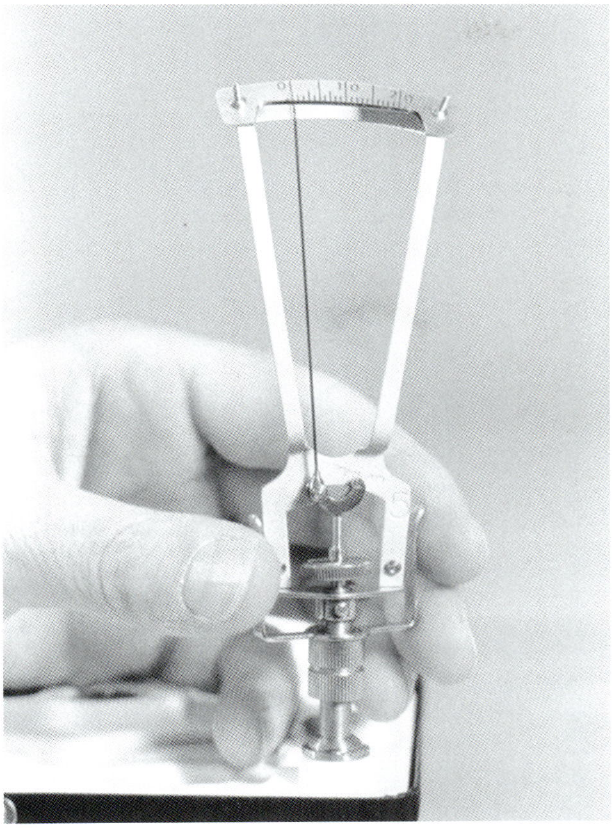

- Check that the calibration is at zero between each use, using the zero test block.
- Be careful not to damage the delicate indicator needle. Never bend it if the calibration is not at zero. This adjustment must be made at the factory.
- Do not interchange weights between two or more separate tonometers because the weights are calibrated specifically for each individual tonometer.

Direct Ophthalmoscope

The direct ophthalmoscope is a hand-held instrument, either battery-powered or electrical, that consists of a light source, built-in dial-up lenses and filters, and a reflecting device to aim light into the patient's eye (Figure A.12). The ophthalmologist uses this instrument to examine the fundus directly. The direct ophthalmoscope is capable of larger magnification (15×) than is the indirect ophthalmoscope, but provides a more restricted view of the fundus. In addition, because only a single eye can be used for viewing at a time, the direct ophthalmoscope does not provide a stereoscopic view.

FIGURE A.12

Direct ophthalmoscope.

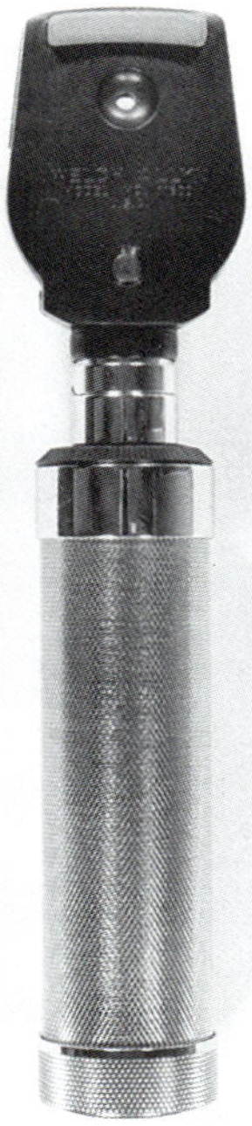

Indirect Ophthalmoscope

The indirect ophthalmoscope is used to examine the complete fundus in stereopsis. The instrument consists of a transformer power source and a headset that fits on the ophthalmologist's head, with a bulb light source and binocular magnifying lenses attached for viewing (Figure A.13). The ophthalmologist uses a hand-held condensing lens (usually +20-diopter) to magnify the image of the fundus. Magnification is usually 2× to 4×, and the image appears as a real, three-dimensional, inverted image of the retina at the focal point of the hand-held lens.

FIGURE A.13

Indirect ophthalmoscope. Transformer (left), hand-held condensing lens and case (center), ophthalmoscope (right).

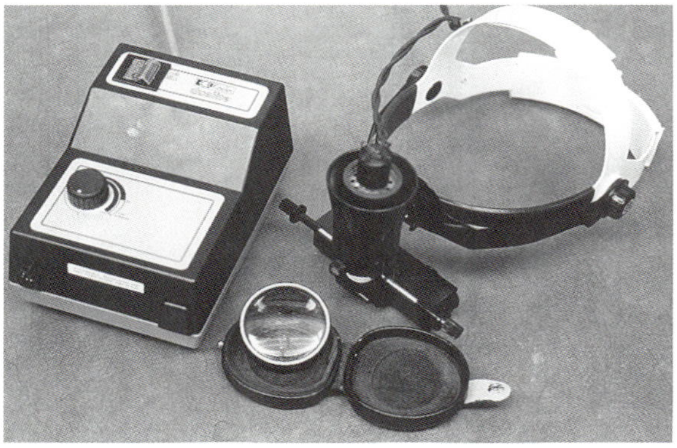

FIGURE A.14

Potential acuity meter.

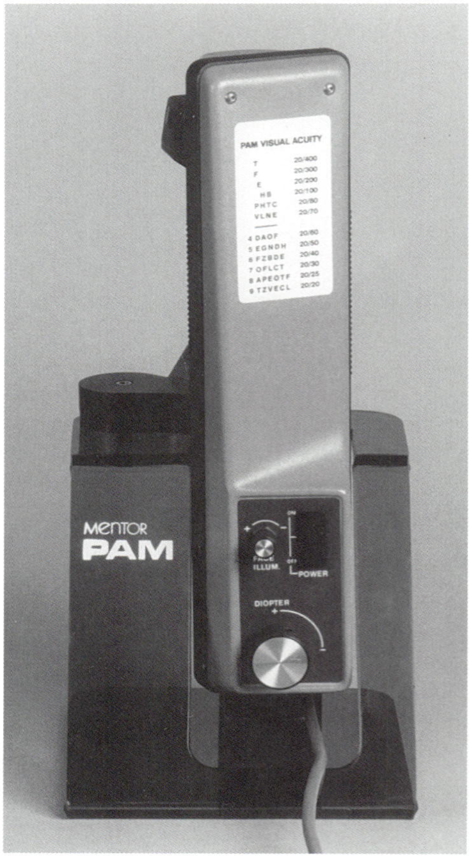

FIGURE A.15

Nd:YAG laser.

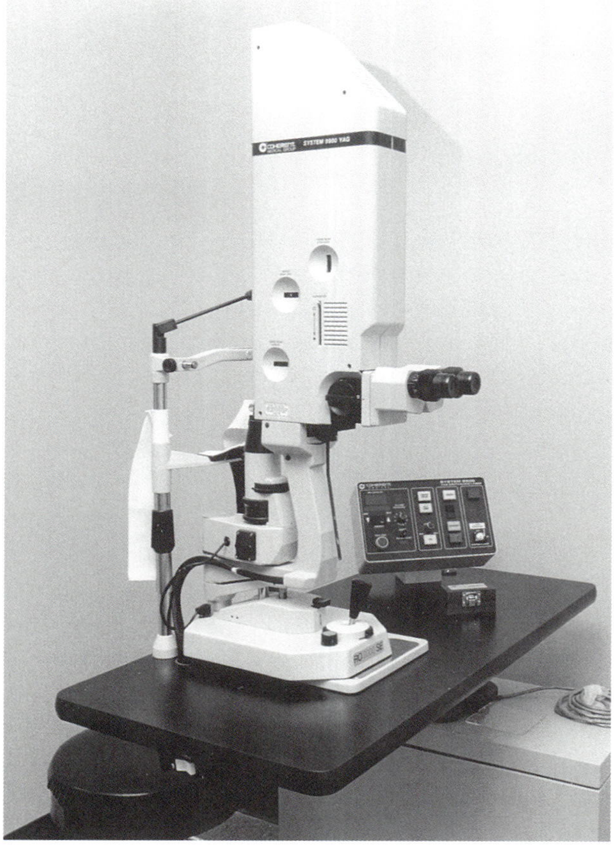

Potential Acuity Meter

The potential acuity meter (PAM) is used to determine potential visual acuities in patients with cataracts. The device consists of a pinpoint light source, a transilluminated Snellen visual acuity chart, and a lens that projects the highly illuminated acuity chart through an opening about 0.1 mm in diameter (Figure A.14).

Lasers

The word *laser* is an acronym for ***l**ight **a**mplification by **s**timulated **e**mission of **r**adiation*. Lasers are a source of an extremely intense form of monochromatic light organized in a concentrated beam that can cut, burn, disrupt, or vaporize tissue (Figure A.15). Common types of ophthalmic lasers include the argon, krypton, CO_2 excimer, and Nd:YAG (neodymium:yttrium-aluminum-garnet).

The ophthalmologist uses lasers in a variety of treatments, including

- Creating multiple burns in the retina of a diabetic patient to decrease the adverse effects of diabetic retinopathy
- Sealing around potential holes or tears associated with retinal detachment
- Cutting a hole in the periphery of the iris to make an outflow channel for aqueous in patients with acute narrow-angle glaucoma
- Cutting the posterior capsule of the lens if it becomes opaque after cataract surgery
- Treating chronic open-angle glaucoma by applying laser treatment to the trabecular meshwork through a gonioprism lens
- Blepharoplasty (eyelid surgery) and skin resurfacing
- Correction of refractive errors and the removal of superficial corneal opacities

Special Care and Cautions

- Maintenance should be performed only by a qualified service technician.
- Because lasers are powerful instruments that can cause damage if improperly focused on the eye (a patient's or your own), review the instruction manuals for specific safeguards before you begin to assist the ophthalmologist in the laser work area.
- Always wear the approved protective eye goggles when assisting the ophthalmologist in the laser work area.
- Never attempt to demonstrate how the laser works without the correct and appropriate knowledge, permission, and supervision.

Appendix B: Systemic Diseases and Ocular Manifestations

Diseases that affect one or more of the major systems of the body are called *systemic diseases*. Examples of systemic diseases are diabetes mellitus, which affects the body's endocrine and cardiovascular systems, and cancers, which can affect various organs and body systems, such as the lungs (respiratory) and brain (nervous). Systemic diseases often create distinctive changes in the eye's external and internal appearance, sometimes without producing visual problems or other troubling symptoms. Because the eye is so readily accessible to both external and internal inspection, an examination of the eye can reveal these changes and help physicians detect the presence of systemic disease. Many systemic disorders also can result in eye disorders that require ophthalmologic treatment in addition to therapy for the other affected bodily functions.

Ophthalmic medical assistants are likely to encounter patients visiting the ophthalmologist for ocular reasons that may relate to their systemic condition. Knowledge of the common ocular manifestations of systemic diseases is helpful in understanding these patients' problems and assisting with their care. The principal systemic diseases that have ocular manifestations may be divided into five categories: inflammatory and autoimmune, metabolic, vascular (including ischemic), infectious, and malignant.

MAJOR BODY SYSTEMS

Important body systems include the cardiovascular, respiratory, endocrine, and nervous systems. The **cardiovascular system** consists of the heart and blood vessels (arteries and veins). The heart functions as a pump for blood, and the arteries and veins are conduits that deliver the blood to and from the heart throughout the body. The **respiratory system** consists of the lungs. This system allows the exchange of oxygen for carbon dioxide in the blood. Oxygen is an essential ingredient for many bodily functions. The **endocrine system** consists of multiple glands that produce substances called *hormones*. Hormones regulate many functions in the body, such as sugar metabolism (the hormone insulin), growth and body metabolism rate (thyroid hormone), and sexual development and function (the hormones estrogen and testosterone). The **nervous system** consists of the brain, spinal cord, and peripheral nerves. It functions as the wiring system of the body. Messages are sent to create certain actions, and messages are received so further action can be taken. The eyes function as an important receptor in this system. These systems, as well as others, work together, allowing smooth functioning of myriad bodily processes. Similarly, a disorder of one system can affect other systems.

INFLAMMATORY AND AUTOIMMUNE DISEASES

Numerous diseases may be characterized as inflammatory, autoimmune, or both. Only the conditions that result in significant ocular involvement are discussed here.

FIGURE B.1

Ptosis in both eyes of a patient with myasthenia gravis.

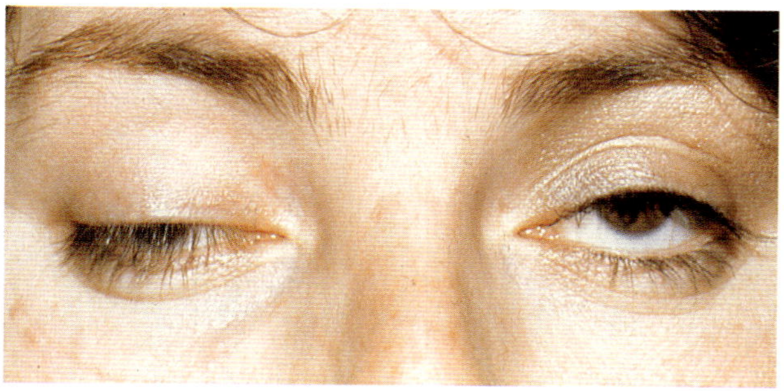

Myasthenia Gravis

Myasthenia gravis is a chronic autoimmune condition that interferes with proper nerve transmission in the skeletal muscles, causing muscle weakness selectively. The disease can occur at any age. The ocular manifestations of myasthenia gravis include ptosis (Figure B.1) and diplopia. Patients may also complain of limited eye movements. Muscle stimulants and other systemic medications may help.

Rheumatoid Arthritis

Rheumatoid arthritis is a chronic disease of unknown origin that causes pain, stiffness, inflammation, swelling, and sometimes destruction of the joints. Dry eyes are common in patients with rheumatoid arthritis. Other ocular manifestations include scleritis (inflammation of the sclera), episcleritis (inflammation of the superficial tissue overlying the sclera), and corneal ulcers (Figure B.2). Treatments vary according to the specific problem: artificial tears, moisture goggles, and lubricating ointments for dry eye; corticosteroids and other potent anti-inflammatory drugs for scleritis; scleral or corneal patch grafts for perforations. Treatment for the more severe systemic manifestations of rheumatoid arthritis requires corticosteroids or even stronger immunologic suppressants.

Sarcoidosis

Sarcoidosis causes inflammation in a number of body systems and organs. The origin of this disease is not completely understood, but sarcoidosis seems to affect blacks and Hispanics more frequently than other population groups. The most common ocular manifestation of sarcoidosis is uveitis (inflammation of the uveal tract), which causes cellular deposits on the cornea (Figure B.3) and damage to the iris. In some patients, sarcoidosis affects the choroid and the vessels of the retina, as well as the optic nerve. Ocular problems related to sarcoidosis are treated with topical or systemic corticosteroids.

Sjögren's Syndrome

Sjögren's syndrome is a combination of dry eyes and dry mouth in the patient. This disorder can appear in the person for no known reason, or it may be associated with other inflammatory or immunologic dis-

FIGURE B.2

Ocular manifestations of rheumatoid arthritis. (A) Scleritis. (B) Corneal ulcer.

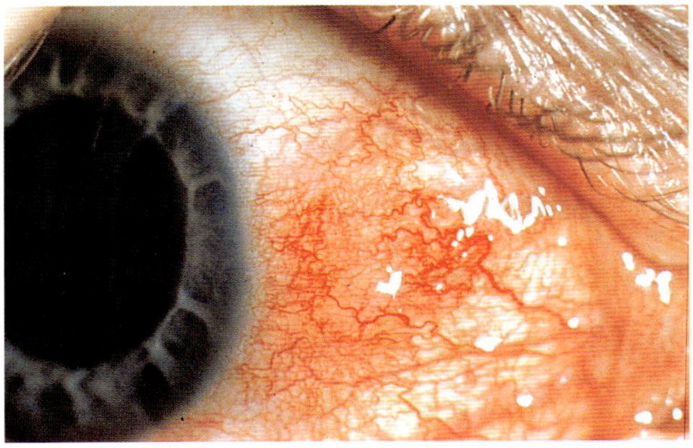

A

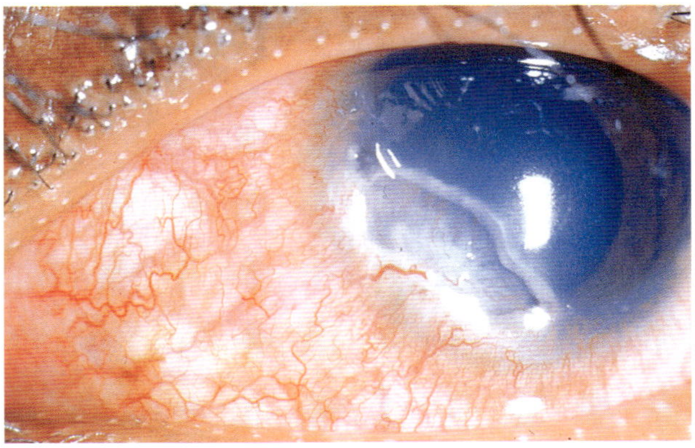

B

FIGURE B.3

Cellular deposits on the cornea resulting from uveitis caused by sarcoidosis.

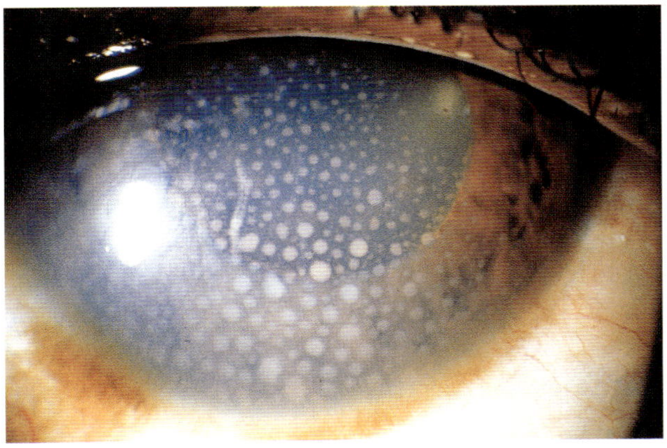

FIGURE B.4

Retinal vasculitis seen in the fundus of a patient with SLE; the characteristic yellowish white patches are known as *cotton-wool spots.*

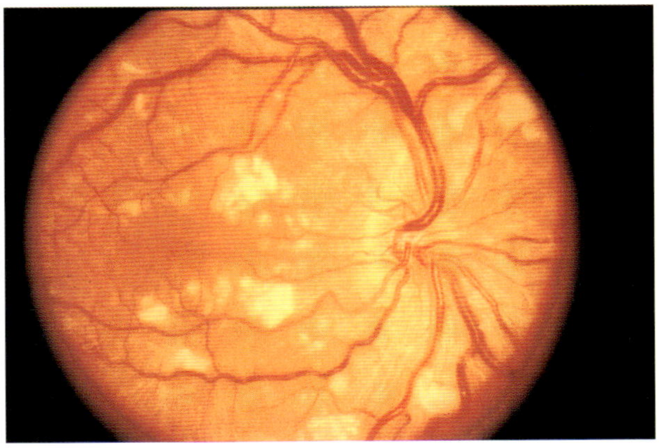

eases, such as arthritic conditions. The dry eyes of Sjögren's syndrome result in the corneal condition keratoconjunctivitis sicca. Symptoms include photophobia and a sensation of burning, grittiness, or foreign body in the eye. The ophthalmologist often treats the ocular symptoms of Sjögren's syndrome with artificial tears and/or lubricating ointment applied at bedtime. Surgical closure of the lacrimal puncta is sometimes necessary.

Systemic Lupus Erythematosus

Systemic lupus erythematosus, or SLE, can affect many body systems and organs, from the skin to the blood vessels, lungs, and kidneys. The disease primarily afflicts women, but the causes are unknown. Dry eyes, scleritis, and corneal ulcers may result from SLE. However, the most common eye conditions produced by SLE are those affecting the vessels of the retina and optic nerve (retinal vasculitis) and the optic nerve itself (Figure B.4). Corticosteroids, administered either topically or systemically, are the usual mode of treatment.

Thyroid Disorders

The thyroid gland, a part of the endocrine system, helps regulate the body's metabolism. The many types

FIGURE B.5

Thyroid ophthalmopathy. (A) Retracted lids and proptosis. (B) Corneal damage.

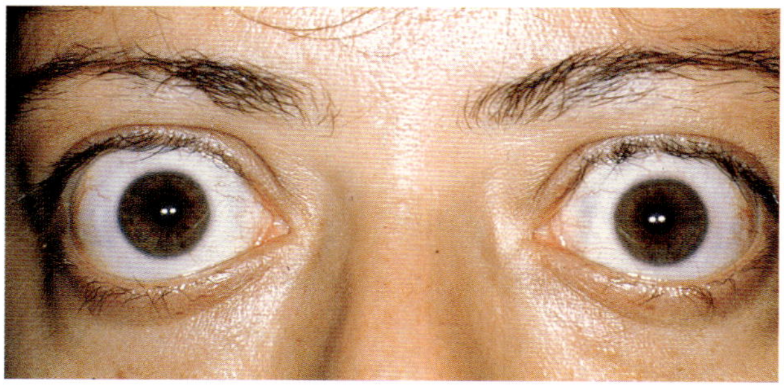

A

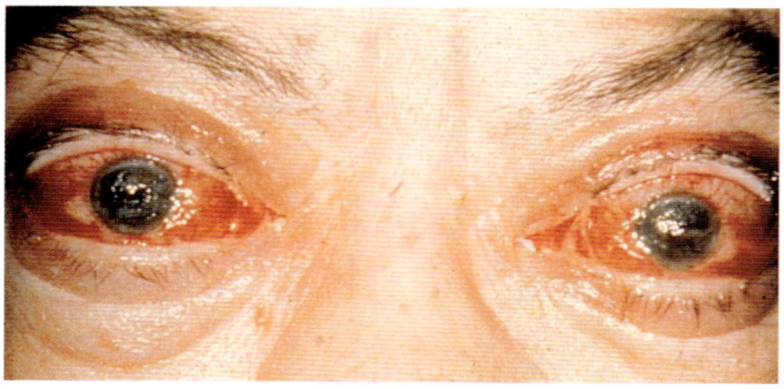

B

of thyroid dysfunction, sometimes manifested as inflammatory disorders, can cause a wide variety of eye problems, known collectively as *thyroid ophthalmopathy* (Figure B.5). This group of conditions produces various degrees of swelling of the eyelids and orbital tissues, which results in proptosis and associated problems with lid and ocular muscle movement and with vision. Severe proptosis, which exposes the delicate outer eye, can lead to dry eyes, corneal damage, and loss of vision. Swelling can lead to compression of the optic nerve, also resulting in visual loss if left untreated.

Treatment for the thyroid condition itself sometimes is effective in relieving the eye problems, but thyroid ophthalmopathy may persist or even progress despite restoration of normal thyroid function. Therapy specifically for the eye conditions ranges from the use of artificial tears for corneal problems to lid and orbital surgery when required.

FIGURE B.6

Fundus of a patient with diabetic retinopathy; new vessels are branching on the optic disc.

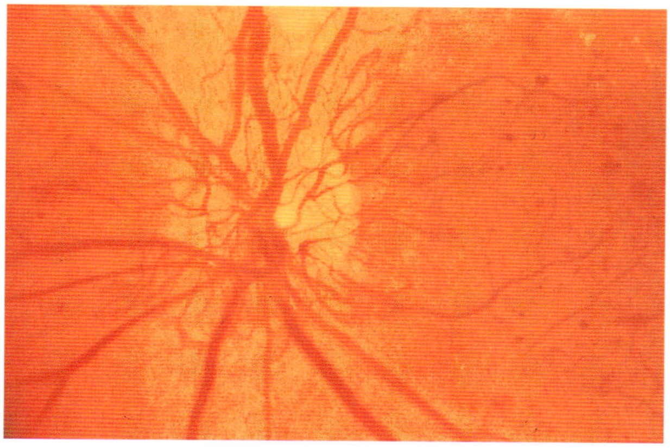

METABOLIC DISORDERS

Of all the metabolic diseases, diabetes is the one that carries the greatest risk for blindness if diabetic retinopathy is neither diagnosed nor treated appropriately.

Diabetes Mellitus

Diabetes mellitus is a metabolic disease that afflicts millions of Americans. It affects a variety of organs and systems, from the nerves to the kidneys. The effects of diabetes on the vascular system can cause *neovascularization* (uncontrolled growth of new blood vessels) in the retina. This proliferation of blood vessels can lead to gradual destruction of the macula and/or the rest of the retina, a condition known as *diabetic retinopathy* (Figure B.6). The occurrence of blindness among people with diabetes is 25 times that of the general population.

Diabetic retinopathy can exist for some time, causing severe damage to retinal structures before patients notice any loss of vision. For this reason, diabetic patients require regular eye examinations by an ophthalmologist to detect possible retinopathy and follow its progression at intervals determined by the type of diabetes they have. Laser surgery has been found to be effective in preventing blindness from diabetic retinopathy. Traditional surgical treatment may be required to remove the vitreous or repair retinal detachments that sometimes occur with diabetic retinopathy.

VASCULAR DISEASES

Problems with the blood vessels—the circulatory system—can lead to a host of diseases, many of them affecting the eye or the visual system.

FIGURE B.7

Emboli due to CVA may become lodged in arteries leading to the eye and cause temporary visual loss.

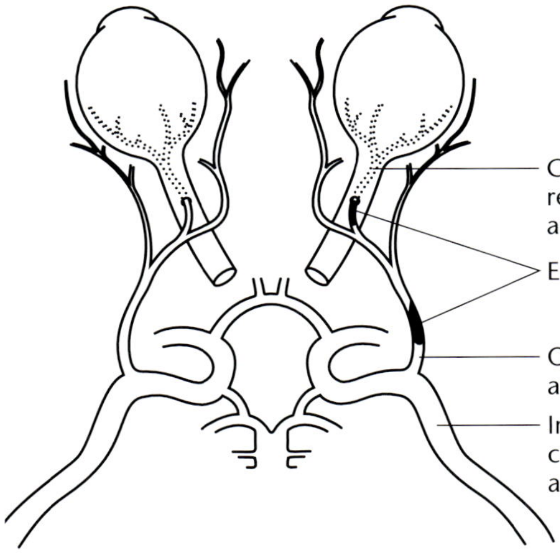

Cerebral Vascular Accident

Stroke and cerebral hemorrhage (bleeding within the brain) are the principal types of cerebral vascular accident (CVA). This is an example of an interaction between the nervous system and the vascular system. A variety of systemic conditions that affect the heart and circulatory system can impair or block blood vessels and lead to a blood loss to the brain, called a *stroke*. Without blood and the oxygen it carries, the brain's tissues quickly die. Unless the blood supply is restored rapidly, damage becomes irreversible.

A primary cause of eye problems associated with CVA is an embolus (plural: emboli), a clot of tissue, fat, or other body matter that plugs tiny vessels of the eye and the optic nerve and blocks blood circulation for a time (Figure B.7). These obstructions can produce a sudden loss of vision, often in just one eye and usually transient. Such incidents of temporary visual loss may be the first indication that a patient has a circulatory problem requiring medical attention. Sometimes the embolus causes a prolonged blockage of the retinal artery, producing permanent visual loss called *central retinal artery occlusion*.

Giant Cell Arteritis

Giant cell arteritis, also known as *temporal arteritis*, affects the circulation of blood in the arteries and is, therefore, considered a vascular disease. But giant cell arteritis can also be classified as an inflammatory or immunologic disorder. It primarily afflicts people over the age of 60. The effects of giant cell arteritis on certain cranial arteries, including those supplying the eye, lead to a number of potential systemic and eye problems. The optic nerve may become severely damaged from reduced blood supply, causing visual loss. Loss of vision can also result when the central retinal artery is deprived of sufficient blood. Eye muscle imbalance also may occur.

Often, eye signs and symptoms serve as the first indication to the doctor that the patient has giant cell arteritis. Urgent blood testing and/or biopsy (surgery to remove and test suspect tissue) of the temporal artery may be required, as well as prompt drug therapy to prevent blindness or death. Treatment of the systemic condition, which may include corticosteroids, can also be effective for the ocular conditions.

Migraine

Migraine usually produces intense headache and possibly nausea, often preceded by scintillations—visual sensations of flashing or whirling lights. Ophthalmic migraine produces only the scintillations and, in some patients, pupillary dilation and temporary partial or complete loss of vision. Although not completely understood, the causes of migraine are thought to involve a problem with the circulatory system of the brain or, in the case of ocular migraine, the eye. Migraine also may stem from a treatable vascular disease. Otherwise, specific systemic drugs may be used to help relieve symptoms and prevent their frequent recurrence.

Hypertension

Also called *high blood pressure*, systemic hypertension impairs blood circulation. In the eye, this circulatory impairment may produce problems in the vessels supplying the retina, choroid, and optic nerve. Hypertension can lead to small hemorrhages and other characteristic changes in the appearance of the retina and its vessels even without creating noticeable visual problems (Figure B.8). An ophthalmologist's fundus examination, therefore, is often important in diagnosing the presence of hypertension and following its course. Various methods of controlling blood pressure, ranging from dietary to drug treatments, can help overcome many of the eye problems associated with systemic hypertension.

FIGURE B.8

Characteristic retinal changes due to hypertension include flame-shaped hemorrhages and whitish cotton-wool patches.

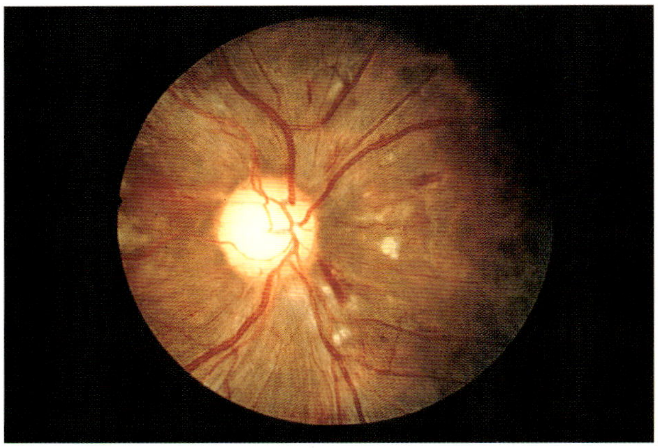

FIGURE B.9

Yellowish lower area of the retina infected with CMV in a patient with AIDS is easily distinguished from upper, uninfected area.

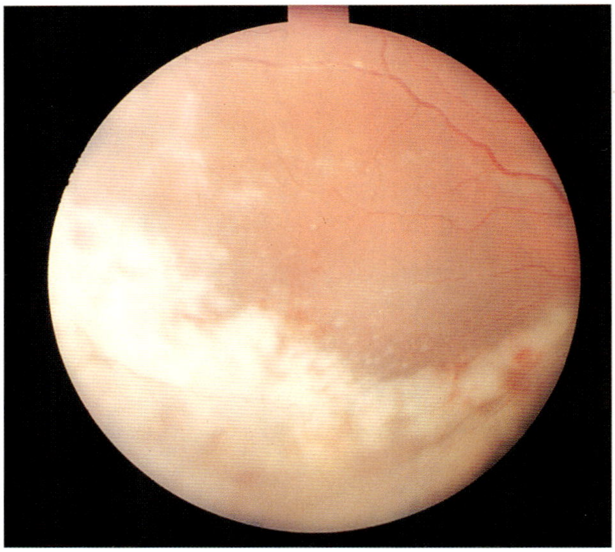

INFECTIOUS DISEASES

Infectious diseases by definition are of special concern because they can be transmitted from one person to another. Several infectious conditions have important ophthalmologic implications.

Acquired Immunodeficiency Syndrome

Acquired immunodeficiency syndrome (AIDS) is an infection caused by the human immunodeficiency virus (HIV). The presence of HIV affects the ability of the body's immune system to combat many different kinds of additional infections. The disease may be present in a variety of increasingly severe forms. Some patients harbor HIV for many years with no extreme effects on their immune systems, while the immune systems of others with HIV are compromised within a year or two of infection. More people with HIV are now able to live in the former state, symptom free, because of the advent of drugs called protease inhibitors.

HIV can be sexually transmitted but also can be acquired through blood transfusions or direct or indirect contact with blood or body fluids from individuals infected with HIV. A fetus can contract HIV during gestation from an HIV-infected mother.

Eye problems frequently occur in patients with AIDS. Retinal infections are common, particularly *cytomegalovirus (CMV) retinitis* (Figure B.9). Growths of malignant cells on the lid and conjunctiva, known as *Kaposi's sarcoma*, also occur, as do nerve conditions affecting the orbital and eyelid muscle movements. Another viral eye infection that may afflict AIDS patients is *herpes zoster ophthalmicus*; it affects numerous parts of the external and internal eye, from the cornea to the retina.

Chlamydial Infections

The bacteria collectively called *chlamydiae* are responsible for this group of infections. One form of chlamydia, which affects the urologic, reproductive, and sexual organs, is easily transmitted through sexual contact. This type of chlamydia occurs commonly among sexually active young people. Infection from the sexual organs can be transmitted to the eye, causing chlamydial, or inclusion, conjunctivitis (see Figure 12.2B).

Symptoms of chlamydial conjunctivitis include eye redness and discharge. Diagnosis of this type of conjunctivitis is usually made through special microbiologic testing. Proper diagnosis is important not only to select the correct treatment, but also to treat the sexual partners of the infected patient and to prevent further spread of the primary disease. Treatment for this condition usually includes use of systemic, and possibly topical, antibiotic drugs.

Herpes Zoster and Herpes Simplex

The viruses varicella zoster and herpes simplex can infect numerous body systems, creating varying effects in each. The varicella-zoster virus, which causes chicken pox, can also affect the central nervous system. When it does, it causes a condition called *shingles*—painful nerve inflammation and swelling and skin eruptions. As the eye infection *herpes zoster ophthalmicus*, the condition causes uveitis, corneal inflammation, and other disease. It is sometimes complicated by opportunistic bacterial eye infection, producing reddened eyes and swollen lids (Figure B.10). The retina and other parts of the eye may also be affected. Treatment for the eye condition usually consists of topical corticosteroids, cycloplegic drops, and/or systemic medications.

Herpes simplex virus type 1 causes fever blisters, while type 2 produces genital infections. Known as *ocular herpes simplex* when it occurs in the eye, type 1 infection can lead to blepharitis, conjunctivitis, keratitis, and other, more severe corneal conditions. Retinal infection, though rare, may also occur. Treatment for ocular herpes simplex may involve oral systemic drugs as well as topical antiviral agents, depending on the area and severity of infection.

FIGURE B.10

Herpes zoster ophthalmicus. (A) Skin eruptions near the eye and swollen lids. (B) Diseased cornea stained with diagnostic fluorescein shows the characteristic branch-like pattern of keratitis.

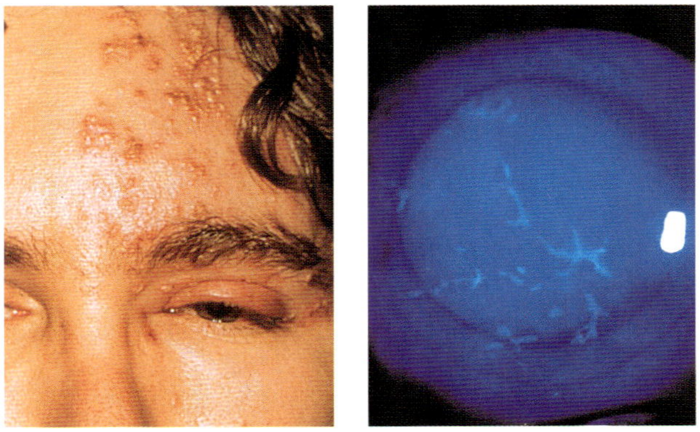

A **B**

Histoplasmosis

Histoplasmosis is a systemic fungal infection contracted by inhaling dust from soil containing spores of the fungus. It is particularly common in the Mississippi River valley and the river valleys of South America, Asia, and Africa. Histoplasmosis principally affects the pulmonary system, causing flu-like symptoms, but can infect a number of other body systems as well. The exact effect of histoplasmosis on the eye is still being debated. Eye conditions related to contact with the fungus, referred to as *ocular histoplasmosis*, involve choroidal and retinal scarring and subretinal hemorrhages.

Syphilis

Syphilis is a highly contagious sexually transmitted disease caused by the bacterium *Treponema pallidum* that can mimic almost any other inflammatory infectious disease. Adults may become infected through sexual activity, while newborns can contract the disease from an infected mother. Uveitis is the principal ocular condition associated with syphilis, but defects in pupillary function and in the optic nerve may also occur. Syphilis is treated with penicillin; untreated syphilis can result in blindness.

Toxoplasmosis

Toxoplasmosis is an infection caused by a protozoan, which may be passed from mother to fetus (congenital toxoplasmosis). It also can be contracted from contact with animal feces (acquired toxoplasmosis), such as when changing cat litter. The congenital form of this disease severely affects the central nervous system of the fetus or newborn (often resulting in death), while the acquired form may cause only mild fever, swollen glands, and general illness. Ocular toxoplasmosis usually occurs as retinal choroiditis, leading to uveitis and vitritis. This infection may also occur in association with AIDS.

MALIGNANT DISEASES

The devastating effects of malignancies on the body as a whole and on the eye in particular are being mitigated in many individuals through recent technologic advances in diagnosis and treatment.

Metastatic Carcinoma

Metastatic carcinoma is the term used to describe cancer that produces tumors (growths that can be malig-

FIGURE B.11

Iris mass in a patient with metastatic lung carcinoma.

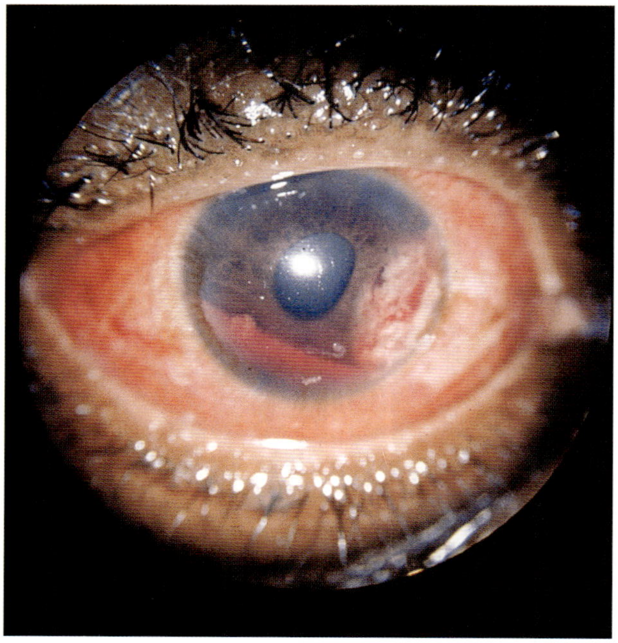

FIGURE B.12

Fundus of a patient with leukemia, displaying preretinal (arrows) and retinal hemorrhages.

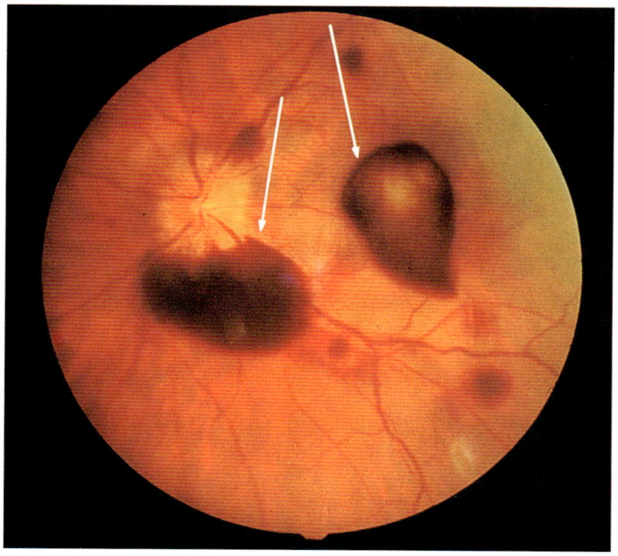

nant and potentially lethal) in more than one part of the body. Tumors in the eye often develop as a result of tumors that have originated elsewhere in the body, notably from cancer in the breast or lungs (Figure B.11). Such metastatic (secondary) carcinoma can lead to loss of vision through invasion by the tumor cells of the choroid, the primary site for metastatic cancer. These tumors may respond to treatment with radiation or chemotherapy.

Blood Dyscrasias

Blood dyscrasias are defined as any abnormal or pathologic conditions of the blood. An example of a serious blood dyscrasia is leukemia, a well-known type of cancer. This disorder can adversely affect the optic disc, optic nerve, retinal blood vessels, and other portions of the retina (Figure B.12). Because changes in retinal appearance may be present before visual symptoms develop, patterns known to have blood dyscrasias often require regular ophthalmologic examinations.

Cerebral Neoplasms

Brain tumors may cause increased intracranial pressure and headaches. Visual field defects and pupillary abnormalities may be the first signs of a brain tumor. Swelling of the optic nerve head, or papilledema, may be detected on funduscopy. Computed tomography (CT) and magnetic resonance imaging (MRI) scans help confirm the diagnosis.

Multiple Sclerosis

Multiple sclerosis (MS) is a chronic disease of the nervous system affecting the white matter of the spinal cord and brain. Optic nerve inflammation (optic neuritis) resulting from MS is frequent in young adults. A positive diagnosis is difficult to establish but may involve examination of spinal fluid, MRI scans, and assessment of the patient's long-term pattern of symptoms.

Appendix C: Universal Precautions

As discussed in Chapter 12, the best way to reduce occupational risk of bloodborne infection is to follow universal precautions. The following list of universal precautions is extracted from the OSHA regulation "Occupational Exposure to Bloodborne Pathogens." Refer to this publication for complete instructions and precautionary guidelines. Ophthalmic medical personnel should regularly review all universal precautions presented there, ensure that they understand them completely, and adhere to them at all times.

1. Hands should be washed before and after patient contact, and immediately if hands become contaminated with blood or other body fluids.
2. Gloves should be worn whenever there is a possibility of contact with body fluids.
3. Masks should be worn whenever there is a possibility of contact with body fluids.
4. Gowns should be worn if exposed skin or clothing is likely to be soiled.
5. During resuscitation procedures, pocket masks or mechanical ventilation devices should be readily available for use.
6. Spills of blood or blood-containing body fluids should be cleaned using a solution of household bleach (sodium hypochlorite) and water in a 1:100 solution for smooth surfaces and a 1:10 solution for porous surfaces.
7. Health care professionals who have open lesions, dermatitis, or other skin irritations should not participate in direct patient care activities or handle contaminated equipment.
8. Contaminated needles should never be bent, clipped, or recapped. Immediately after use, contaminated sharp objects should be discarded into a puncture-resistant "sharps container" designed for this purpose.
9. Contaminated equipment that is reusable should be cleaned of visible organic material, placed in an impervious container, and returned to central hospital supply or some other designated place for decontamination and reprocessing.
10. Instruments and other reusable equipment used in performing invasive procedures should be disinfected and sterilized as follows:
    - Equipment and devices that enter the patient's vascular system or other normally sterile areas of the body should be sterilized before being used for each patient.
    - Equipment and devices that touch intact mucous membranes but do not penetrate the patient's body surfaces should be sterilized when possible, or undergo high-level disinfection if they cannot be sterilized, before being used for each patient.
    - Equipment and devices that do not touch the patient or that only touch intact skin need only be cleaned with a detergent or as indicated by the manufacturer.
11. Body fluids to which universal precautions always apply are as follows: blood, serum/plasma, semen, vaginal secretions, cerebrospinal fluid, vitreous fluid, synovial fluid, pleural fluid, pericardial fluid, peritoneal fluid, amniotic fluid, and wound exudates.
12. Body fluids to which universal precautions apply only when blood is visible in them are as follows: sweat, tears, sputum, saliva, nasal secretions, feces, urine, vomitus, and breast milk.

Answers to Review Questions

Chapter 1

1. a, e, d, b, f, c
2. certified ophthalmic assistant (COA), certified ophthalmic technician (COT), certified ophthalmic medical technologist (COMT)
3. d
4. ethics
5. e

Chapter 2

1. Light rays reflected from an object are focused by the cornea and the lens to produce an upside-down image of the object on the light-sensitive retina. The retina converts the image to electric impulses, which are carried by the optic nerve to the brain's visual cortex, where they produce the sensation of sight.
2. Orbit, extraocular muscles, eyelids, and lacrimal apparatus
3. The bony cavity in the skull that houses the globe, extraocular muscles, blood vessels, and nerves; protects the globe from major injury by a rim of bone
4. d, a, b, c, f, e
5. To protect the eye from injury, to exclude light, to aid in lubricating the ocular surface
6. Outer layer of skin, middle layer of fibrous tissue and muscle, inner layer of tissue (conjunctiva)
7. To produce and drain tears
8. Any two of: Ocular comfort, clear vision, provide moisture, nourish eye
9. Tears are produced by the lacrimal gland; tears are collected in the lacrimal sac; tears drain into the nasal cavity by means of the nasolacrimal duct.
10. Outer, oily layer helps prevent evaporation of moisture from the middle, aqueous layer; middle layer provides moisture, oxygen, and nutrients to the cornea; inner, mucinous layer promotes even spread of the tear film.
11.

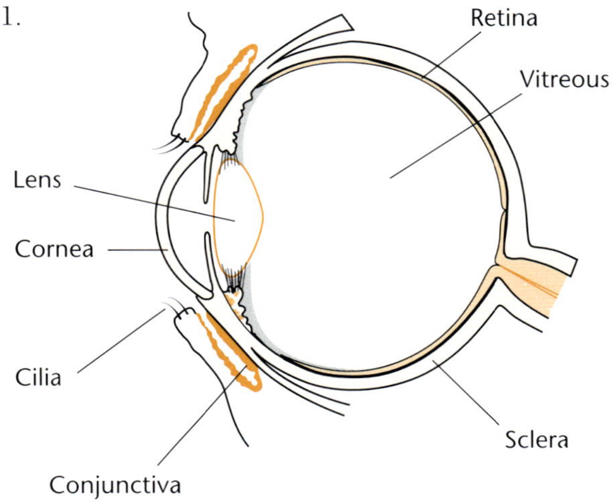

12. To focus light rays reflected to the eye, contributing about two thirds of the focusing power of the eye
13. d, a, c, b, b
14. To protect intraocular contents
15. To maintain intraocular pressure
16. Aqueous humor enters the eye from behind the iris, flows across the back of the iris, through the pupil, and into the anterior chamber; it leaves the anterior chamber at the filtration angle and passes through the trabecular meshwork, the canal of Schlemm, and into the blood vessels.
17. Iris, ciliary body, choroid
18. Fibers of the dilator muscle that extend from the pupil to the boundary of the iris contract to dilate the pupil; contraction of the sphincter muscle that encircles the pupil makes the pupil smaller.
19. To secrete aqueous humor
20. To supply blood (nourishment) to the outer layers of the retina
21. Lens
22. The curvature of the lens can change, becoming rounder, to focus images of objects that are closer to the eye.
23. Zonules
24. Acts as a shock absorber for the eye and helps maintain the spherical shape of the globe
25. The retinal rods and cones receive light rays and, in turn, generate electric (nerve) impulses. These impulses are transmitted to the brain, where the visual messages they carry are converted to the sensation of sight.
26. Rods, cones
27. Rods are largely responsible for vision in dim light ("night vision") and for peripheral vision; cones provide sharp central vision and color perception.
28. Cone
29. The optic nerves from each eye merge at the optic chiasm. Axon fibers from the nasal retina of each eye cross to the opposite side of the chiasm, while axons from the temporal retina of each eye continue on the same side. The realigned axons emerge from the chiasm as the left and right optic tracts, ending in the left and right lateral geniculate bodies. There the axons synapse (connect) to the optic radiations, which travel to the right and left halves of the visual cortex of the brain.

Chapter 3

1. Infectious, inflammatory, allergic, ischemic, metabolic, congenital, developmental, degenerative, neoplastic, traumatic
2. *Sign*: a change that can be observed by a physician. *Symptom*: a change experienced by a patient. (A sign is usually more objective; a symptom, more subjective.) *Syndrome*: a group of signs or symptoms characteristic of a particular condition.
3. Proptosis, exophthalmos
4. Grossly swollen lids, red eyes
5. Misalignment of the eyes; greater than normal tissue bulk in orbit, loss of muscle elasticity from scarring, muscle paralysis due to nerve damage, congenital weakness of one or more extraocular muscles
6. a, c, d, g, b, h, i, e, f
7. Dry eyes; artificial tears in the form of eyedrops
8. Dacryocystitis
9. *Bacterial*: mucopurulent discharge. *Viral*: watery discharge, palpebral conjunctiva is covered with small bumps. *Allergic*: tearing, itching, redness, swelling.
10. Rupture of a conjunctival blood vessel, allowing blood to flow under the conjunctival tissue; may occur after violent sneezing or coughing
11. *Pinguecula*: small, benign yellow-white mass of degenerated tissue beneath bulbar conjunctiva that does not cross onto the cornea and that can cause minor eye irritation. *Pterygium*: wedge-shaped growth of abnormal tissue on bulbar conjunctiva that can cross onto the cornea and can cause irritation, redness, foreign-body sensation, sensitivity to light.
12. Pain, sensitivity to light, tearing; antibiotics
13. Symptoms are not as severe; dense corneal opacity; branch-shaped figure on cornea
14. Center of cornea thins and acquires a cone shape, which affects vision
15. Abnormal rise in intraocular pressure, with eventual damage to the optic nerve and sight loss; glaucoma
16. c, d, b, a

17. Opacification, or loss of transparency
18. Aging, injury, disease, congenital
19. Small particles of dead cells and other debris in vitreous and collagen fibers from vitreous degeneration; experienced by patient as spots or cobwebs
20. Endophthalmitis
21. Separation of sensory and pigment layers of retina
22. Patient notices stars or flashes of light at corner of eye, followed some hours later by sensation of a curtain moving across eye and by painless loss of vision
23. Sensory cells of macula deteriorate, causing loss of central vision
24. Swelling of optic disc with engorged blood vessels, causing enlargement of the normal physiologic blind spot
25. Tumor, stroke, trauma, inflammation

Chapter 4

1. *Refractive index*: the ratio of the speed of light in a vacuum to its speed in a specific substance. *Focal point*: the point somewhere along the principal axis of a lens at which the paraxial rays converge or diverge. *Focal length*: the distance between the focal point and the lens. *Diopter*: the unit of measure of the power of a lens.
2. A convex lens converges light rays; a concave lens diverges light rays.
3. *Emmetropia*: the normal refractive state of an eye, in which light rays from distant objects are focused clearly on the retina by the relaxed lens without any accommodative effort. *Ametropia*: the abnormal refractive state of the eye, in which light rays from distant objects cannot be focused clearly on the retina due to refractive error.
4. *Myopia*: nearsightedness; the cornea and lens have too much plus power for the length of the nonaccommodating eye, so that the light rays from distant objects are focused in front of the retina. *Hyperopia*: farsightedness; the cornea and lens have too little plus power for the length of the nonaccommodating eye, so that light rays from distant objects are focused theoretically behind the retina. *Astigmatism*: blurred vision of both distant and near objects due to a toric cornea or one whose surface is irregular, so that light rays are not brought to a single focal point.
5. Progressive loss of accommodative ability of the crystalline lens due to natural processes of aging
6. Eyeglasses, contact lenses, intraocular lens implants, refractive surgery
7. Lower segment(s) of a multifocal lens; used to provide near vision to patients with presbyopia
8. Lens that has different curvatures in each of two perpendicular meridians (like a football), each of which possesses refractive power
9. Refracts light rays toward its base
10. To correct diplopia caused by visual misalignments
11. Prism diopters
12. 2
13. *Myopia*: concave, or minus, sphere. *Hyperopia*: convex, or plus, sphere. *Astigmatism*: spherocylinder, or cylinder.
14. Process of measuring a person's refractive error and determining the optical correction required to provide clear vision.
15. Refractometry and clinical judgment
16. Retinoscopy (objective refractometry), refinement (subjective refractometry), binocular balancing
17. *Cycloplegic refraction* uses cycloplegic drops to temporarily paralyze the ciliary muscle and block accommodation. *Manifest refraction* is obtained without cycloplegia.
18. *Objective refractometry* is retinoscopy, which does not require responses from the patient. *Subjective refractometry* is refinement, which requires the patient to participate by choosing the lens (usually presented by means of a phoropter or trial frame and lenses) that provides the better clarity.
19. Retinoscope, refractor (or phoropter), trial lens set and trial frame, cross cylinder
20. *With motion*: the retinoscopic reflex of the eye that moves in the same direction as the retinoscope streak of light. *Against motion*: the retinoscopic reflex of the eye that moves in the opposite direction from the retinoscope streak of light.
21. a. Sign and power of sphere b. Sign and power of cylinder c. Axis of cylinder
22. $+5.75 -1.50 \times 45$
23. Measurement of the prescription of eyeglass lenses or the power of contact lenses

24. Power in diopters, axes of cylinder component, presence and direction of prism, optical centers
25. Sphere
26. +1.75
27. Measurement of a patient's corneal curvature; provides an objective, quantitative measurement of corneal astigmatism.
28. a. The reticle is in the center of the bottom-right circle. b. The instrument is focused with fusion of the bottom-right circles. c. The pluses between the circles are in the same plane and are fused. d. The minuses between the circles are in the same plane and are fused.

Chapter 5

1. To reveal both existing and potential eye problems, even in the absence of specific symptoms
2. Certain eye diseases cause no symptoms until they are too advanced for effective treatment. Eye health is an important indicator of general health. Individuals who are at high risk for developing certain eye diseases can be monitored.
3. Chief complaint, ocular history, medical history, family ocular and medical history, allergies
4. Refer the patient to the ophthalmologist for a diagnosis or medical advice, even if you think you know the answer.
5. The ability to discern fine visual detail
6. The first number represents the distance in feet at which the test was performed (distance of patient from chart). The second number indicates that the patient can read at 20 feet what a normal eye can read at 40 feet.
7. V OD 20/60 OS 20/40 $\overline{sc}$
8. Can reveal whether a patient's below-normal visual acuity is the result of a refractive error or is due to some other cause
9. The patient complains that reading or other close work is difficult. There is reason to believe that the patient's ability to accommodate is insufficient or impaired.
10. Eye movement (motility), eye alignment, fusional ability
11. Right and up, right, right and down, left and up, left, left and down
12. To measure the extent of a misaligned eye's deviation
13. To determine whether the eyes are perfectly aligned and, if so, whether the brain acknowledges the visual information from both eyes or suppresses the information from one eye; the test will also reveal diplopia
14. To determine whether the patient has fine depth perception and to qualify it in terms of binocular cooperation
15. Direct and consensual pupillary reaction
16. To measure the expanse and sensitivity of vision surrounding the direct line of sight (peripheral vision)
17. On each other's uncovered eye
18. The presence and location of defects in the central portion of the visual field
19. For early detection of abnormal intraocular pressure and glaucoma, which may be present long before patients notice any symptoms such as visual loss
20. Applanation and indentation
21. c
22. To assess the ocular adnexa, external globe, and anterior chamber
23. To estimate the depth of the anterior chamber and the chamber angle; the test helps screen for the presence of narrow-angle glaucoma and can alert the physician to avoid using drugs that would dilate the patient's pupil
24. To obtain a magnified view of the patient's ocular adnexa and anterior segment structures; to perform applanation tonometry with the Goldmann tonometer; to examine the fundus; to perform gonioscopy
25. A noncontact lens attached to the slit lamp; used to examine the optic nerve head and small areas of the posterior retina and vitreous
26. A special viewing method for examination of the anterior chamber angle; employs a mirrored or high-plus contact lens
27. Direct and indirect
28. Pseudoisochromatic color plates; 15-hue (Farnsworth-Munsell D-15) test
29. To measure the patient's tear output
30. To test the structural and physiologic integrity of the corneal epithelium and to check for corneal abrasions or lesions and for dry eye

31. The examiner touches the central portion of the cornea with a sterile wisp of cotton to determine whether the patient has normal corneal sensation.
32. To measure the prominence of the eyeball in relation to the bony orbital rim surrounding it and record the existence and extent of proptosis

Chapter 6

1. To determine the potential visual status of a patient with a media opacity and the extent to which surgery or other types of therapy may improve vision
2. Potential acuity meter, super pinhole, interferometer
3. To determine whether a patient's visual complaints are due to cataract and whether the patient requires surgery for cataract
4. To determine whether sensitivity to glare is contributing to a patient's visual symptoms
5. Corneal thickness, that is, the distance between the epithelium (front layer of cells) and the endothelium (back layer of cells) of the cornea
6. To diagnose the cause and determine the extent of corneal swelling and thickening and to help estimate the cornea's ability to withstand the stress of an operation
7. To photograph the cornea's endothelial cells at great magnification for cell counting to assess the health of the cornea and its ability to withstand certain intraocular surgical procedures
8. b
9. d
10. Fluorescein, a fluorescent dye, is injected into a vein in the patient's arm; the dye is delivered to the retinal blood vessels by the vascular system; the fundus camera photographs the appearance of the vessels in rapid sequence.
11. Temporary nausea, a severe allergic reaction
12. The reflection (echo) of high-frequency sound waves defines the outlines of ocular and orbital structures, measures the distance between these structures, and determines the size, composition, and position of intraocular abnormalities.
13. a
14. e

Chapter 7

1. Testing procedures for measuring the expanse and sensitivity of a patient's peripheral vision and visual field and for pinpointing possible defects
2. Retina
3. Because of the high concentration of cone cells
4. The physiologic blind spot, located close to the fovea on the nasal side of the retina, corresponds to the point at which the optic nerve exits the eye; sight is not possible there because of the absence of rods and cones at the head of the optic nerve.
5. To relate the scope of a patient's visual field to locations in the eye and to express locations in normal and defective visual fields in words and numbers
6. Fovea
7. Circles of eccentricity, radial meridians
8. About 15° eccentricity on the 0° or 180° (horizontal) meridian in the temporal field
9. About 90° temporally; 60° nasally, superiorly, and inferiorly
10. Inferior nasal
11. To detect abnormalities in the peripheral visual field and to monitor changes in the normal or defective field
12. *Kinetic perimetry*, which uses a moving test object (target) of predetermined size and brightness. *Static perimetry*, which employs a stationary target that can be changed in size, brightness, and position within the visual field but is not displayed until it has stopped moving.
13. A contour of the visual field obtained with a single target of a particular size and brightness, representing a line of equal sensitivity to the stimulus
14. A scotoma is an area of reduced sensitivity in the visual field. A shallow scotoma is a mild visual defect; a deep scotoma, a serious defect; and an absolute scotoma, a totally blind spot.
15. Confrontation field test, tangent screen test, Goldmann perimetry. Simplicity of the confrontation field test makes it useful for screening patients with major defects, particularly children, the very old, and the mentally impaired. The tangent screen test is more sensitive than the confrontation test, but still relatively simple to perform. Goldmann

perimetry is more sensitive and reproducible than the other two procedures; it is also able to measure the entire visual field.

16. Simple to understand for both the patient and the examiner; produces a pictorial result that is easy to interpret
17. The patient is slow to respond, either because of a long reaction time or because of a poor understanding of the test. The examiner moves the target too fast or too slow.
18. Suprathreshold perimetry, threshold perimetry
19. More sensitive at detecting small or shallow defects in the visual field; can eliminate certain technician- and environment-induced errors
20. Takes longer to perform; is more tedious; is more difficult for patients to understand; is less reliable for use with patients with limited mobility, attention span, or knowledge of the examiner's spoken language
21. General defects, focal defects
22. Glaucoma, retinal ischemia, optic nerve atrophy, media opacity (cataract or corneal scarring)
23. In kinetic perimetry, too rapid movement of the test object, poor understanding of the test by the patient, and patient slowness in signaling that the target has been seen; also, small pupils, interference with vision by eyeglass rims, aphakia, or a target that seems to be out of focus due to refractive error
24. Location, size, shape, depth, slope of margins
25. *Hemianopia*: the right or left half of the visual field is missing. *Homonymous hemianopia*: the right or left half of the visual field is defective or missing in both eyes.
26. Bjerrum scotoma, paracentral scotoma, nasal step
27. Loss of the entire upper or lower visual field
28. Environment-, device-, patient-, and examiner-related factors
29. *Environment*: room too hot or cold; room lights too bright or fluctuate; intrusion, movement, noise, and other distractions. *Device*: perimeter illumination not calibrated; paper, pencils, and other markers are unavailable; if computer-controlled, incorrect disk or door of disk drive not closed. *Patient*: misunderstanding the test, slow reaction time, poor physical condition, distractibility, boredom, anxiety, discomfort, abnormal pupil size, visual acuity, refractive error. *Examiner*: failure to calibrate perimeter illumination or to ensure that environmental conditions are suitable for testing, failure to properly cover eye not being tested, failure to instruct the patient properly in the test procedure, moving or presenting test targets too rapidly or too slowly.

Chapter 8

1. b, c, d, a
2. b, a, e, d
3. e
4. Glass
5. b
6. The curve of the lens surface from which the other curves necessary for sight correction are calculated
7. Black
8. 6 diopters
9. The angle by which the front of an eyeglass frame deviates from the vertical plane of the wearer's face
10.

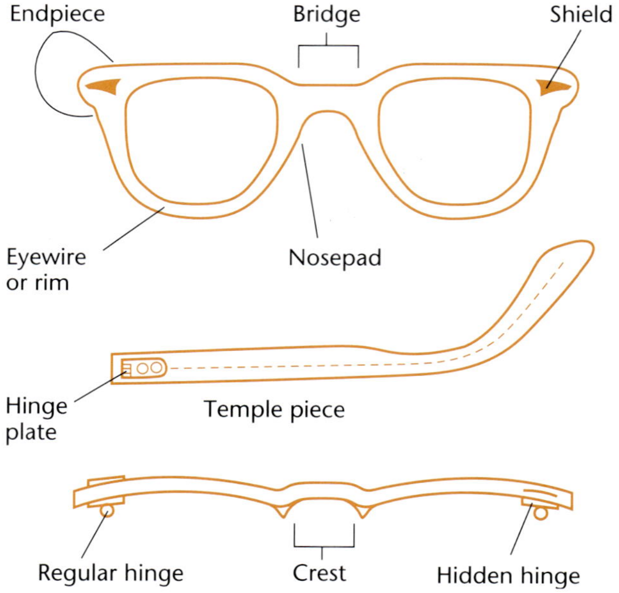

11. Cover the tips of the temple pieces of the frames with your fingers until you have moved them past the patient's eyes.
12. Lower lid margin
13. c, d, e, b, a

Chapter 9

1. A preliminary interview with a patient to determine the urgency of the situation and to schedule a visit with the doctor accordingly
2. What is the basic medical complaint or symptom? How did the complaint or symptom originate? When did the complaint or symptom start?
3. Acid, alkali, organic solvents
4. Irrigate the affected eye immediately by holding it open either under a continuous flow of running tap water or in a basin filled with water for at least 15 to 20 minutes before proceeding to the office or emergency facility
5. c, d
6. If possible, get the patient's head below the heart.

Patient Screening Exercises

1. b, c, e, f, h *Discussion*: Any screening evaluation requires you to obtain the most important information in the shortest time. The principal questions to ask in assessing the urgency of a complaint of visual disturbance are how long the symptom has been present (b), how rapidly it has occurred (c), how severe it is (f), and whether one or both eyes are affected (e). For any complaint, it is useful to document any noticeable associated symptoms (h). The other questions might be useful in a more detailed history, but they do not help to establish the urgency of the patient's complaint.
2. a, c, d, e, i *Discussion*: A chemical injury should always be considered an emergency, and the screening evaluation should seek only the most crucial pieces of information. For injuries that have just occurred, immediate irrigation should always supersede all other instructions or inquiries (a). Timing of the accident (c) is relevant because the more recent the occurrence, the greater the benefit of immediate irrigation and prompt medical attention. This information tells the doctor how far, if at all, damage has progressed and helps in patient evaluation. Impaired vision (d) may suggest a more serious injury, and knowing the chemical involved (e) can provide information about the potential for serious eye damage. Both of these facts help the ophthalmologist make the most informed treatment decisions. It can help to know whether a patient can see well enough with at least one eye to get to the water faucet or drive to the doctor's office, although it may not ordinarily matter which eye was involved (h). Always ask patients with potential emergencies if they have transportation to the office or a medical facility (i); if not, an ambulance or a taxicab may have to be summoned. The presence or absence of glasses (b) is usually critical only if there was an explosion that may have caused fragments from the glasses to penetrate the eye. History of glaucoma (f) and presence of tearing (g) are not considered crucial information in this case.
3. b, c, e, f, h *Discussion*: All patients should be questioned about the duration of their symptoms (b). Mild symptoms of long duration, such as burning eyes over a 3-month period, typically do not represent an emergency. However, a patient with sudden, unexplained burning and/or redness (e) of previously normal eyes may be experiencing an acute reaction to an environmental irritant and should be handled expeditiously. Knowing whether and when symptoms seem most noticeable (c), whether and what other symptoms are present (f), and what activities relieve the patient's symptoms (h) can better indicate the nature of the problem and may allow the doctor to recommend relief measures until the patient can be seen. Questions a, d, and g are not necessarily inappropriate but may be better left for a more detailed history at the time of the visit.
4. a, b, d, e *Discussion*: Whenever a patient reports visual impairment, such as this one and the patient reporting blurred vision in exercise 1, it is important to define the nature of the visual loss precisely. This includes the time of onset (a) and whether one or both eyes are affected (b). If the patient had not volunteered that the episodes were transient, it would be appropriate to ask if the visual loss was intermittent or persistent. This information, as well as the length of time of each episode (d), gives the doctor important diagnostic clues that would bear on the urgency. For patients such as this one with repeated episodes, identifying associated symptoms can be important (e). Specifically asking about discharge and tearing

(c) or headaches (g) is not usually useful in determining the nature of the visual loss itself. These questions and questions about family history (f) may be asked during a more detailed history-taking at the office.

Chapter 10

1. d
2. No peripheral vision but good central vision, no central vision, less than 20/200 visual acuity, only portions of the visual field perceived, light perception only, no light perception, fluctuations in vision
3. Either proceed to a room with the patient or have another office staff member take over guiding the patient for you.
4. 8/200
5. See and count fingers, detect hand movements, perceive light
6. c
7. c
8. Hypoglycemia

Chapter 11

1. Topical, injectable, oral
2. Solutions, suspension, ointments and gels, inserts
3. Redness, tearing, pain
4. Drug remains in contact with eye or lid longer
5. Registered nurse or doctor
6. c, a, d, b, e
7. a
8. d
9. a
10. b
11. d
12. c
13. b
14. a

Chapter 12

1. Bacteria, viruses, fungi, protozoa
2. Airborne droplets and particles; direct contact with an infected person; indirect contact with a contaminated person or object; common vehicles; vector-borne spread
3. To prevent the spread of infectious microbes to or from patients and medical office personnel
4. (1) Wash hands between contacts with patients. (2) Wear disposable gloves to avoid contact with body fluids or contaminated objects. (3) Use special receptacles ("sharps containers") for disposal of contaminated needles, blades, and other sharp objects. (4) Properly dispose of, disinfect, or sterilize contaminated objects between uses with patients. (5) Wear a fluid-impermeable gown and mask when there is the potential for splash of bloody or contaminated body fluids. (6) Dispose of eye patches, gauze, and the like that are saturated with blood (blood that can be wrung or squeezed out) in a special red impermeable isolation bag.
5. (1) Assistants with a fever blister should be excused from hands-on contact with patients until recovery. (2) If the patient has a fever blister, assistants should avoid touching the patient near the mouth with fingers or instruments. Assistants should wash their hands after completing any tests and be certain instruments used with the patient are properly disinfected or sterilized.
6. (a) Turn on the faucets and adjust the water to the warmest comfortable temperature. (b) Wet your hands, wrists, and about 4 inches of the forearms. (c) Apply antiseptic soap from a dispenser, and wash your hands with circular strokes for at least 15 seconds. (d) Rinse your hands and forearms. (e) Hold dry paper towels to close the faucets, discarding the paper towels when finished. (f) Dry your hands with clean paper towels.
7. *Disinfection* inactivates or eliminates most disease-causing microorganisms. *Sterilization* destroys all microorganisms.
8. Moist heat, ethylene oxide gas
9. Handle the sterile item only by a nonfunctional part (a part that does not come in contact with the patient or other sterile materials).
10. Avoid finger contact with the lip, tip, or inner lid of the bottle. Never permit the tip of the dropper bottle to touch the patient's eyelashes, lid, or eye. Check the liquid in the bottle for cloudiness or particulate matter and discard if present. Discard single-dose containers after one use.

11. Contaminated sharp objects are placed in a rigid, puncture-proof biohazard container (a "sharps container"), and when the container is full, it is disposed of according to standard procedures.

Chapter 13

1. Informed consent
2. d
3. Topical eyedrops and infiltrative injection
4. Forceps, scissors, needle holder
5. Taper point, cutting, reverse-cutting, spatula
6. *Absorbable*: surgical gut, collagen, polyglactin 910. *Nonabsorbable*: silk, nylon, polypropylene, polyester.
7. Chalazion surgery, other lid-lesion removal, lacrimal-system probing
8. To minimize postsurgical bleeding and immobilize the eyelid
9. To reduce the number of microorganisms that come in contact with the surgical wound, thus minimizing the chance of infection
10. Instrument sterilization, germicidal prepping of the operative site, scrubbing and gloving (also gowning and masking if required), handling materials in a way that prevents contamination
11. Cleansing the patient's operative site with germicidal solution
12. Sterile table and trays containing instruments, portions of the patient that have been prepped and draped, portions of the surgical personnel that have been cleansed and gloved
13. To provide a clean operating field and a sterile area on which personnel may rest their hands and instruments during surgery
14. Sharps must be re-counted to ensure that none remains near the patient; disposable sharps are placed in safety containers so that they will not injure office personnel or waste collectors.

Chapter 14

1. A layer of tears lies between the contact lens and the cornea, filling out corneal irregularities and converting the interface between the contact lens and the cornea into a smooth, spherical surface; the contact lens provides a radius of curvature different from that of the cornea, allowing light to focus on the retina.
2. Allow adequate oxygen to reach all of the cornea, promote flushing of metabolic waste from underneath the lens, sustain the integrity of the corneal epithelium, sustain normal corneal temperature
3. Spherical power, keratometry readings, lens diameter, base curve, lens thickness, lens material, water content (soft lens), specific brand or type of lens, edge blends or peripheral curves, tint, wearing instructions
4. b, c, f, a
5. Soft lenses diffuse oxygen and carbon dioxide through the lens material, with a minimal tear pump; PMMA lenses deliver oxygen only by pumping oxygenated tears under the lens; RGP lenses provide oxygen and carbon dioxide diffusion through the lens material and a tear pump.
6. Cleaning removes protein deposits and other debris that can blur vision or irritate the eye and act as a reservoir for microorganisms; disinfection prevents the growth of bacteria, viruses, and fungi on the lens.
7. Chemical, heat
8. To keep the lens surface hydrophilic and to provide a lubricating cushion between the contact lens and the cornea and between the contact lens and the eyelid
9. Wash hands and dry them with a lint-free towel; be sure all traces of soap are rinsed off.
10. Irritation, fogging, redness, tearing, decreased wearing time
11. Warping is a semipermanent change in the corneal curvature; it is caused by an improperly fit rigid contact lens
12. Edema, vascularization, ulcer, abrasion, infection
13. The conjunctiva, which lines both the globe and the inner lid, prevents the lens from disappearing behind the eye.
14. Pathologic conditions such as allergies, chronic blepharoconjunctivitis, pterygium, seventh-nerve paresis, anesthetic cornea; inappropriate nervous and emotional temperament; poor or no blink reflexes; dry eyes; disabilities such as parkinsonism or arthritis; ongoing exposure to dust, dirt, particles, or caustic chemicals

Glossary

This glossary includes pronunciations for many ophthalmic technical terms. Accented syllables are indicated by CAPITAL LETTERS; in words of five or more syllables, a secondary accent is indicated by an Initial Capital Letter. Vowel sounds are indicated and pronounced as shown in the table below. Pronunciations are approximate, and alternative pronunciations are often acceptable.

Vowel	Written	Pronounced as in
A	ay	may
	a + consonant	tap
	ah	father
	uh	about
	ae	pair
E	ee	bee
	e + consonant *or* eh	bet
	ur	term
I	iy	eye
	consonant + y	dye
	i + consonant + e	bite
	i, ih	bit
O	oh	oh
	uh	mother
	o + consonant	hot
	ah	fog
	oo	do
U	yoo	cute
	u + consonant, *or* uh	hut
Y	ee	happy
	ih	myth
	y	my

abduction (ab-DUK-shun) The movement of the eye outward toward the temple.

abrasion A scratch.

abscess (AB-sehs) A localized collection of pus surrounded by inflamed tissue.

absolute scotoma (skoh-TOH-muh) A severe visual field defect in which the largest and brightest stimulus cannot be seen; blindness at that location.

accommodation The change in the curvature of the crystalline lens that helps to focus images of objects close to the eye.

acquired immunodeficiency syndrome (AIDS) A viral infection characterized by a compromised immune system.

acute Refers to a condition that flares up suddenly and persists for only a short time.

add The portion of the multifocal lens (usually the lower part) that provides near vision. Also called *segment* or *near add*.

adduction (uh-DUK-shun) The movement of the eye inward toward the nose.

adenovirus (Ad-een-oh-VY-rus) A family of viruses involved primarily in respiratory infections; can cause highly contagious forms of conjunctivitis.

adnexa (ad-NEK-suh) The tissues and structures surrounding the eye; includes the orbit, extraocular muscles, eyelids, and lacrimal apparatus.

against motion The retinoscopic reflex movement that is in the opposite direction from the streak of light; typical of the myopic eye.

age-related macular degeneration (MAK-yoo-lahr) A disease in which sensory cells of the macula degenerate, resulting in a loss of central vision; affects older people.

AIDS *See* **acquired immunodeficiency syndrome**.

allergic reaction A condition in which the body produces antibodies to foreign materials such as food, plant pollens, or medications.

altitudinal scotoma (skoh-TOH-muh) The joining and enlargement of a nasal step visual field defect and an arcuate scotoma to cause loss of the entire upper or lower visual field.

amblyopia *See* **strabismic amblyopia.**

ametropia (Am-eh-TROH-pee-uh) The refractive state of an eye that is unable to focus correctly due to refractive error.

A-mode ultrasonography *See* **A-scan ultrasonography**.

Amsler grid test (AHM-zler) A test for determining the presence and location of defects in the central portion of the visual field.

anatomy The structure of an organism.

anesthetic A drug that causes a temporary deadening of a nerve, resulting in loss of feeling in the surrounding tissue.

anisocoria (an-Ih-so-KOH-ree-uh) A condition in which the pupils are of unequal size.

anterior Front.

anterior chamber The small compartment between the cornea and the iris that is filled with a clear, transparent fluid called *aqueous humor*.

anterior chamber angle The junction of the cornea and the iris, from which aqueous humor leaves the eye. Also called *filtration angle*.

anterior segment The front of the eye; includes the structures between the front surface of the cornea and the vitreous.

antibiotic A drug that combats a bacterial infection.

antibody The type of chemical that the body manufactures to neutralize an infecting microorganism.

antifungal A drug that combats a fungal infection.

antiviral A drug that combats a viral infection.

apex The top, as of a prism.

aphakia (ah-FAY-kee-uh) Absence of the lens, usually because of cataract extraction.

aphakic correction(ah-FAY-kik) The use of a contact lens, eyeglasses, or an intraocular lens for more normal vision in aphakic patients.

applanation (ap-lah-NAY-shun) A form of tonometry in which the force required to flatten a small area of the central cornea is measured.

aqueous humor (AY-kwee-us) The clear, transparent fluid that fills the anterior chamber.

arc perimeter A perimetric device that can test the entire field of vision.

arcuate scotoma (AHR-kyu-at skoh-TOH-muh) The enlargement of a Bjerrum scotoma to become an arc-shaped area of reduced sensitivity.

arcus senilis (AR-kus sih-NIL-us) A common degenerative change in which the outer edge of the cornea gradually becomes opaque, generally in both eyes; affects people over the age of 50.

A-scan ultrasonography (Ul-trah-son-OG-ruh-fee) A diagnostic procedure in which sound waves traveling in a straight line are used to reveal the position of, and distances between, structures within the eye and orbit. Also called *A-mode ultrasonography*.

aseptic technique (ay-SEP-tik) A range of procedures used in medical environments to prevent the spread of infectious microbes.

astigmatism (uh-STIG-muh-tizm) The refractive error of an eye whose corneal surface curvature is greater in one meridian than another; both distant and near objects appear blurred and distorted.

autoclave A metal chamber equipped to use steam or gas under high pressure and temperature to destroy microorganisms.

Autoplot A refined version of the tangent screen (kinetic perimetric device) for measuring the central 30° of vision.

axial ray (AK-see-al) A light ray that strikes the center of a lens of any shape and passes undeviated through the lens material. Also called *principal ray*.

axis The meridian perpendicular to the meridian with curvature in a cylindrical lens.

axon The long fiber-like portion of a ganglion cell that courses over the surface of the retina and converges at the optic disc.

bacteria (singular: *bacterium*) Single-celled microorganisms, widely dispersed in nature; some bacteria are capable of causing disease in humans.

balancing A procedure performed on both eyes at once to ensure that the optical correction determined by refractometry for distance vision does not include an uneven overcorrection or undercorrection. Also called *binocular balancing*.

basal cell carcinoma (kar-sih-NOH-muh) The most common malignant lid tumor; has a characteristic appearance of a pit surrounded by raised "pearly" edges.

base The bottom, as of a prism.
base curve The curve of the lens surface, usually the outer or front side of the lens, from which the other curves necessary for sight correction are calculated.
benign (beh-NINE) Refers to any tumor that is not dangerous to the well-being of the individual.
bifocal lens One that has two powers: usually one for correcting distance vision and one for correcting near vision.
binary fission The form of reproduction by a bacterium, by splitting in two.
binocular balancing *See* **balancing**.
binocular vision The blending of the separate images seen by each eye into one image; occurs when both eyes are directed toward a single target and perfectly aligned.
biomicroscope *See* **slit lamp**.
bipolar cell A type of retinal cell that accepts electric (nerve) impulses from the photoreceptors and passes them to the ganglion cells.
bitemporal hemianopia (Hem-ee-uh-NOH-pee-uh) A visual field defect affecting the temporal field of both eyes.
Bjerrum scotoma (BYER-oom skoh-TOH-muh) A small, relatively blind area in the visual field.
blended bifocal *See* **invisible bifocal**.
blepharitis (blef-ah-RY-tis) A common inflammation of the eyelid margin.
blowout fracture An injury due to blunt trauma, in which orbital bones are broken.
B-mode ultrasonography *See* **B-scan ultrasonography**.
Bowman's membrane A layer of the cornea, located between the corneal epithelium and the corneal stroma; acts as an anchor for the corneal epithelium.
B-scan ultrasonography (Ul-trah-son-OG-ruh-fee) A diagnostic procedure that provides two-dimensional reconstruction of ocular and orbital tissues, using radiating sound waves. Also called *B-mode ultrasonography*.
bulbar conjunctiva (kon-junk-TY-vuh) The globe portion of the conjunctiva.

calibration The testing of any device against a known standard; for example, the illumination of a perimetric device.
canaliculus (Kan-ah-LIK-yu-lus; plural: *canaliculi*) One of two tubes (*upper canaliculus* and *lower canaliculus*) through which tears pass into the lacrimal sac.
canal of Schlemm (SHLEM) A structure that drains the aqueous humor from the anterior chamber after it has flowed through the trabecular meshwork.
cannula (KAN-yu-luh) A blunt needle-like tube used during surgery for injecting or extracting fluid or air.
canthus (KAN-thus; plural: *canthi*) The point where the upper and lower eyelids meet on the nasal (inner) side (*medial canthus*) and the temporal (outer) side (*lateral canthus*).
cardinal positions of gaze The six points to which a patient's eyes are directed to test extraocular muscle function; the positions are right and up, right, right and down, left and up, left, and left and down.
cardiovascular system The body system consisting of the heart and blood vessels (arteries and veins).
cataract (KAT-ah-rakt) An opacified (clouded) lens.
cautery (KAW-ter-ee) The application of an electric current by means of a specialized instrument; used to destroy a lesion and prevent bleeding.
central scotoma (skoh-TOH-muh) A visual field defect in the center of the field.
chalazion (kah-LAY-zee-on) A nontender lump that may become visible on the outer lid; due to long-term inflammation and infection of a meibomian gland.
chemical trauma (TRAW-muh) Refers to injury caused by a chemical, such as an acid or an alkali.
chief complaint The principal reason for the patient's visit to the doctor, defined by the nature and duration of the patient's symptoms and by whether the problem is worsening.
chlamydiae (klah-MID-ee-ee; singular: *chlamydia*) A type of bacteria.
choroid (KOR-oyd) A layer of tissue, largely made up of blood vessels, that nourishes the retina; it lies between the sclera and the retina in the uveal tract.
chronic Refers to a condition that has persisted for some time.
cilia (SIL-ee-ah; singular: *cilium*) The eyelashes.
ciliary body (SIL-ee-ehr-ee) A band-like structure of muscle and secretory tissue that extends from the edge of the iris and encircles the inside of the sclera.
ciliary muscle (SIL-ee-ehr-ee) The muscle fibers in the ciliary body of the uveal tract that are involved in accommodation.

ciliary process (SIL-ee-ehr-ee) A finger-like extension of the ciliary body that produces aqueous humor.

cilium *See* **cilia**.

circles of eccentricity A series of concentric circles at intervals of 10° from the point of central visual fixation, providing coordinates for mapping the visual field.

common-vehicle transmission The form of infection transmission involving the transfer of infectious microbes from one reservoir to many people.

complication A problem that occurs during or after medical or surgical treatment.

concave lens A piece of glass or plastic in which one or both surfaces are curved inward. Also called *negative lens* or *minus lens*.

concave mirror effect The lighting effect of a retinoscope that produces convergent rays.

cone The retinal photoreceptor largely responsible for sharp central vision and for color perception.

confrontation field test A test comparing the boundaries of the patient's field of vision with that of the examiner, who is presumed to have a normal field.

congenital Refers to any disease process or effect that is present from birth.

congenital glaucoma (glaw-KOH-muh) A rare disease that occurs in infants; due to a malformation of the anterior chamber angle.

conjunctiva (kon-junk-TY-vuh) The thin, translucent mucous membrane that lines the inner surface of the eyelids and outer surface of the globe, except for the cornea.

conjunctivitis (Kon-junk-tih-VY-tis) A swelling of the small conjunctival blood vessels, making the conjunctiva appear red. Also called *pink eye*.

contraindication Any condition that renders a particular treatment, medication, or medical device inadvisable for a particular patient.

contrast-sensitivity test A procedure for determining the ability to distinguish between light and dark areas; useful in the diagnosis of cataract.

converge To come together.

convex lens A piece of glass or plastic in which one or both surfaces are curved outward. Also called *positive lens* or *plus lens*.

cornea (KOR-nee-uh) The clear tissue at the front of the globe that begins the process of focusing light the eye receives.

corneal abrasion (KOR-nee-uhl) A scratch of the corneal epithelium.

corneal endothelium (KOR-nee-uhl En-doh-THEE-lee-um) The layer of cells that covers the inner surface of the cornea and maintains proper fluid balance within the cornea.

corneal epithelium (KOR-nee-uhl Ep-ih-THEE-lee-um) The outermost layer of the cornea, providing defense against infection and injury.

corneal stroma (KOR-nee-uhl STROH-muh) The main body of the cornea; contributes rigidity to the cornea.

corneal topography (KOR-nee-uhl top-OG-rah-fee) A photographic procedure that produces a color-coded "map" of the surface of the cornea, used in evaluating patients for contact lens wear or refractive or cataract surgery.

corneal ulcer (KOR-nee-uhl) A lesion after an infection of or injury to the corneal epithelium.

corticosteroid (Kor-tih-koh-STEER-oyd) A drug, either a natural or a synthetic hormone, that combats an allergic or inflammatory condition. Also called *steroid*.

cover–uncover test A test performed by alternately covering and uncovering each eye to determine if a patient's eyes are misaligned.

cross cylinder A special lens consisting of two cylinders of equal power, one minus and one plus, with their axes set at right angles to each other; used for determining the axis and power of an astigmatic correction.

cryopexy (kry-oh-PEKS-ee) Freezing by surgical means.

crystalline lens *See* **lens**.

cul-de-sac (KUL-deh-Sahk) *See* **fornix**.

cycloplegia (Sy-kloh-PLEE-jee-uh) Temporary paralysis of the ciliary muscle (preventing accommodation) and of the iris sphincter muscle (preventing dilation of the pupil).

cycloplegic refraction (sy-kloh-PLEE-jik) Refractometry performed with the use of a drug that temporarily paralyzes the ciliary muscle, thus blocking accommodation.

cylinder *See* **spherocylinder**.

cylindrical lens A lens that has curvature in only one meridian.

cytomegalovirus (CMV) (sy-toh-Meg-ah-loh-VY-rus) A member of the herpesvirus family; causes CMV retinitis.

dacryocystitis (Dak-ree-oh-sis-TY-tis) Inflammation of the lacrimal sac; usually caused by blockage or obstruction of the nasolacrimal duct.

daily-wear lenses Rigid and soft contact lenses intended to be worn for fewer than 24 consecutive hours while awake.

DBC *See* **distance between optical centers**.

decibel The unit (one tenth of a log) of measure of the brightness of a test object.

decongestant A drug that constricts the superficial blood vessels in the conjunctiva to reduce eye redness; a cosmetic effect only.

deep scotoma (skoh-TOH-muh) A visual field defect more serious than a shallow scotoma; appears as a pit or well in the island of vision.

degenerative Refers to any process in which the structure or function of body tissues gradually deteriorates.

dendritic (den-DRIT-ik) Branch-shaped, such as the corneal ulcers seen after infection with the herpes simplex virus.

density Compactness, with reference to the structure of a particular substance.

depression The type of visual field defect that is like an indentation in the surface of the island of vision.

Descemet's membrane (des-eh-MAYZ) The thin, elastic layer between the corneal stroma and the corneal endothelium; contributes rigidity to the cornea.

developmental Refers to any disease process or effect that results from faulty development of a structure or system.

diabetes mellitus (dy-uh-BEE-tis MEL-it-us) A condition in which the body is unable to produce enough insulin, the hormone required for the metabolism of sugar.

diabetic retinopathy (dy-uh-BET-ik Reh-tin-OP-uh-thee) A progression of pathologic changes in the retina; produced by long-standing diabetes mellitus.

diagnosis (dy-ag-NOH-sis) Determination of a medical condition.

diffuse *See* **infection**.

dilator muscle The iris muscle that dilates the pupil in reduced light conditions; fibers from this muscle stretch from the pupil to the boundaries of the iris.

diopter (dy-OP-tur) The unit of measure of the power of a lens.

diplopia (dih-PLOH-pee-uh) Double vision.

direct and consensual pupillary reaction (PYU-pih-lehr-ee) The response of the pupils when light is shone in one eye: that eye constricts (*direct reaction*) and the other eye also constricts, even when light does not reach it (*consensual reaction*).

direct-contact transmission The form of infection transmission between people usually requiring body contact.

direct ophthalmoscope (ahf-THAL-muh-skohp) A hand-held instrument with a light-and-mirror system that affords an upright, monocular view of a narrow field of the fundus, magnified 15-fold.

disease A specific process in which abnormal changes result in malfunction of a particular part or system of the body.

disinfection The process of inactivating or eliminating pathogenic microorganisms.

disposable lenses Soft contact lenses designed for either daily or extended wear and then disposal after 1 week to 1 month.

distance between optical centers (**DBC**) The distance between the optical center of the right lens and that of the left; corresponds to the patient's interpupillary distance.

distometer (dis-TOM-eh-ter) An instrument for measuring vertex distance.

diverge To spread apart.

double-D segment A multifocal lens with the distance correction in the middle, a traditional near-power D segment at the bottom, and an intermediate-power inverted D segment at the top.

D segment A portion of a bifocal or trifocal lens; so called because it is shaped like the capital letter D lying on its side.

eccentricity, circles of *See* **circles of eccentricity**.

ectropion (ek-TROH-pee-on) A condition in which the lower eyelid margin is pulled away from the eye; caused by malformation of or damage to the eyelid tissues.

edema (eh-DEE-mah) Swelling caused by a large amount of fluid in a part of the body.

electromagnetic radiation The spectrum of rays from invisible cosmic, gamma, and x-rays, through visible light waves, to invisible radio and television signals.

emergency A medical situation that requires immediate attention.

emmetropia (em-eh-TROH-pee-uh) The refractive state of an eye that is able to focus correctly.

empiric treatment The institution of medical treatment based on probable cause, before test results or other time-consuming procedures confirm a diagnosis.

endocrine system The body system consisting of multiple glands that produce chemicals called hormones, which regulate various bodily functions.

endophthalmitis (En-dahf-thal-MY-tis) A serious ocular bacterial infection with inflammation of the vitreous and adjacent tissues.

endothelium, corneal *See* **corneal endothelium**.

entropion (en-TROH-pee-on) A condition in which the upper or lower lid margin is turned inward.

enzyme cleaner A specially designed detergent for removing protein deposits from contact lenses.

epiphora (eh-PIF-oh-ruh) Excessive tearing.

episcleritis (Ep-ih-skleh-RY-tis) Inflammation of the surface layer of the sclera.

epithelium, corneal *See* **corneal epithelium**.

eso deviation The inward deviation of the eye.

esophoria (Ees-oh-FOR-ee-uh) The inward deviation of the eye that is present only when one eye is covered.

esotropia (Ees-oh-TROH-pee-uh) The inward deviation of the eye in which the eyes are misaligned even when uncovered.

etiology (Ee-tee-OL-oh-jee) Literally, the study of the causes of a disease; informally, the causes themselves.

executive Refers to a bifocal lens consisting of a top distance band and a bottom near band that divide the entire width of the lens into two parts.

exo deviation The outward deviation of the eye.

exophoria (Ek-soh-FOR-ee-uh) The outward deviation of the eye that is present only when one eye is covered.

exophthalmometer (Ek-sahf-thal-MOM-uh-tur) An instrument that measures the prominence of the eyeball in relation to the bony orbital rim surrounding it.

exophthalmometry (Ek-sahf-thal-MOM-uh-tree) The measurement of the prominence of the eyeball in relation to the bony orbital rim surrounding it.

exophthalmos (ek-sahf-THAL-mohs) *See* **proptosis**.

exotropia (Ek-soh-TROH-pee-uh) The outward deviation of the eye in which the eyes are misaligned even when uncovered.

extended-wear lenses Soft contact lenses that are approved for overnight wear for up to 7 days.

external hordeolum *See* **stye**.

extraocular muscles The six muscles that attach to the outside of the globe and control its movements.

eyeball *See* **globe**.

eyelid The moving fold of skin that covers the outer portion of the globe.

Farnsworth-Munsell D-15 test *See* **15-hue test**.

15-hue test A test that can identify color vision deficits by asking the patient to arrange 15 pastel-colored chips of similar brightness but subtly different hues in a related color sequence. Also called *Farnsworth-Munsell D-15 test*.

filtration angle *See* **anterior chamber angle**.

fixate To gaze steadily at something.

flashlight test A simple test for estimating the depth of the anterior chamber and the chamber angle.

floaters Small particles of dead cells or other debris that become suspended in vitreous, or particles of the vitreous itself that degenerate in the normal aging process; they cast shadows on the retina and appear as spots or cobwebs.

fluorescein (FLOOR-uh-seen) A dye solution that is used in applanation tonometry; also used intravenously in fluorescein angiography to identify abnormal blood vessels.

fluorescein angiography (FLOOR-uh-seen An-jee-OG-ruh-fee) Diagnostic photography of retinal vessels that requires injection of fluorescein dye.

focal defect The type of visual field defect in which a local pit or well in the field of vision occurs.

focal length The distance between the focal point and the lens.

focal point The point somewhere along the principal axis at which the paraxial rays from a distant source are refracted by a lens and converge in the case of a convex lens and diverge in the case of a concave lens.

foreign-body sensation A feeling of eye irritation or grittiness.

fornix (FOR-niks) The loose pocket of conjunctival tissue where the eyelid and globe portions of the conjunctiva meet beneath the upper and lower lids. Also called *cul-de-sac*.

fovea (FOH-vee-uh) The center of the macula.

fundus (FUN-dus) A collective term for the retina, optic disc, and macula.

funduscopic examination (fun-du-SKOP-ik) Examination of the vitreous and fundus by ophthalmoscope. Also called *posterior segment examination*.

fungus (plural: *fungi*) A multicelled microorganism that differs from a bacterium in that it has a more complex structure; includes yeasts and molds. Some can live inside the body and cause infection.
fusion The blending by the brain of the separate images received by the two eyes so that a single view is perceived even when the eyes move.

ganglion cell (GANG-glee-on) The type of retinal cell that accepts electric (nerve) impulses from the bipolar cells and sends the impulses via axons through the optic disc to the brain.
gel *See* **ointment**.
general defect The type of visual field defect in which the field of vision shrinks symmetrically or is depressed evenly across the entire retina.
genetic Refers to a trait that is inherited from either or both parents.
Geneva lens clock An instrument for measuring the base curve of an eyeglass lens.
genus (plural: *genera*) A category of biologic classification ranking immediately higher than the species; the general name for a type of organism.
geometric optics The area of optics that deals with the transmission of light as rays and is concerned with the effect of lenses on light and the production of images.
germicide (JER-mih-side) A chemical that kills germs.
giant papillary conjunctivitis (**GPC**) (PAP-ih-lehr-ee Kon-junk-tih-VY-tis) Inflammation of the tarsal conjunctiva, characterized by large raised bumps.
gimbal (GIM-buhl) The ring-like frame in the lensmeter.
glare testing A procedure for assessing a patient's vision in the presence of a bright light source to determine whether sensitivity to glare is contributing to visual symptoms.
glaucoma (glaw-KOH-muh) An eye disease in which the intraocular pressure is high enough to cause damage to the optic nerve, resulting in visual loss; caused by impaired drainage of the aqueous fluid out of the eye.
globe The eye, without its surrounding structures. Also called *eyeball*.
goblet cell The type of cell in the conjunctiva that produces the sticky fluid that comprises the innermost tear-film layer.
Goldmann goniolens (GOH-nee-oh-lenz) A mirrored contact lens used in gonioscopy; reflects an image of the anterior chamber, which is seen through a slit lamp.
Goldmann perimeter A bowl-like instrument for testing visual fields in which targets (lights) of different sizes and intensities are projected onto a standardized background illumination.
Goldmann tonometer (toh-NOM-eh-ter) An applanation tonometer that measures corneal flattening to determine intraocular pressure.
gonioscopy (Goh-nee-OS-koh-pee) A method of viewing the chamber angle through a special contact lens placed on the anesthetized eye.
GPC *See* **giant papillary conjunctivitis**.
Gram staining The procedure for identifying bacteria and certain other microbes according to their reaction to a dye—either *Gram-positive* or *Gram-negative*.
granuloma (gran-yu-LOH-mah) A firm collection of a specific kind of inflammatory cell.
Graves' disease A condition of unknown origin that involves the thyroid gland and causes the soft tissues surrounding the globe to swell.

hemianopia (Hem-ee-uh-NOH-pee-uh) The type of visual field defect in which the right or left half of the field in one eye is missing.
hemorrhage (HEM-or-ij) The accumulation of blood from a broken vessel.
hemostasis (hee-moh-STAY-sis) The control of bleeding.
herpes simplex virus (HER-peez SIM-pleks) In ophthalmology, a type of virus that infects the cornea, producing branch-like ulcers (dendritic keratitis).
herpes simplex virus type 1 (**HSV-1**) (HER-peez SIM-pleks) A herpesvirus that causes recurrent fever blisters on the lips and mouth and, if introduced to the eye, blepharokeratoconjunctivitis.
herpes simplex virus type 2 (**HSV-2**) (HER-peez SIM-pleks) Similar to HSV-1, except that it more commonly infects the genital region and is spread by sexual contact.
herpesvirus (her-peez-VY-rus) A family of viruses.
HIV *See* **human immunodeficiency virus**.
homonymous hemianopia (hoh-MON-ih-mus Hem-ee-uh-NOH-pee-uh) The type of visual field defect in which the right or left half of the field in both eyes is missing.
hordeolum (hor-DEE-oh-lum) *See* **internal hordeolum**; **stye**.

horizontal and vertical meridians The radial meridians that divide the circular visual field mapping device into quarters.
host The animal or plant from which a microbe gains nutrients and the conditions necessary for its survival and reproduction.
Hruby lens (HRU-bee) A noncontact lens attached to the slit lamp; useful for examining the optic nerve head and small areas of the posterior retina and vitreous.
HSV-1 *See* **herpes simplex virus type 1**.
HSV-2 *See* **herpes simplex virus type 2**.
human immunodeficiency virus (HIV) A virus that causes a deficiency of the immune system, making the patient susceptible to a variety of infections of various tissues, including the retina.
hydrophilic (hy-droh-FIL-ik) Refers to the property of combining with or attracting water.
hydrophobic (hy-droh-FOH-bik) Refers to the property of resisting or repelling water.
hyperopia (Hy-per-OH-pee-uh) Farsightedness; the eye is too short for its optical system.
hyphema (hy-FEE-muh) The pooling of blood in the anterior chamber as a result of trauma or certain diseases.
hypoglycemia (Hy-poh-gly-SEE-mee-uh) Low blood sugar level, common among patients with diabetes.
hypopyon (hy-POH-pee-on) The accumulation of pus in the anterior chamber.
hypoxia (hy-POK-see-uh) A loss of oxygen.

immune reaction The body's response to infection, in which antibodies are manufactured to neutralize the infecting microorganism and perhaps prevent recurrence of the infection.
incision A cut produced by a sharp instrument.
indentation A form of tonometry in which the amount of corneal indentation produced by a fixed weight is measured.
indirect-contact transmission The form of infection transmission involving an intermediate, inanimate object.
indirect ophthalmoscope (ahf-THAL-muh-skohp) An instrument that affords an inverted but wider view of the fundus than does the direct ophthalmoscope.
infection The invasion and multiplication of harmful microorganisms in the body tissues: a *local* bacterial or fungal infection begins in the tissues immediately surrounding the microorganism's point of entry; if unchecked, the infection may spread to surrounding tissues, thereby becoming *diffuse*.
inferior oblique muscle The extraocular muscle that rotates the eye upward and toward the nose.
inferior rectus muscle The extraocular muscle that is primarily responsible for turning the eye downward.
inflammation A local protective tissue response to infection, in which specialized cells move to the affected area to destroy the injurious agent, while other cells release fluids to dilute any toxic substances produced by the infectious agent and wall off both the offender and the damaged tissue.
informed consent The process by which, after discussion with the physician about the risks and benefits of a proposed procedure, the patient agrees to undergo a treatment.
injection The delivery system by which a drug is injected into the body with a hypodermic needle.
injury Damage to or destruction of cells that compose a tissue, organ, or system.
insert The delivery system by which a drug-containing wafer is placed on the conjunctiva under the upper or lower eyelid; releases the drug slowly and steadily over a period of time.
insulin (IN-suh-lin) A hormone the body uses to metabolize sugar.
interferometer (In-ter-Feer-OM-uh-ter) A laser instrument for determining visual acuity in the presence of an opacity, such as a cataract.
internal hordeolum (hor-DEE-oh-lum) A lump on the inner or outer eyelid; caused by inflammation and infection of a meibomian gland.
interpupillary distance (IPD *or* PD) (In-ter-PYU-pih-Lehr-ee) The distance from the center of the pupil of one eye to the center of the pupil of the other eye.
intraocular pressure (In-trah-OK-yu-lur) Fluid pressure within the eye.
invisible bifocal A bifocal lens with a softened or blended transitional zone between the segment and the distance portion. Also called *seamless bifocal* or *blended bifocal*.
IPD *See* **interpupillary distance**.
iridotomy (Ihr-ih-DOT-oh-mee) A type of laser surgery used to open the anterior chamber angle of patients with glaucoma.

iris The colored circle of tissue that controls the amount of light entering the eye by enlarging or reducing the size of its aperture, the pupil.
iritis (iy-RY-tis) Inflammation of the iris.
irregular astigmatism (uh-STIG-muh-tizm) The less common form of astigmatism, in which the cornea resembles a football tipped to one side.
ischemia (is-KEE-mee-uh) A condition in which the supply of blood to a part of the body is severely reduced.
isopter (iy-SOP-ter) In visual field tests, a line connecting the points denoting areas of equal sensitivity to a stimulus; similar to contour lines denoting equal elevations of a topographic map.

keratitis (kehr-ah-TY-tis) Inflammation of the cornea.
keratoconjunctivitis sicca (Kehr-ah-toh-kon-Junk-tih-VY-tis SIHK-uh) Dry eyes.
keratoconus (Kehr-ah-toh-KOH-nus) An uncommon degenerative corneal disease in which the center of the cornea thins and assumes the shape of a cone, seriously affecting vision.
keratometer (Kehr-ah-TOM-eh-tur) An instrument used to measure corneal curvature. Also called *ophthalmometer*.
keratometry (Kehr-ah-TOM-eh-tree) The measurement of corneal curvature.
kinetic perimetry (kih-NET-ik peh-RIM-eh-tree) The type of perimetry that uses a moving test object of a predetermined size and brightness.
Koeppe lens (KEP-ee) A high-plus contact lens used in gonioscopy to examine the angle structures directly with a hand-held light source and microscope.

laceration A cut.
lacrimal apparatus (LAK-ri-mul) The structures of the eye that produce tears and the ducts that drain the excess fluid from the front of the eyes into the nose.
lacrimal gland (LAK-ri-mul) The gland that produces the watery substance making up the middle layer of the tear film; located in the lateral part of the upper lid.
lacrimal needle (LAK-ri-mul) *See* **cannula**.
lacrimal probe (LAK-ri-mul) An instrument for exploring and clearing an obstruction of the tear duct.
lacrimal sac (LAK-ri-mul) The sac that holds tears after they pass through the canaliculi, which empty through the nasolacrimal duct into the nasal cavity.
lacrimal set (LAK-ri-mul) A group of instruments for clearing an obstruction of the tear duct.
lagophthalmos (lag-ahf-THAL-mos) A condition in which the globe is not completely covered when the eyelids are closed; may be caused by facial-nerve paralysis or by an enlarged or protruding eye.
lateral canthus *See* **canthus**.
lateral geniculate body (jeh-NIK-yu-let) The part of the brain where optic fibers synapse to the optic radiations and transmit visual impulses.
lateral rectus muscle The extraocular muscle that rotates the eye outward toward the temple.
legal blindness A best-corrected visual acuity of 20/200 or less or a visual field reduced to 20° or less in the better-seeing eye.
lens Part of the optical focusing system of the eye, immediately behind the iris. Also called *crystalline lens*.
lensmeter (LENZ-mee-tur) An instrument for measuring the prescription of eyeglass lenses or the power of rigid contact lenses.
lensometry (lenz-OM-eh-tree) The measurement of certain qualities of lenses by the use of a lensmeter.
lesion An abnormal tissue or a break in a normal tissue.
levator palpebrae (leh-VAY-tor PAL-peh-bree) The muscle attached to the tarsal plate in the middle layer of the upper and lower eyelids that raises the eyelid when it contracts.
limbus The junction between the sclera and the cornea.
local *See* **infection**.
lower canaliculus *See* **canaliculus**.
lower punctum *See* **punctum.**
lubricant A medication that helps maintain an adequate tear-film balance or keeps the external eye moist.

macula (MAK-yoo-luh) The specialized area of the retina close to the center of the back of the eye that provides detailed central vision.
malignant (mah-LIG-nant) Refers to any tumor that is cancerous and has the potential of spreading to other parts of the body.
manifest reaction Refraction performed without the use of cycloplegic drugs.
medial canthus *See* **canthus**.
medial rectus muscle The extraocular muscle that rotates the eye inward toward the nose.
media opacities (oh-PASS-ih-teez) The general term used to describe a variety of conditions that

cloud, obscure, or otherwise affect the ocular media and, ultimately, may disrupt vision.

meibomian gland (my-BOH-mee-an) A specialized gland that secretes the oily part of the tear film that lubricates the outer surface of the globe; located on the inner margin of the eyelid (the edge closest to the globe).

meridian (meh-RID-ee-an) Plane.

metabolism (meh-TAB-uh-lizm) The physical and chemical processes by which the body converts food into energy and new body tissues.

metastasis (meh-TAS-tuh-sis) The process by which cancerous cells move to other parts of the body and produce new tumors.

microbe *See* **microorganism**.

microorganism An extremely small life form invisible to the unaided eye. Also called *microbe*.

minus lens *See* **concave lens**.

miotic (my-OT-ik) A drug that causes the iris sphincter muscle to contract, producing *miosis* (pupillary constriction), which reduces the amount of light entering the eye.

mires (MERZ) The perpendicular crossed lines in a lensmeter, keratometer, and Goldmann tonometer.

mold A form of fungus that produces a woolly, fluffy, or powdery growth.

mucinous (MYU-sih-nus) Sticky.

mucopurulent discharge (Myu-koh-PYUR-yu-lent) A thick fluid containing mucus and pus; symptomatic of bacterial infection.

multifocal lens *See* **bifocal lens**; **trifocal lens**.

mydriasis (mih-DRY-ah-sis) Dilation of the pupil.

mydriatic (mid-ree-AT-ik) A drug that dilates the pupil.

myopia (my-OH-pee-uh) Nearsightedness; the eye is too long for its optical system.

nasal step The type of visual defect that, when plotted, appears as a step-like loss of vision at the outer limit of the nasal field.

nasolacrimal duct (Nay-zoh-LAK-rih-mal) The duct through which tears pass from the lacrimal sac into the nasal cavity.

near add *See* **add**.

near visual acuity (uh-KYU-ih-tee) The ability to see clearly at a normal reading distance.

negative lens *See* **concave lens**.

neoplasm (NEE-oh-plazm) A new growth of different or abnormal tissue, such as a tumor or wart.

neovascularization (Nee-oh-Vas-kyu-lar-ih-ZAY-shun) The abnormal growth of new blood vessels.

nervous system The body system consisting of the brain, spinal cord, and peripheral nerves.

neutralization *See* **lensometry**.

neutralization point The lens power that is the approximate correction for a refractive error.

nevi (NEE-vy; singular: *nevus*) Literally, freckles; common tumors involving the bulbar conjunctiva and appearing as yellowish pink or brown areas on the conjunctiva or skin.

nystagmus (nis-TAG-mus) A condition in which the eyes continually shift in a rhythmic side-to-side or up-and-down motion and then snap back to the normal position.

objective refractometry *See* **retinoscopy**.

occlusion Blockage.

ocularist (ok-yu-LEHR-ist) A professional who measures and fits patients with an artificial eye (prosthesis) to replace an absent eye or cover an unsightly one.

ocular media The three transparent optical structures that transmit light: cornea, lens, and vitreous.

oculomotor nerve (Ok-yu-loh-MOH-ter) The third cranial nerve, which supplies the impulses that activate the superior, medial, and inferior rectus muscles, the inferior oblique muscle, and the levator superioris muscle.

OD (*oculus dexter*) Latin for right eye.

ointment *or* **gel** The form of a drug in which the drug is dissolved or suspended in an oily or greasy vehicle.

opacification (oh-Pass-ih-fih-KAY-shun) Clouding of the lens; occurs in many people over age 65.

opaque Refers to a substance that completely blocks light.

ophthalmia neonatorum (ahf-THAL-mee-uh Nee-oh-nay-TOH-rum) Conjunctivitis in the newborn.

ophthalmic medical assistant (ahf-THAL-mik) A professional who assists the ophthalmologist in a variety of diagnostic and administrative tasks, including performing certain tests, administering certain topical medications or diagnostic drugs, and helping with office surgical procedures.

ophthalmic photographer (ahf-THAL-mik) A professional who photographs eye structures for diagnosis and documentation.

ophthalmic registered nurse (ahf-THAL-mik) A registered nurse with special training in problems related to the eye; frequently functions as a surgical assistant to an ophthalmologist, a director of an ophthalmic surgery service, or a director of clinical services.

ophthalmologist (Ahf-thal-MOL-uh-jist) A medical doctor (MD or DO) who specializes in the prevention, diagnosis, and medical as well as surgical treatment of vision problems and diseases of the eye.

ophthalmology (Ahf-thal-MOL-uh-jee) The medical and surgical specialty concerned with the eye and its surrounding structures, their proper function, eye disorders, and all aspects of vision.

ophthalmometer (Ahf-thal-MOM-uh-ter) *See* **keratometer**.

ophthalmoscope (Ahf-THAL-muh-skohp) An instrument for examining directly or indirectly the vitreous and fundus.

optical center The point of optimal vision; the single point of a lens through which light may pass without being bent or changed.

optical centers, distance between *See* **distance between optical centers**.

optic chiasm (KY-azm) The point behind the eyes in the brain where the two optic nerves merge and the axon fibers from the nasal retina of each eye cross to the opposite side.

optic disc The location where the central retinal artery enters and the central retinal vein, as well as the nerve fibers, exits. Also called *optic nerve head.*

optician An independent professional licensed to dispense eyeglasses and contact lenses from the prescription of an ophthalmologist or optometrist.

optic nerve The nerve that carries electric impulses to the brain's visual cortex, where they are integrated to produce the sensation of sight.

optic nerve head *See* **optic disc**.

optic neuritis (noo-RY-tis) Inflammation of the optic nerve; can produce a sudden, but reversible, loss of sight.

optic radiation The nerve cell that transmits visual information from the lateral geniculate body to the visual cortex.

optics The branch of physical science that deals with the properties of light and vision.

optic tract The part of the brain between the optic chiasm and the lateral geniculate body.

optometrist An independent practitioner trained in the prescription of eyeglasses and contact lenses as well as in the detection of eye disease.

optotypes, Snellen *See* **Snellen chart**.

oral drug delivery The delivery system by which a drug is taken by mouth.

orbicularis oculi (or-Bik-yu-LEHR-is OK-yu-liy) The circular muscle, located in the middle layer of the eyelids, that closes the eye when it contracts, as in winking.

orbit The bony cavity in the skull that houses the globe, extraocular muscles, blood vessels, and nerves.

orbital cellulitis A diffuse infection of tissues in the orbit, causing grossly swollen eyelids and red eye, sometimes without proptosis.

orthophoric (or-thoh-FOR-ik) Refers to the absence of ocular deviation; normal alignment.

orthoptist (or-THOP-tist) A professional who works under the direction of an ophthalmologist to help with the diagnosis, management, and nonsurgical treatment of eye muscle imbalance and related visual impairments.

OS (*oculus sinister*) Latin for left eye.

pachymeter (pah-KIM-eh-ter) An instrument, attached to a slit lamp, that measures the distance between the corneal epithelium and the corneal endothelium. Sometimes spelled *pachometer*.

pachymetry (pah-KIM-eh-tree) The measurement of corneal thickness by the use of a pachymeter. Sometimes spelled *pachometry*.

palpation Medical examination by touch.

palpebral conjunctiva (PAL-peh-bruhl kon-junk-TY-vuh) The eyelid portion of the conjunctiva.

palpebral fissure (PAL-peh-bruhl) The almond-shaped opening between the upper and lower eyelids.

palsy (PAWL-zee) Paralysis.

pantoscopic angle (pan-toh-SKOP-ik) The angle of an eyeglass frame by which the frame front deviates from the vertical plane when the glasses are worn.

papilledema (Pap-il-eh-DEE-muh) A swelling of the optic disc with engorged blood vessels; caused by increased fluid pressure within the skull.

papoose board A padded board with Velcro straps; used for immobilizing an infant during an ophthalmologic examination.

paracentral scotoma (skoh-TOH-muh) A relatively blind area in the visual field, smaller than a Bjerrum scotoma, near the fixation point above or below the horizontal.

parallax (PAER-ah-laks) An optical distortion that occurs when the measurer's line of sight is not parallel to that of the patient.

parallel Refers to rays that travel side by side in the same direction, neither diverging nor converging.

paraxial (paer-AK-see-ahl) Refers to parallel light rays from a distant source that enter the lens at any point other than the center.

pathologic Abnormal.

PD *See* **interpupillary distance**.

perimetry (peh-RIM-eh-tree) The measurement of the expanse and sensitivity of peripheral vision and the visual field to pinpoint possible defects.

peripheral vision The visual perception of objects and space that surround the direct line of sight.

pharmacology (Fahr-mah-KOL-uh-jee) The study of the medicinal use and actions of drugs (medications).

phoria (FOH-ree-uh) The tendency of the eyes to deviate; usually prevented by the brain's effort to fuse the two images.

phoropter (foh-ROP-ter) *See* **refractor**.

photochromic (foh-toh-KROH-mik) Refers to lenses made of crown glass that is specially manufactured to be sensitive to ultraviolet light, so that it darkens in sunlight and lightens when not in sunlight.

photocoagulation (Foh-toh-koh-Ag-yu-LAY-shun) Surgical welding with laser light beams.

photoreceptor (Foh-toh-ree-SEP-tor) A light-sensitive cell.

photorefractive keratectomy (Foh-toh-ree-FRAK-tiv Kehr-uh-TEK-tuh-mee) A type of refractive surgery that employs laser light instead of surgical knives to reshape the corneal curvature; also referred to as PRK.

physical optics The area of optics that describes the nature of light in terms of its wave properties.

physiologic blind spot The sightless "hole" in the normal visual field corresponding to the optic disc.

physiology The function and operation of an organism.

pigment epithelium (Ep-ih-THEE-lee-um) The outer layer of the retina; lies against the choroid.

pinguecula (ping-GWEK-yu-luh) A small, benign, yellow-white mass of degenerated tissue beneath the bulbar conjunctiva, just nasal or temporal to the limbus.

pinhole occluder The hand-held device that completely covers one eye and allows the other to view a chart through a tiny central opening; often used to confirm a diagnosis of refractive error.

"pink eye" *See* **conjunctivitis**.

Placido disk (plah-SEE-doh) A flat disk with alternating black and white rings encircling a small central aperture, used in evaluating the regularity of the anterior curvature of the cornea. With a normal corneal curvature, the rings are reflected without distortion.

plane Flat.

planned-replacement lenses Contact lenses that are designed to be replaced on a regular schedule determined by the ophthalmologist according to patient wearing characteristics and other factors.

plano mirror effect (PLAY-noh) The flat lighting effect of a retinoscope that produces slightly divergent rays.

pledget (PLEJ-eht) A small tuft of cotton soaked in an anesthetic solution for application to the conjunctiva and punctum.

plus lens *See* **convex lens**.

PMMA *See* **polymethylmethacrylate lenses**.

pneumatoretinopexy (Noo-mah-toh-Reh-tih-NOP-pek-see) A surgical procedure for correcting retinal detachment by injecting gas into the eye.

polymethylmethacrylate (PMMA) lenses (Pol-ee-Meth-il-meh-THAK-ril-ayt) Hard contact lenses that provide oxygen by means of a tear pump only; no oxygen or carbon dioxide diffuses through the lens.

positive lens *See* **convex lens**.

posterior Back.

posterior chamber The space between the back of the iris and the front of the vitreous; the crystalline lens is suspended in this chamber, which is filled with aqueous fluid.

posterior segment The rear portion of the eye; includes the vitreous and the retina.

posterior segment examination *See* **funduscopic examination**.

potential acuity meter (uh-KYU-ih-tee) A device for determining visual acuity in the presence of media opacities.

power *See* **vergence power**.

prepping Short for *preparing*; the routines for cleansing a patient's surgical site prior to surgery.

presbyopia (Prez-bee-OH-pee-uh) The progressive loss of the accommodative ability of the lens, due to natural processes of aging.

primary angle-closure glaucoma A form of glaucoma in which the natural age-related increase in the size of the lens blocks the flow of aqueous through the pupil, gradually bowing the iris forward until its outer edge blocks the aqueous outflow channels in the anterior chamber angle.

primary open-angle glaucoma A form of glaucoma in which the pressure inside the eye is elevated because of increased resistance to aqueous drainage in the outflow channels; accounts for 60% to 90% of all adult glaucomas.

principal axis The pathway of a light ray that strikes the center of a lens of any shape and passes undeviated through the lens material.

principal meridians The meridians of maximum and minimum corneal curvature.

principal ray *See* **axial ray**.

prism A triangular piece of glass or plastic with flat sides, an apex, and a base.

prism and alternative cover test A test for measuring the extent of an eye's deviation.

prismatic effect (priz-MAT-ik) An optical distortion in which images are displaced from their normal position; can occur if the distance between optical centers (DBC) does not correspond to the interpupillary distance (IPD).

prism diopter (dy-OP-tur) The unit of measure of the refractive power of a prism.

PRK *See* **photorefractive keratectomy**.

prognosis (prog-NOH-sis) Prediction of the outcome of a medical condition.

progressive addition multifocals Multifocals in which no discrete, visible line divides the distance and near segments; rather, the optical power is added progressively in a transitional zone. Also called *progressive-add multifocals*.

proptosis (prop-TOH-sis) A condition characterized by a protruding eyeball; caused by an increase in volume of the orbital contents. Also called *exophthalmos*.

protozoan (proh-toh-ZOH-an; plural: *protozoa*) A large, single-celled microbe found in fresh and salt water, soil, plants, insects, and animals.

pseudoisochromatic color plates (Soo-doh-Iy-soh-kroh-MAT-ik) A book of plates that display patterns of colored and gray dots; used for evaluating color vision.

pseudophakia (Soo-doh-FAY-kee-uh) The use of an intraocular lens to correct the vision of an aphakic patient.

pterygium (teh-RIJ-ee-um) A wedge-shaped growth on the bulbar conjunctiva.

ptosis (TOH-sis) Drooping of and inability to raise the upper eyelid; caused by the levator muscle's inability to function.

punctum (PUNK-tum; plural: *puncta*) The tiny opening on the upper eyelid margin (*upper punctum*) and lower eyelid margin (*lower punctum*) near the nose, from which tears pass.

punctum dilator (PUNK-tum) Part of the lacrimal set; the instrument used for enlarging the punctum.

pupil The opening in the center of the iris that enlarges (admitting more light) and reduces (admitting less light).

quadrant One of four quarters of the visual field: upper left, upper right, lower left, and lower right.

radial keratotomy (Kehr-uh-TOT-uh-mee) A type of refractive surgery in which radial incisions are made in the cornea to flatten its curvature and reduce nearsightedness; also referred to as RK.

radial meridians Dividing sections radiating from the point of central fixation on a visual field chart.

reagent (ree-AY-jent) A special solution designed to react with a specific type of microorganism or chemical; used in microbiologic testing.

refinement The second step in refractometry, requiring patient participation and responses, which confirms the information produced by retinoscopy. Also called *subjective refractometry*.

refracted Refers to a light ray that bends when it passes at an angle from one transparent medium to another.

refraction (1) In physics, the bending of a light ray as it passes through substances of different densities. (2) In eye care, the process of measuring a patient's refractive error and the clinical judgment to determine the optical correction needed.

refractive error A nonpathologic deficiency in the eye's optical system.

refractive index The ratio of the speed of light in a vacuum to its speed through a specific substance.

refractive state The relative ability of the refractive components of the eye to bring objects into focus on the retina.

refractive surgery A type of corneal surgery that modifies the shape of the cornea to correct some types of myopia, hyperopia, and astigmatism.

refractometry (Ree-frak-TOM-eh-tree) The measurement of refractive error with a variety of instruments and techniques.

refractor An instrument for determining a corrective lens prescription; stores a range of trial lenses that can be dialed into position. Also called *Phoroptor*.

regular astigmatism (uh-STIG-muh-tizm) The most common form of astigmatism, in which the cornea resembles a football standing on one end or on its side.

reservoir An animate or inanimate object that provides a microorganism the means for survival and opportunity for transmission.

respiratory system The body system consisting of the lungs, which process the exchange between needed oxygen and waste carbon dioxide in the blood.

retina (RET-in-uh) The inner lining of the posterior segment of the eyeball; consists of a layer of light-sensitive cells that convert images from the optical system into electric impulses sent along the optic nerve for transmission to the brain.

retinal detachment The separation of the sensory layer from the pigment layer of the retina.

retinitis pigmentosa (ret-ih-NY-tis pig-men-TOH-suh) A hereditary, progressive retinal degeneration that may lead to blindness.

retinoscope (ret-TI-nuh-skohp) An instrument for measuring refractive error; consists of a light source and a viewing component.

retinoscopy (Ret-tih-NAHS-kuh-pee) The use of a retinoscope to determine a refractive error; the first step in refractometry. Also called *objective refractometry*.

retrobulbar (ret-roh-BUL-bar) Behind the eye.

retrobulbar visual pathway (ret-roh-BUL-bar) *See* **visual pathway**.

retroscopic tilt (ret-roh-SKOP-ik) The tilt of an eyeglass frame adjusted so that the lower rim tilts away from the face.

RGP *See* **rigid gas-permeable lenses**.

rigid gas-permeable (RGP) lenses Contact lenses that permit oxygen and carbon dioxide diffusion through both the lens material and a tear pump.

RK *See* **radial keratotomy**.

rod The retinal photoreceptor largely responsible for vision in dim light ("night vision") and for peripheral vision.

round-top segment A portion of a circle fused or ground into a distance lens; may be used in bifocals and trifocals.

routine situation A medical situation that usually can be scheduled for the next available routine office appointment time, within a few days or weeks.

rubeosis iridis (ru-bee-OH-sis IY-rid-is) A condition in which the iris develops a reddish color due to neovascularization.

Schiøtz tonometer (SHEE-ets) An indentation contact tonometer that uses weights to determine intraocular pressure and detect glaucoma.

Schirmer test (SHIR-mer) A test that uses filter paper to measure the patient's tear output and helps to confirm the diagnosis of a dry-eye condition.

Schlemm's canal *See* **canal of Schlemm**.

sclera (SKLEH-rah) The outer fibrous tissue of the globe, which surrounds the cornea and forms the wall of the eye; protects intraocular contents.

scleral buckle (SKLEH-ral) A surgical procedure for correcting retinal detachment that involves placing a block of silicone or other material on the eye to indent the wall.

scleritis (skleh-RY-tis) Inflammation of the sclera.

scotoma (skoh-TOH-muh) An area within the contours of the visual field where vision is reduced.

seamless bifocal *See* **invisible bifocal**.

secondary glaucoma (glaw-KOH-muh) Glaucoma that occurs secondary to another, primary disease.

segment *See* **add**.

segment height The distance between the lowest part of an eyeglass rim and the top of the multifocal lens segment.

shallow scotoma (skoh-TOH-muh) A mild visual field defect that appears as a depression in the island of vision.

sign An abnormal change observed objectively by the physician on examination of the patient.

single lines The closely spaced mires in a lensmeter.

sinus A bony cavern of the skull that contains air and connects with the nasal passages.

slit lamp An instrument used for close examination of the lids and lashes, cornea, lens, membranes, and clear fluids within the eye; consists of a microscope of low magnifying power and a light source that projects a rectangular beam that changes in size and focus. Also called *biomicroscope*.

Snellen acuity test (uh-KYU-ih-tee) A measurement of visual acuity by testing the ability to read characters at a standard distance on a special target called the *Snellen chart*.

Snellen chart A printed visual acuity chart consisting of *Snellen optotypes*—specially formed letters of the alphabet arranged in rows of decreasing letter size.

soft lenses Flexible contact lenses that permit oxygen and carbon dioxide diffusion through the lens material itself, with a minimal tear pump.

solution The form of a drug in which the drug is completely dissolved in an inert liquid.

species (plural: *species*) A category of biologic classification ranking immediately below the genus; the specific name for a type of organism.

spectacle blur Temporary blurred vision upon switching from contact lenses to eyeglasses.

specular microscopy/photography A method of microscopically photographing the cornea's endothelial cells at great magnification and producing photographs on which the cells can be counted.

sphere *See* **spherical lens**.

spherical cornea (KOR-nee-uh) A cornea (of the normal eye and most myopic and hyperopic eyes) whose curvature is uniform.

spherical lens Also simply *sphere*. A concave or convex lens whose curvature is uniform, allowing it to focus light rays to a single point.

spherocylinder (Sfee-roh-SIL-in-der) Also simply *cylinder*. A combination of a spherical lens and a cylindrical lens. Sometimes called *toric lens*.

sphincter muscle (SFINGK-ter) The muscle that encircles the pupil and makes the pupil smaller in response to bright light.

spore A resting state of bacterium, protected by a heavy cell wall that permits the bacterium to survive for a long period of time until suitable conditions for growth occur.

standard precautions A program of sanitation and microbial control in the medical office, intended to reduce the opportunity for harmful microbes to flourish and threaten patients and medical personnel. Includes the provisions of universal precautions and body substance isolation precautions.

static perimetry (peh-RIM-eh-tree) The type of perimetry that uses a stationary target that can be varied in size, brightness, and position within the visual field but is not displayed until it has stopped moving.

stereopsis (stehr-ee-OP-sis) The ability to perceive depth visually in three dimensions.

sterile drapes Large, sterilized protective sheets or cloths placed around the part of the body that is to undergo surgery.

sterile operating field The surgical area and the materials within that area that have undergone sterilization. Also called simply *sterile field*.

sterilization The destruction of all microorganisms by various methods.

steroid *See* **corticosteroid**.

strabismic amblyopia (struh-BIZ-mik Am-blee-OH-pee-uh) The tendency of a child's brain to suppress the image from the deviating eye.

strabismus (struh-BIZ-mus) A misalignment of the eyes that may cause vision to be disturbed; occurs when the extraocular muscles do not work in a coordinated manner.

stroma, corneal *See* **corneal stroma**.

stye (STY) A reddened, sore lump near the outer edge of the eyelid; caused by an inflamed lash follicle. Also called *external hordeolum*.

subconjunctival hemorrhage (Sub-kon-junk-TY-vul HEM-or-ij) A rupture of a conjunctival blood vessel that allows blood to flow under the tissue and produces a bright-red flat area on the conjunctiva.

subjective refractometry *See* **refinement**.

superior oblique muscle The extraocular muscle that rotates the eye both downward and inward toward the nose in primary position.

superior rectus muscle The extraocular muscle that is primarily responsible for turning the eye upward.

super pinhole A pinhole occluder that helps to determine macular function in a patient with an opacity, such as a cataract.

suprathreshold static perimetry (soo-prah-THRESH-hold peh-RIM-eh-tree) The type of static perimetry in which a light or target of a specific size is chosen so that the patient should be able to see it when it is placed at a particular site in the visual field.

surfactant cleaner (sur-FAK-tant) A specially manufactured detergent for removing superficial dirt from contact lenses.

suspension The form of a drug in which particles of the drug are suspended in a liquid vehicle.

suture (SOO-chur) To stitch a wound closed; the pattern of the stitch; or the thread-like material used to make the stitch.

symptom A change in vision, pain, or other subjective effect that indicates a disease process.

synapse (SIN-aps) The connection between nerves, where electric (nerve) impulses are transmitted.
syndrome A set of signs or symptoms that is characteristic of a specific condition or disease.
syringe (sih-RINJ) An instrument for injecting or withdrawing liquid from a vessel or cavity.
systemic drug delivery Intravenous, intramuscular, or subcutaneous injection or oral intake into the circulatory system.

tangent screen test A type of kinetic perimetry used for qualifying visual field defects within 30° of a fixation point.
tarsal plate (TAHR-sal) *See* **tarsus**.
tarsus (TAHR-sus) The dense, plate-like framework within the middle layer of each eyelid that gives the eyelids their firmness and shape. Also called *tarsal plate*.
tear film The moist coating composed of 3 layers that covers the anterior surface of the globe.
thermal trauma (TRAW-muh) Refers to injury that results in the burning or freezing of tissues.
threshold static perimetry (peh-RIM-eh-tree) The type of static perimetry in which the threshold is that level of brightness at which the patient can just detect a test object about half the time.
Titmus stereopsis test (stehr-ee-OP-sis) A test for determining whether the patient has fine depth perception in terms of binocular cooperation.
tonometer (toh-NOM-eh-ter) An instrument for measuring intraocular pressure.
tonometry (toh-NOM-eh-tree) The measurement of intraocular pressure by means of a tonometer; useful in the diagnosis of glaucoma.
topical application The delivery system by which a drug is applied directly to the surface of the eye or surrounding skin.
toric cornea (TOH-rik KOR-nee-uh) A cornea whose surface curvature is not uniform.
toric lens *See* **spherocylinder**.
toxin (TOK-sin) A poison.
trabecular meshwork (trah-BEK-yu-lar) The sponge-like structure that filters the aqueous humor from the anterior chamber and controls its rate of flow out of the eye.
translucent Refers to a substance that transmits light but significantly interferes with its passage.
transparent Refers to a substance that permits the passage of light without significant disruption.
transposition The conversion of a lens prescription from plus-cylinder form to minus-cylinder form or vice versa.
trauma (TRAW-muh) A sudden wound or injury to the body, often from outside the body.
triage (tree-AHZH) The screening of patients (in person or by telephone) to ensure that the patients with the most serious complaints are seen promptly.
trial frame The frame into which various trial lenses are placed; used during refractometry.
trial lens set A set of various lenses introduced before a patient's eye to select the appropriate corrective lens.
trichiasis (trih-KY-ah-sis) An abnormality of the eyelid caused by an eyelash that grows in the wrong direction and rubs against the surface of the eye.
trifocal lens One that has three powers: one for correcting distance vision, one for correcting intermediate range of sight, and one for correcting near vision.
triple lines The widely spaced perpendicular mires in a lensmeter.
tropia (TROH-pee-uh) A condition in which misalignment of the eyes is present even when the eyes are uncovered.

ultrasonography (Ul-trah-son-OG-ruh-fee) A method of examination that uses the reflection (echo) of high-frequency sound waves to define the outline of ocular and orbital structures, measure the distance between structures, and identify abnormal tissues inside the eye or orbit.
universal precautions Standards set by OSHA to minimize the risk to health care workers of infection by bloodborne pathogens.
upper canaliculus *See* **canaliculus**.
upper punctum *See* **punctum.**
urgent situation A medical situation that requires attention within 24 to 48 hours.
uveal tract (YU-vee-al) The pigmented layers of the eye (iris, ciliary body, and choroid) that contain the majority of the blood vessel supply. Also called *uvea*.

varicella-zoster virus (**VZV**) (vahr-ih-SEL-uh ZOS-ter) A herpesvirus that produces chicken pox and the skin disease zoster, or shingles.
vehicle The inert liquid in which a drug is dissolved to form a solution.

vergence power (VER-jens) Also simply *power*. The measure of a lens's ability to converge or diverge light rays.

vertex distance (VER-teks) The distance from the back surface of an eyeglass lens to the front surface of the cornea.

vertical meridians *See* **horizontal and vertical meridians**.

virtual image The image formed by a concave lens when the paraxial rays from a distant source are refracted and diverge.

virus (plural: *viruses*) A microorganism smaller than the smallest bacterium that has no cellular structure and can cause infectious disease.

visual acuity (uh-KYU-ih-tee) The ability to discern fine detail.

visual cortex The area of the brain responsible for the initial conscious registration of visual information; the designation of electric (nerve) impulses from the retina.

visual field The height and breadth of space seen by the eye when the gaze is fixated straight ahead.

visual pathway The route that is taken by light-generated nerve impulses after they leave the eye. Also called *retrobulbar visual pathway*.

vitreous (VIH-tree-us) The clear, jelly-like substance that fills the space behind the lens. Also called *vitreous body*.

VZV *See* **varicella-zoster virus**.

with motion The retinoscopic reflex movement that is in the same direction as the streak of light; typical of the hyperopic eye.

Worth four-dot test A test for determining whether the eyes are perfectly aligned and whether the brain suppresses information from one eye.

yeast A form of fungus that produces creamy or pasty colonies.

zonule (ZOHN-yul) A transparent fiber that supports the lens by attaching to the ciliary body.

Index

NOTE: A *t* following a page number indicates tabular material; an *f* following a page number indicates a figure; and a *b* following a page number indicates a performance box. Drugs are listed under their generic names. When a drug trade name is listed, the reader is referred to the generic name.

AAO. *See* American Academy of Ophthalmology
Abduction, lateral rectus muscle in, 13
Abrasions, corneal, 18, 33
  contact lenses causing, 230
Abscess, eyelash follicle (stye/external hordeolum), 14, 29–30, 31*f*
Absolute scotoma, 112, 113*f*, 119, 119*f*
Absorbable sutures, 204
Abuse (physical), eye trauma and,147
Acanthamoeba species, 191, 191*f*, 230
Accommodation, 20, 47–48, 48*f*
  age affecting (presbyopia), 20, 36, 47–48
Acetazolamide, for glaucoma, 178
Acid burns, 147, 150
Acquired immunodeficiency syndrome. *See* HIV infection/AIDS
Actinomyces species, 189*t*
Acuity. *See* Visual acuity
Acular. *See* Ketorolac
Acute inflammation, 26
Acyclovir, 179
Add, in multifocal lenses, 49, 128, 128*f*
Adduction, medial rectus muscle in, 13
Adenoviruses, 191
Adjunctive tests and procedures, 97–106
Admission (hospital), for patient emergency, 153
Adnexa of eye, 12–16. *See also specific structure*
  abnormalities of, 28–33. *See also specific disorder*
Adrenergic-blocking agents, for glaucoma, 177
Adrenergic-stimulating agents, for glaucoma, 178
Against motion movement, of retinoscopic reflex, 53, 53*f*, 54
Age/aging
  degenerative disorders and, 27
  dry eye and, 33
  lens accommodation affected by (presbyopia), 20, 36, 47–48
  vision changes associated with, 165–166
  vitreous detachment and, 37
Age-related macular degeneration, 37
AIDS. *See* HIV infection/AIDS
Air, refractive index of, 43*t*
Airborne transmission of disease, 192
Air-puff tonometer, 86
Alamast. *See* Pemirolast potassium
Alcaine. *See* Proparacaine
Alcohol (ethyl), for glaucoma, 178
Alignment of eyes, assessment of, 70, 79–82
Alkali burns, 147, 149–150
Allen chart, for acuity testing in children, 164, 164*f*
Allergic conjunctivitis, 30
Allergic response/allergies, 26–27
  to anesthetics, 177
  contact lens preservatives/disinfectants causing, 227–228
  to drugs, first aid for, 182, 182*b*
  drugs for management of, 179, 180
  to fluorescein, 102–103, 176
  history of, 74
Alocril. *See* Nedocromil sodium
Alomide. *See* Lodoxamide
Alpha agonists, for glaucoma, 178
Alphagan. *See* Brimonidine
Altitudinal scotoma, 120, 122*f*
Amblyopia, 29, 79
American Academy of Ophthalmology (AAO)
  code of ethics of, 7
  continuing education courses and, 5
  Extended Wear of Contact Lenses published by, 221
American Optical (Reichert) Phoroptor, care of, 240–241
Ametropia, 46–48, 46*f*
Amphotericin, 179
Amsler grid testing, 83, 84, 85*f*
  procedure for, 85*b*
Anacel. *See* Tetracaine

Anesthetics, 176–177
administration of before office surgery, 202–203, 203*f*
for chalazion surgery, 207
for lacrimal-system probing, 208
for lid-lesion surgery, 208
allergic reaction to, 177
topical, 176, 177
Angiogram, fluorescein, 102, 102*f*
Angiography, fluorescein, 102–103, 102*f*, 176
Angle-closure glaucoma
mydriatics simulating attack of, 175
primary, 35, 35*f*
Anisocoria, 36
Anterior chamber, 18, 19*f*
abnormalities of, 34–36
evaluation of, 89, 90*b*
Anterior chamber angle (filtration angle), 18, 18*f*
assessment of, 89, 90*b*
mydriatics and, 175
Anterior segment, 16. *See also* Cornea; Vitreous
Antiallergic agents, 179
Antibiotics, 178
postsurgical, 207, 209
Antibodies, 26
Antifungals, 178, 179, 191
Antihistamines, 180
Anti-inflammatory agents, 179
Antimicrobials, 178
Antivirals, 178, 179, 190
Apex of prism, 43
Aphakia, 36
perimetry accuracy affected by, 124
Aphakic correction, 36
Applanation tonometer, 86–88, 87*f*, 243, 244*f*
care of, 243–244
Applanation tonometry, 85, 86–88, 87*f*
indentation tonometry compared with, 89
procedure for, 86–87*b*
Appointments (patient), scheduling, 148–149
for diabetic patient, 168
triage procedure and, 147–148
waiting periods and, 158
Apraclonidine, for glaucoma, 178
Aquasite, 180
AquaTears, 180
Aqueous flow, 18, 18*f*
blockage of, glaucoma and, 18, 34, 35, 84
Aqueous humor, 17, 18
refractive index of, 43*t*
Arc perimeter, 114
Arcuate scotoma, 120
Arcus senilis, 34
Argon laser, 247
Arteritis, giant cell (temporal), ocular manifestations of, 253
Arthritis, rheumatoid, ocular manifestations of, 250, 251*f*
Artificial tears, 180
A-scan (A-mode) ultrasonography, 103, 103*f*
Aseptic technique, 195–196, 210
office surgery and, 210
Aspherical cornea, 47
Aspheric (condensing) lenses, 236, 236*f*
care of, 236–237, 237*b*
Astigmatism, 47, 47*f*
irregular, 47
keratoconus lenses for, 223
regular, 47, 47*f*
retinoscopic reflex in, 54
toric contact lenses for, 222
Atropine, 176
Autoclave, 195, 195*f*
for lens sterilization, 238
Autoimmune disorders, ocular manifestations of, 250–252
Automated lensmeter, 58, 60*f*
Automated refractors, 56–57, 57*f*
Automated static perimeter, 115, 115*f*
Autoplot, 114
Axial (principal) ray, 44, 44*f*
Axis of cylinder, 50, 50*f*
Axis of lens, principal, 50, 50*f*
Axons, of retinal ganglion cells, 21
Azopt. *See* Brinzolamide

Bacillus cereus, 189*t*
Bacitracin, 178
Bacteria/bacterial infections, 26, 188, 188–189, 188*f*, 189*f*, 189*t*
conjunctivitis, 30, 188, 189*f*
drugs for treatment of, 178
"Bandage lenses," 223
Basal cell carcinoma, eyelid, 30, 31*f*
Base curve of lens, 131, 135–137
Geneva lens clock for measurement of, 136–137, 136*b*, 137*f*
Base of prism, 43
Benign epithelial cyst of eyelid, surgical removal of, 207–208, 208*f*
Benign neoplasms/tumors, 27–28
eyelid, 30
Benoxinate plus fluorescein, 177
Betagan. *See* Levobunalol
Betamethasone, 179
Betaxolol, for glaucoma, 177
Betimol. *See* Timolol
Betoptic. *See* Betaxolol
Bifocal contact lenses, 222–223, 223*f*
Bifocals, 49, 49*f*, 128, 128*f*
D segment, 128, 129*f*
executive, 128, 128*f*
invisible, 128, 129*f*
measuring power of, 61*b*
prescription for, 56
progressive add, 60–61, 60*f*
round-top, 128, 128*f*
segment placement and, 139, 140*f*
Bimatoprost, for glaucoma, 178
Binocular balancing, 52, 55
Binocular distance IPD, 132
procedure for measuring, 133*b*
Binocular near IPD, 132
procedure for measuring, 134*b*
Binocular vision, 14
Biometry (ultrasonography), ophthalmic, 103–104, 103*f*, 104*f*
Biomicroscope (slit lamp), 71, 90, 90*f*, 242, 242*f*
care of, 242
in tonometry, 86–87*b*, 87*f*, 243, 243*f*
Biomicroscopy, 71, 90–91, 90*f*, 91*f*
Bion Tears, 180
Bipolar cells, retinal, 21, 21*f*
Bitemporal hemianopia, 119, 121*f*
Bjerrum scotoma, 120, 122*f*
Blades (scalpel), 206, 206*f*
on instrument tray, 211
Bleach (hypochlorite), for disinfection, 194
Bleeding, clamps for control of, 206
Blepharitis, 14, 30, 31*f*
Blindness. *See also* Visual impairment; Visual loss
assisting patient and, 160–161, 161*f*
diabetes and, 252
history-taking and, 160
legal, 159, 161
patient greeting and, 160
patient interaction and, 159–160
Blind spot, physiologic, 21, 108, 108*f*, 109
Blinking, 16
Blood dyscrasias, 256
Blood pressure, high (hypertension), ocular manifestations of, 253, 254*f*
Blood sugar/glucose, monitoring levels of in diabetes, 167, 167*f*
Blowout fracture, 29
Blunt trauma
as emergency, 147
as urgent situation, 148
Body substance isolation precautions, 193, 258
Boiling water, for disinfection, 194
Borrelia burgdorferi, 189
Bowman's membrane, 17*f*, 18
Brimonidine, for glaucoma, 178

Brinzolamide, for glaucoma, 178
B-scan (B-mode) ultrasonography, 103–104, 104*f*
Bulbar conjunctiva, 15, 15*f*
  nevi of, 32
Burns, 28
  chemical, 28, 147, 149–150

Calibration, of perimeter, accuracy affected by, 123
Canaliculi, 16, 17*f*
Canal of Schlemm, 18, 18*f*
Cancer
  of eyelid, 30, 31*f*
  metastatic, 255–256, 256*f*
  ocular manifestations of, 255–256, 256*f*
Candida albicans, 191
Cannulas, 207, 207*f*
  lacrimal (lacrimal needle), 206–207, 206*f*
Carbachol, 177
Carbon dioxide excimer laser, 247
Carbonic anhydrase inhibitors, for glaucoma, 178
Carboxyquinolone, fluorinated, 178
Cardinal positions of gaze, 80, 80*f*
Cardiopulmonary resuscitation (CPR), 150
Cardiovascular system, 250
Carteolol, for glaucoma, 177
Cataracts, 20, 36, 36*f*
  vision tests for patients with, 98–99
Cautery, 207*t*
  after lid-lesion surgery, 207*t*, 208, 208*f*
Cellufresh, 180
Cellulitis, orbital, 28
Cellulose sponges/spears, for office surgery, 211, 212*f*
Celluvisc, 180
Centers for Disease Control and Prevention, infection control procedures of, 193
Central retinal artery, 20
  embolus causing occlusion of, 253, 253*f*
Central scotoma, 120, 123*f*
Cerebral hemorrhage, ocular manifestations of, 253
Cerebral vascular accident (CVA), ocular manifestations of, 253, 253*f*
Certification levels, for ophthalmic medical personnel, 4–5
Certified ophthalmic assistant (COA), 4. *See also* Ophthalmic medical assistant
Certified ophthalmic medical technologist (COMT), 4
Certified ophthalmic technician (COT), 4
Chalazion, 14, 30, 31*f*, 207
  surgery for removal of, 207, 207*t*, 208*f*
Chalazion clamp, 207, 207*f*
Chemical burns/trauma, 28, 147, 149–150
Chemical disinfection, 194
  for contact lenses, 224
Chiasm, optic, 21, 22*f*
Chicken pox, 190, 255
  airborne transmission of, 192
Chief complaint, 72–73
Children. *See also* Infants; Toddlers
  assistant's interaction with, 161–165
  cycloplegic refraction in, 175, 176
  greeting, 161–162
  positioning for examination, 162–163, 162*f*
  visual acuity and ability testing in, 163, 164–165
    charts for, 164, 164*f*
    tips for, 164–165, 165
Chlamydial infections, 188–189, 189*f*
  ocular manifestations of, 188–189, 189*f*, 254
Chlamydia trachomatis, 188–189, 189*f*
Chloramphenicol, 178
Chlorhexidine, prepping for office surgery with, 211
Choroid, 19, 19*f*
Chronic inflammation, 26
Cilia (eyelashes), 14, 15*f*
  as protective barrier, 192
Ciliary body, 19, 19*f*
Ciliary muscle, 19, 19*f*
  cycloplegics affecting, 175
  miotics affecting, 177
Ciliary processes, 19, 19*f*
Ciprofloxacin, 178
Circle of least confusion, 51, 51*f*
Circles of eccentricity, 108, 109*f*
Clamps, surgical, 205–206, 206*f*, 207*t*
  chalazion, 207, 207*f*
Cleaning/cleaning solutions
  for contact lenses, 223, 224
    interaction of with lens materials, 230–231
  for ophthalmic (diagnostic) lenses, 236–238
    for lenses that contact eye, 237–238, 238*b*
    for lenses that do not contact eye, 236–237, 237*b*
    standard care guidelines for, 236
Clear Eyes, 180
Clērz, 180
Cloudy corneas, vision tests for patients with, 98–99
CMV retinitis, 190, 254, 254*f*
CO_2 excimer laser, 247
COA. *See* Certified ophthalmic assistant
Coatings, lens, 130–131
Code of ethics, of American Academy of Ophthalmology, 7
Color plates, pseudoisochromatic, for color vision testing, 92, 93*f*
Color vision
  cones in, 20
  tests of, 92, 93*f*
Common-vehicle transmission of disease, 192, 193
Complications, of office surgery, informed consent and, 202
Comprehensive eye examination. *See* Eye examination
Computerized static threshold perimetry, 115–116, 116*f*
COMT. *See* Certified ophthalmic medical technologist
Concave (negative/minus) lenses, 43, 44*f*
  corrective, 48*t*
  passage of light rays through, 44, 44*f*, 45
  spherical, 48*t*, 49
Concave mirror effect, 53
Condensing lenses, 236, 236*f*
  care of, 236–237, 237*b*
Cones, 20, 21*f*
Confidentiality (right to privacy), 6, 158
Confrontation field test, 83, 84, 84*f*, 111
  procedure for, 84*b*
Congenital cataracts, 36
Congenital disorders, 27
Congenital glaucoma, 36
Congenital ptosis, 30
Conjunctiva, 14, 15–16, 15*f*
  abnormalities of, 29–32. *See also* Conjunctivitis
  collecting specimen from, 197, 197*f*
  HIV isolated from, 190
  mucous layer of, as protective barrier, 192
Conjunctivitis, 16, 30, 32*f*. *See also* Keratoconjunctivitis
  bacterial, 188–189, 188*f*, 189*f*
  chlamydial, 188–189, 189*f*, 254
  giant papillary, contact lens wear and, 230
  hyperacute, 188, 188*f*, 189*f*
  in newborn, 30, 188–189, 189*f*
  pharyngoconjunctival fever form of, 191
  viral, 30, 191

Consensual pupillary reaction, 82
  procedure for checking, 82, 83*b*
Consent, informed, 202
Constricted visual field, 117–118, 117*f*
Contact lens care, 223–224
  Acanthamoeba infection and, 191, 191*f*, 230
  cleaning and, 223, 224, 224*f*
  disinfection and, 223, 224
  lubrication and, 223, 224
  solution–lens interaction and, 230–231
  storage and, 224
Contact lenses, 217–233
  Acanthamoeba infection and, 191, 191*f*, 230
  advantages and disadvantages of, 219, 220, 221
  allergic reactions to, 227–228
  "bandage," 223
  basic principles of, 218–219, 218*f*
  bifocal, 222–223, 223*f*
  care of. *See* Contact lens care
  contraindications to use of, 231
  corneal problems associated with, 229–230, 229*f*
  cosmetic
    fashion, 222, 222*f*
    restorative, 222, 222*f*
  daily-wear, 221
  debris on, 224, 224*f*
  diagnostic, care of, 237–238, 238*b*
  displacement of, 231
  disposable, 221
  extended-wear, 221
  eyeglasses compared with, 219
  giant papillary conjunctivitis associated with, 230
  HIV isolated from, 190
  improper fit and, 228–229
  insertion and removal of, 225–226, 225*b*, 226*b*, 227*b*, 228*b*
    difficulties with, 231
  irritation caused by, 229
  keratoconus, 223
  loose-fitting, problems associated with, 229
  "lost" in eye, 231
  materials for, 219–222
  optician dispensing, 3
  optometrist prescribing, 3
  overwearing syndrome and, 228
  planned-replacement, 221
  polymethylmethacrylate, 219, 220
  prescription of, information needed for, 218, 219
  problems with, 226–231. *See also specific type*
  Pseudomonas aeruginosa infection and, 189, 230
  rigid gas-permeable, 219, 220, 220*f*
    advantages and disadvantages of, 220
    insertion and removal of, 226, 227*b*, 228*b*
  soft (hydrophilic), 218, 219–220, 220–221, 220*f*
    advantages and disadvantages of, 221
    insertion and removal of, 225–226, 225*b*, 226*b*
  solutions for, interactions and, 230–231
  special-purpose, 222–223
  storage of, 224
  tearing caused by, 229
  therapeutic, 223
  tight-fitting, problems associated with, 229
  tinted, 222, 222*f*
  toric, 222
  types of, 219–222
Contamination
  of equipment, handling and decontamination of, 196, 258
  of gowns or gloves for office surgery, 211
  of medical instruments, transmission of disease and, 192–193
  of medications, 193
Continuing education, in professional development, 5, 5*f*
Contracted visual field, 117–118, 117*f*
Contraindications, to contact lens use, 231
Contrast sensitivity, 99
  testing, 79, 99, 99*f*
Convergence, 43, 43*f*, 44
Convex (positive/plus) lenses, 43, 44, 44*f*
  corrective, 48*t*
  passage of light rays through, 44, 44*f*
  spherical, 49, 49*t*
Convulsions, first aid for, 182*b*
Cornea, 12, 12*f*, 16–18
  abnormalities of, 33–34. *See also* Keratitis
    contact lenses causing, 229
    tests for, 99–101
    in thyroid disorders, 252, 252*f*
  Acanthamoeba infection of, 191, 230
  aspherical, 47
  cloudy, vision tests for patients with, 98–99
  curvature of
    keratometry for measurement of, 61, 62*f*, 63–65*b*
      contact lens prescription determination and, 218
    warping of, improperly fitted contact lenses causing, 229
  HIV isolated from, 190
  layers of, 17, 17*f*
  light rays focused by, 17
  mucous layer of, as protective barrier, 192
  Pseudomonas aeruginosa infection of, 189, 230
  refractive index of, 43*t*
  sensitivity of, testing, 93–94
  toric, 47
Corneal abrasion, 18, 33
  contact lenses causing, 230
Corneal dystrophies, pachymetry in, 100
Corneal edema, contact lenses causing, 229, 229*f*
Corneal endothelium, 17*f*, 18
  specular microscopy/photography in evaluation of, 101, 101*f*
Corneal epithelium, 17, 17*f*
  evaluation of, 93, 94*f*
Corneal infections, in contact lens wearers, 189, 191, 230
Corneal sensitivity test, 93–94
Corneal stroma, 17*f*, 18
Corneal topography, 70, 79, 100, 100*f*
Corneal ulcers, 18, 33
  contact lenses causing, 221, 230
  extended-wear lenses and, 221
  herpetic, 33–34, 34*f*, 190, 190*f*
  in rheumatoid arthritis, 250, 251*f*
Corneal vascularization, contact lenses causing, 229, 230*f*
Corrective lenses, 48–52, 48*t*. *See also* Contact lenses; Eyeglasses; Intraocular lenses
  cylinders, 48*t*, 50, 50*f*
  fitting, measurements for, 131–137
  making (opticianry), 127–144
  materials made from, 129–131
  multifocal, 49, 49*f*, 128–129, 128*f*, 129*f*
  optical center of, lensmeter for verification of position of, 61
  during perimetry, 124
  plastic, 130
  prisms, 48*t*, 51–52, 51*f*, 52*f*
  safety standards and treatments for, 130, 130*f*
  single-vision, 128
  spheres, 48*t*, 49, 49*f*
  spherocylinders, 48*t*, 50–51, 50*f*, 51*f*
  treatments/tints/coatings for, 130–131
  types of, 128–129
Corticosteroids, 179
  in combination preparations with antibiotics, 178

Cortisone, 179
Corynebacterium species, 189*t*
Cosmetic contact lenses
fashion, 222, 222*f*
restorative, 222, 222*f*
COT. *See* Certified ophthalmic technician
Cotton-tipped applicators, for office surgery, 211, 212*f*
Cotton-wool patches, in hypertension, 254*f*
Cover–uncover test, 80
CPR. *See* Cardiopulmonary resuscitation
CR-39 plastic, refractive index of, 130
Crolom. *See* Cromolyn
Cromolyn, 180
for giant papillary conjunctivitis, 230
Cross cylinder, for refinement, 54, 55*f*
Crown glass
photochromic lenses made from, 130–131
refractive index of, 43*t*, 130
Cryopexy, for retinal detachment, 37
Crystalline lens, 12, 12*f*, 20
abnormalities of, 36
refractive index of, 43*t*
Cul-de-sac (fornix), 15, 15*f*
Cultures, for microorganism identification, 197
Curettes, 206, 206*f*, 207*t*
Curvature of cornea
keratometry for measurement of, 61, 62*f*, 63–65*b*
contact lens prescription determination and, 218
warping of, improperly fitted contact lenses causing, 229
Cushioning/wetting solutions, for contact lenses, 223, 224
Cutting suture needles, 204, 204*f*
CVA. *See* Cerebral vascular accident
Cyclogel. *See* Cyclopentolate
Cyclopentolate, 176
for cycloplegic refraction in children, 176
Cycloplegia, 175
Cycloplegic refraction, 52, 175
Cycloplegics, 175–176
Cylinders/cylindrical lenses, 48*t*, 50, 50*f*
measuring power of, 58–59*b*, 59
Cytomegalovirus (CMV) retinitis, 190, 254, 254*f*

Dacryocystitis, 16, 32–33, 33*f*
Daily-wear lenses, 221
DBC. *See* Distance between optical centers
Decibels, in static perimetry, 114
Decongestants, 180
Deep scotoma, 112, 113*f*, 119*f*
Degenerative disorders, 27
Dendritic corneal ulcer, herpetic, 34, 34*f*
Density, definition of, 43
Department of Labor, Occupational Safety and Health Administration (OSHA), regulations of for prevention of infection transmission, 193
Depression (visual field), 118, 118*f*
Descemet's membrane, 17*f*, 18
Developmental disorders, 27
Dexamethasone, 179
in combination products, 178
Diabetes mellitus, 27, 167–168
blood glucose level monitoring and, 167, 167*f*
ocular manifestations of, 37, 167, 168, 252, 252*f*
Diabetic retinopathy, 37, 167, 252, 252*f*
Diagnosis, informing patient about, as physician responsibility, 6
Diagnostic lenses. *See* Ophthalmic lenses
Diagnostic medications, 173–177
Diamox. *See* Acetazolamide
Diclofenac, 179
Dilator muscle of iris, 18, 19*f*
Diopters, 45
prism, 51, 52*f*
Dipivefrin, for glaucoma, 178
Diplopia (double vision), 29, 29*f*, 79
in myasthenia gravis, 250
as urgent situation, 148
Worth four-dot test for, 81, 81*f*
Direct and consensual pupillary reaction, 82
procedure for checking, 82, 83*b*
Direct-contact transmission of disease, 192
Direct ophthalmoscope/ophthalmoscopy, 91, 92*f*, 245, 245*f*
Discharge (eye), collecting specimen from, 197, 197*f*
Disease, definition of, 26
Disinfection, 194, 258
of contact lenses, 223, 224
allergic reactions and, 227–228
Dispensing optician. *See* Optician
Disposable lenses, 221
Disruptive patients, management of, 159
Distance acuity test, 74–77. *See also* Visual acuity examination
procedure for performing, 76*b*
Distance between optical centers (DBC), 132
measuring, 139, 140*b*
prismatic effect and, 132, 133*f*
Distance equivalent, 78
Distometer, 135
procedure for use of, 136*b*
Divergence, 43, 43*f*, 44
Dizziness, change in base curve causing, 135
Doctor-patient relationship, professional behavior by assistant and, 7–8
Dorzolamide, for glaucoma, 178
Double-D segment multifocal lens, 129, 129*f*
Double vision (diplopia), 29, 29*f*, 79
in myasthenia gravis, 250
as urgent situation, 148
Worth four-dot test for, 81, 81*f*
Downward gaze, extraocular muscles in, 13
Draping, for office surgery, 211
Dressings, postsurgical, 209, 209*b*
Drugs (medications), 171. *See also specific type*
allergic reactions to, first aid for, 182, 182*b*
contaminated, 193
delivery systems for, 172–173, 172*f*
diagnostic, 173–177
injectable, 172, 173
oral, 172
purposes and actions of, 173–180
systemic delivery of, 173
therapeutic, 177–180
topical, 172, 172–173
administration of, 173, 174*b*, 175*f*
for conjunctivitis, 30
miotics as, 177
Dry eye (keratoconjunctivitis sicca), 16, 33
in rheumatoid arthritis, 250
in Sjögren's syndrome, 250–251
D segment, 128, 129*f*
Dyes, 176. *See also* Fluorescein; Rose bengal dye
for corneal epithelium evaluation, 93, 94*f*
in tonometry, 86

Eccentricity, circles of, 108, 109*f*
Echothiophate, 177
Ectropion, 15, 30, 31*f*
Edema
corneal, 229
orbital, 28
E game chart (tumbling E), 75, 75*f*, 164, 164*f*
difficulties with use of, 164–165

EKC. *See* Epidemic keratoconjunctivitis
Elderly patients, 165–166
Electromagnetic radiation, spectrum of, 42, 42*f*
Emboli, cerebral vascular accident causing, ocular manifestations of, 253, 253*f*
Emergencies, 147–148, 149–153
  general patient assistance and, 150–152
  hospital admission and, 153
  triaging patients with, 147–148
Emergency cart, 150–152, 152*f*
Emergency procedures, 149–153
Emmetropia, 46, 46*f*
Empiric treatment, 197
Endocrine system, 250
Endophthalmitis, 37
Endothelium, corneal, 17*f*, 18
  specular microscopy/photography in evaluation of, 101, 101*f*
Entropion, 15, 30, 31*f*
Environment, for perimetry, accuracy affected by, 121
Enzyme cleaners, for contact lenses, 224
Epidemic keratoconjunctivitis (EKC), 191
Epinephrine, for glaucoma, 178
Epiphora (tearing)
  contact lenses causing, 229
  lacrimal-system probing for, 208–209
Epiphrin. *See* Epinephrine
Episcleritis, 34
  in rheumatoid arthritis, 250
Epithelial cyst of eyelid, benign, surgical removal of, 207–208, 208*f*
Epithelium, corneal, 17, 17*f*
  evaluation of, 93, 94*f*
Epitrate. *See* Epinephrine
Eppy. *See* Epinephrine
Equipment. *See also* Instruments; Ophthalmic lenses
  contaminated, handling and decontaminating, 196, 258
  disinfection and sterilization of, 194–195, 195*f*, 258
    aseptic technique and, 195–196
  in indirect-contact transmission of disease, 192–193
  preparation of for office surgery, 211–212, 211*f*
Equipment failure, troubleshooting, 239
Eso deviation, 29
Esophoria, 29
Esotropia, 29, 29*f*
Essilor Pupilometer, 134, 135*f*
Ethics, 5–7
Ethyl alcohol, for glaucoma, 178
Ethylene oxide gas, for sterilization, 195
  of ophthalmic lenses, 238
Etiology, definition of, 26
Examination equipment. *See also* Instruments; Ophthalmic lenses
  contaminated, handling and decontaminating, 196
  disinfection and sterilization of, 194–195, 195*f*, 258
    aseptic technique and, 195–196
  in indirect-contact transmission of disease, 192–193
Examination of eye. *See* Eye examination
Examiner, perimetry accuracy affected by factors related to, 124
Excimer lasers, 247
  for refractive surgery, 48
Executive multifocal lenses, 128, 128*f*
Exo deviation, 29
Exophoria, 29
Exophthalmometer, 94, 94*f*
Exophthalmometry, 89, 94, 94*f*
Exophthalmos (proptosis), 28, 28*f*
  assessment of (exophthalmometry), 89, 94, 94*f*
  in thyroid disorders, 252, 252*f*
Exotropia, 29, 29*f*
Extended Wear of Contact Lenses, 221
Extended-wear lenses, 221
External eye examination, 70, 89, 90*b*
External hordeolum (stye), 14, 29–30, 31*f*
Extraocular muscles, 12–14, 13*f*. *See also specific muscle*
  assessment of function of, 70, 79–82
  disorders of, 29
Eye. *See also* Globe
  abnormalities of, 33–37
  adnexa of, 12–16
    abnormalities of, 28–33
  allergic processes affecting, 26–27
  anatomy and physiology of, 11–24. *See also specific structure*
  congenital processes affecting, 27
  degenerative processes affecting, 27
  developmental processes affecting, 27
  dry (keratoconjunctivitis sicca), 16, 33
    in rheumatoid arthritis, 250
    in Sjögren's syndrome, 250–251
  examination of. *See* Eye examination
  infectious processes affecting, 26, 187–199, 254–255. *See also* Ocular infections
    specimen collection for identification of microorganisms and, 197, 197*f*
    transmission of, 192–193
  inflammatory processes affecting, 26, 250–252
  irrigation of, 149–150, 151*b*
  irritation of, contact lenses causing, 229
  ischemic processes affecting, 27, 252–253, 253*f*, 254*f*
  mechanisms of disease and injury of, 26–28
  metabolic processes affecting, 27, 252
  neoplastic processes affecting, 27–28, 255–256, 256*f*
  as optical system, 12, 12*f*
  protective barriers of, 192
  redness of
    decongestants for, 180
    as urgent situation, 148
  refractive states of, 45–48
  signs/symptoms/syndromes and, 28
  systemic diseases affecting, 249–256
  traumatic processes affecting, 28, 147, 150
    physical abuse and, 147
Eye alignment, testing, 70, 79–82
Eyeball. *See* Globe
Eye care, providers of, 2–4
Eyedrops
  anesthetic, 202
  instilling, 174*b*, 175*f*
  maintaining sterility of, 196
  solutions applied as, 172
  suspensions applied as, 172
Eye examination, 69–96
  adjunctive tests and procedures and, 97–106
  alignment and motility examination in, 70, 79–82
  biomicroscopy in, 71, 90–91
  color vision tests in, 92, 93*f*
  corneal disease screening and, 99–101
  corneal epithelium evaluation in, 93, 94*f*
  corneal sensitivity testing in, 93–94, 94*f*
  exophthalmometry in, 94, 94*f*
  external, 70, 89, 90*b*
  frequency of, 71
  intraocular pressure measurement in, 70, 84–89
  ophthalmic and medical history in, 71–74, 72*f*, 73*t*
    visually impaired/blind patients and, 160
  ophthalmic photography in, 101–103

ophthalmoscopy in, 71, 91–92, 92*f*
overview of parts of, 70–71
patients with opacities and, 98–99
pupillary examination in, 70, 82, 83*b*
tear output tests in, 93, 93*f*
ultrasonography in, 103–104, 103*f*, 104*f*
visual acuity examination in, 70, 74–79
visual field examination in, 70, 83–84, 84*b*
Eyeglasses. *See also* Corrective lenses
adjustment of, 139–140
care of, 138–139
contact lenses compared with, 219
fitting, measurements for, 131–137
in lensometry, positioning, 58*b*, 59
optician dispensing, 3, 127–144
prescription of
information needed for, 219
by optometrist, 3
protective, 130, 130*f*
in infection control, 194, 212
Eyeglass frames
adjustment of, 139–140
care of, 138–139
fitting, 137–138
parts of, 137, 137*f*
patient comfort and, 138
Eyelashes (cilia), 14, 15*f*
as protective barrier, 192
Eyelids, 13–16, 15*f*
abnormalities of, 29–32
margin of
collecting specimen from, 197, 197*f*
infection of, 30, 31*f*
lashes on, 14, 15*f*
meibomian glands on, 14, 14*f*
infection of, 14, 29–30, 31*f*
as protective barrier, 192
surgical removal of lesions of, 207–208, 208*f*
Eye movements
abnormal, 29, 29*f*
assessment of (ocular alignment and motility testing), 70, 79–82
extraocular muscles in, 12–14, 13*f*
Eye muscles. *See* Extraocular muscles
Eye pads, 207*t*
Eye pain
as emergency, 148
as urgent situation, 148
Eye physician. *See* Ophthalmologist
Eyepiece, focusing, for lensometry, 58*b*, 59
Eye protection, 130, 130*f*
in infection control, 194, 212
Eye surgery, in office, 201–215. *See also* Office surgery

Fainting
patient
assisting, 152, 152*f*
office surgery and, 210
assistant during first surgical experience, 210
Falling patient, guidelines for handling, 152
Family history, 74. *See also* History, ophthalmic and medical
Family members (of patient)
consideration of, 158
with infant or young child, 161
Farnsworth-Munsell D-15 test, of color vision, 92, 93*f*
Farsightedness (hyperopia), 46–47, 46*f*
prescription for, 56
retinoscopic reflex in, 53, 53*f*, 54
spherical plus-power (convex) lenses for, 48*t*, 49
Fever blisters, 190, 255
hygienic practices in infection control and, 197
Fields of vision. *See* Visual fields
15-hue test, of color vision, 92, 93*f*
Filtration angle (anterior chamber angle), 18, 18*f*
assessment of, 89, 90*b*
mydriatics and, 175
First aid, administering, 150–152, 182*b*
for acute drug reactions, 182, 182*b*
Fixation, in retinoscopy, 53
Flashes of light, as urgent situation, 148
Flashlight test, 89, 90*b*
Flint glass, refractive index of, 43*t*, 130
Floaters, vitreous, 20, 36–37
as urgent situation, 148
Fluoracaine. *See* Fluorescein, with proparacaine
Fluorescein, 176. *See also* Dyes
allergic reaction to, 102–103, 176
for angiography, 102, 176
with benoxinate, 177
for corneal epithelium evaluation, 93, 94*f*
for overwearing syndrome evaluation, 228
with proparacaine, 177
for tonometry, 86
precautions with use of, 86*b*
Fluorescein angiogram, 102, 102*f*
Fluorescein angiography, 102–103, 102*f*, 176
Fluorinated carboxyquinolone, 178
Fluoromethodone, 179
Fluoroquinolones, 178
Flurbiprofen, 179
Fluress. *See* Benoxinate plus fluorescein

Focal length, 45
relationship of to lens power, 45, 45*f*
Focal lines
of cylinders, 50, 50*f*
of spherocylinders, 50–51, 51*f*
Focal point, 44, 44*f*
Focal visual field defects, 118–119, 118*f*, 119*f*
Forceps, 205, 205*f*, 207*t*
Foreign body, as emergency, 147
Foreign-body sensation, 16
Formaldehyde, for disinfection, 194
Fornix (cul-de-sac), 15, 15*f*
Four-dot test, Worth, 81, 81*f*
Fovea, 20, 20*f*
Frames. *See* Eyeglass frames; Trial frame
Frame screws, adjusting, 139, 139*f*
Frequent- (planned-/programmed-) replacement lenses, 221
Functional surface, aseptic technique and, 196
Fundus camera, 101–102, 102*f*
Fundus contact lenses, 237, 237*f*
care of, 237–238, 238*b*
Funduscopic examination, 90, 91–92, 91*f*, 92*f*. *See also* Biomicroscopy; Ophthalmoscopy
mydriasis for, 173–175
Funduscopic lenses, hand-held noncontact, 236
care of, 236–237, 237*b*
Fundus photography, 101–103, 102*f*
Fungi/fungal infections, 26, 191, 191*f*
drugs for treatment of, 179, 191
Fusion, 14
failure to achieve, 79
testing (ocular alignment and motility testing), 70, 79–82
Worth four-dot test for, 81, 81*f*

Ganglion cells, 21, 21*f*
Gas sterilization, 195
Gaze, cardinal positions of, 80, 80*f*
Gel, for topical drug administration, 172
General visual field defects, 117–118, 117*f*
Genetic disorders, 27
cataracts as, 36
Geneva lens clock, 136–137, 137*f*
procedure for using, 136*b*
Gentamicin, 178
Genteal, 180
Geometric optics, 42
Germicides, 194
prepping for office surgery with, 211
Giant cell (temporal) arteritis, ocular manifestations of, 253
Giant papillary conjunctivitis (GPC), contact lens wear and, 230

Gimbal, in measuring bifocal power, 61
Glare testing, 79, 99, 100*f*
Glass
crown
photochromic lenses made from, 130–131
refractive index of, 43*t*, 130
flint, refractive index of, 43*t*, 130
Glass lenses, 130. *See also* Corrective lenses
cleaning, 139
safety treatments for, 130
ultraviolet protection and, 131
Glass target slides, 242, 243*f*
care of, 242
Glaucoma, 18, 34–36, 35*f*
congenital, 36
drug therapy for, 177–178
miotics for, 177
primary angle-closure, 35, 35*f*
mydriatics simulating attack of, 175
primary open-angle, 35, 35*f*
secondary, 35–36
testing for, 34–35, 70, 84–89
visual field defects in, 35, 120, 122*f*, 123*f*
Globe (eyeball), 12, 16–21. *See also* Eye
muscles controlling movement of, 12–14, 13*f*
Gloves
in infection control, 194, 194*t*, 258
sterile, for office surgery, 210–211
wearing during instrument cleaning, 212
Glucose, blood levels of, monitoring in diabetes, 167, 167*f*
Glutaraldehyde, for disinfection, 194
Glycerine, for glaucoma, 178
Glyrol. *See* Glycerine
Goblet cells, 16
Goggles, protective, 130, 130*f*
Goldmann goniolens, 91, 91*f*. *See also* Goniolens
Goldmann perimeter, 113–114, 113*f*
Goldmann tonometer, 86–88, 87*f*, 243, 244*f*
care of, 243–244
Goldmann tonometry, 86–88, 87*f*
procedure for, 86–87*b*
Goniolens, 237, 237*f*
care of, 237–238, 238*b*
Goldmann, 91, 91*f*
Koeppe, 91, 237, 237*f*
Gonioscopy, 90–91, 91*f*
Gowns
in infection control, 194, 194*t*
for office surgery, 211
GPC. *See* Giant papillary conjunctivitis
Gradual defect, 118*f*, 119
Gramicidin, in combination products, 178
Gram-negative bacteria, 188, 188*f*, 189*t*
Gram-positive bacteria, 188, 188*f*, 189*t*
Gram staining, 188, 188*f*, 189*t*
Graves' disease, 28
Green's manual refractor, care of, 241
Greeting patients, 146
children, 161–162

Haemophilus influenzae, 189*t*
Handling tint, for contact lenses, 222
Hand movement, low vision testing and, 162*b*
Hand washing
in infection control, 194, 194*t*, 195*b*, 196, 197, 258
scrubbing for office surgery and, 210–211
Hard lenses, 219, 220. *See also* PMMA lenses; RGP lenses
advantages and disadvantages of materials used for, 220
insertion and removal of, 226, 227*b*, 228*b*
Heat
for contact lens disinfection, 224
moist, for sterilization, 195, 195*f*
Hemianopia, 119, 120*f*, 121*f*
Hemorrhages
orbital, 28
retinal, in hypertension, 253, 254*f*
subconjunctival, 16, 32, 32*f*
Hemostasis, clamps for, 206
Herpes simplex virus
corneal infection caused by, 33–34, 34*f*, 190, 190*f*, 255
ocular, 33–34, 34*f*, 190, 190*f*, 255
type 1, 190, 190*f*, 255
type 2, 190, 255
Herpesviruses, 190, 255. *See also specific type*
Herpes zoster ophthalmicus, 190, 255, 255*f*
in HIV infection/AIDS, 254
Herplex. *See* Idoxuridine
Hexachlorophene, prepping for office surgery with, 211
High blood pressure, ocular manifestations of, 253, 254*f*
Hi-index glass, refractive index of, 130
Hi-index plastic, 130
refractive index of, 130
Histoplasma capsulatum, 191
Histoplasmosis, 191, 255
History, ophthalmic and medical
in comprehensive eye examination, 71–74, 72*f*, 73*t*
guidelines for taking, 74
with visually impaired/blind patient, 160
HIV infection/AIDS, 190, 254
contact lens cleaning guidelines and, 224
cytomegalovirus retinitis in, 190, 254, 254*f*
ocular manifestations of, 37, 190, 254
toxoplasmosis in, 191, 255
Homatropine, 176
Homonymous hemianopia, 119, 120*f*
Hordeolum
external (stye), 14, 29–30, 31*f*
internal, 14, 30, 31*f*
Horizontal meridians, in visual field mapping, 108, 109*f*
Hormones, 250
Hospital admission, 153
Host, of microorganism, 192
Hruby lens, 90, 236, 236*f*
care of, 236–237, 237*b*
HSV-1. *See* Herpes simplex virus, type 1
HSV-2. *See* Herpes simplex virus, type 2
Human immunodeficiency virus. *See* HIV infection/AIDS
Hydrocortisone, 179
in combination products, 178
Hydrogen peroxide, for disinfection, 194
Hydrophilic contact lenses. *See* Soft (hydrophilic) contact lenses
Hydrophobic nature of eye, topical drug solutions and, 172
Hyoscine. *See* Scopolamine
Hyperacute conjunctivitis, 188, 188*f*, 189*f*
Hyperopia (farsightedness), 46–47, 46*f*
prescription for, 56
retinoscopic reflex in, 53, 53*f*, 54
spherical plus-power (convex) lenses for, 48*t*, 49
Hyperosmotics, for glaucoma, 178
Hypersensitivity reactions. *See also* Allergic response/allergies
contact lens preservatives/disinfectants causing, 227–228
Hypertension, ocular manifestations of, 253, 254*f*
Hyphema, 34, 34*f*
Hypochlorite (bleach), for disinfection, 194

Hypoglycemia, 168
Hypoglycemic reaction, treatment of, 168
Hypopyon, 33, 33*f*, 34
Hypotears, 180
Hypoxia, 27

Idoxuridine, 179
Immune response/immunity, 26–27
Inclusion conjunctivitis, 189
Indentation tonometer, 88–89, 88*f*, 244, 245*f*
  care of, 244–245
Indentation tonometry, 85, 88–89, 88*f*
  applanation tonometry compared with, 89
Index of refraction. *See* Refractive index
Indirect-contact transmission of disease, 192, 192–193
Indirect ophthalmoscope/ophthalmoscopy, 91–92, 92*f*, 245, 246*f*
Infants
  assistant's interaction with, 161–165
  greeting parent/caregiver and, 161
  positioning, 162–163
  visual acuity and ability testing in, 163, 163*b*
Infection control, 193–197
  aseptic technique and, 195–196
  body substance isolation precautions and, 193, 258
  decontaminating materials and, 196
  disinfection and sterilization and, 194–195, 195*f*, 258
  handling contaminated materials and, 196
  hand washing and, 194, 195*f*, 258
  hygienic practices for potentially infectious situations and, 197, 258
  personal protective equipment and, 194, 194*t*, 212
  standard precautions and, 187, 193–194, 194*t*
  universal precautions and, 193, 257–258
Infection/infectious diseases, 26, 187–199, 254–255. *See also specific type*
  bacterial, 26, 188–189, 188*f*, 189*f*, 189*t*
  fungal, 26, 191, 191*f*
  ocular manifestations of, 254–255
  protozoan, 191, 191*f*
  specimen collection for microorganism identification and, 197, 197*f*
  transmission of, 192–193
  viral, 26, 189–191, 190*f*
    herpes simplex causing, 33–34, 34*f*, 190, 190*f*, 255
Inferior oblique muscle, 13, 13*f*
Inferior rectus muscle, 13, 13*f*
Inflammation/inflammatory response, 26. *See also specific structure affected*
  acute, 26
  chronic, 26
  drugs for management of, 179
  ocular manifestations of, 250–252
Informed consent, 202
Injections, for medication administration, 172, 173
Injury, 26. *See also* Trauma
Inserts, for topical drug administration, 173
Instrument failure, troubleshooting, 239
Instruments. *See also specific type*
  care of, 239–247
    standard guidelines for, 239–240
  contaminated, handling and decontaminating, 196, 212–213, 258
  disinfection and sterilization of, 194–195, 195*f*, 212–213, 258
    aseptic technique and, 195–196
  in indirect-contact transmission of disease, 192–193
  for office surgery, 203–207
    care of, 212–213, 258
    disposition of after procedure, 212–213, 258
    passing to surgeon, 212, 212*f*
    preparation of, 211–212, 211*f*
  troubleshooting failure of, 239
Instrument tray, for office surgery, preparation of, 211–212, 211*f*
Insulin
  for diabetes control, 167
  lack of in diabetes mellitus, 27
Interferometer, 98–99, 99*f*
Internal hordeolum, 14, 30, 31*f*
Interpupillary distance (IPD), 131, 131–134, 131*f*, 131*t*
  binocular measurement of, 131, 131*f*
    distance, 132, 133*b*
    near, 132, 134*b*
  errors in measurement of, 132–134
  instruments for measurement of, 134, 135*f*
  monocular measurement of, 131, 131*f*, 132*t*
    distance, 132, 132*t*, 134*b*
    near, 132, 132*t*
Intramuscular injections, 173
Intraocular lens implantation, 36
Intraocular pressure
  drugs reducing, 177–178
  in glaucoma, 18, 34–35
  measurement of, 34–35, 70, 84–89. *See also* Tonometry
  miotics affecting, 177
Intraocular surgery, suture material for, 204
Intravenous injections, 173
Intravitreal injections, 173
Invisible bifocal, 128, 129*f*
Iodine solution, prepping for office surgery with, 211
IPD. *See* Interpupillary distance
Iridotomy, for angle-closure glaucoma, 35
Iris, 12, 12*f*, 18, 19*f*
  abnormalities of, 36
  color of, contact lenses tinted to change, 222
Iris sphincter muscle, 18, 19*f*
  cycloplegics affecting, 175
  miotics affecting, 177
Iritis, 36
Irregular astigmatism, 47
Irrigation (eye)
  for chemical burns, 149–150
  of lacrimal area, in lacrimal-system probing, 208–209
  procedure for, 151*b*
  solutions for, 180
Irritation, contact lenses causing, 229
Ischemia, 27
Island of vision, 108, 110, 111*f*. *See also* Visual fields
  defects of, 112–113, 113*f*, 117–120
    focal, 118, 118*f*, 119*f*
    general, 117, 117*f*
  normal, 117*f*
Isomotic. *See* Isosorbide
Isopters, from tangent screen testing, 112, 112*f*
Isosorbide, for glaucoma, 178

Jaeger notation, 78
Joint Commission on Allied Health Personnel in Ophthalmology (JCAHPO), 4, 5
  certification by, 4–5

Kaposi's sarcoma, in HIV infection/AIDS, 254
Keratectomy, photorefractive (PRK), 48
Keratitis, 33
  Acanthamoeba, 191, 191*f*, 230
  extended-wear lenses and, 221
Keratoconjunctivitis. *See also* Conjunctivitis
  epidemic (EKC), 191
  sicca (dry eye), 16, 33
    in rheumatoid arthritis, 250
    in Sjögren's syndrome, 250–251

Keratoconus, 34
contact lenses for, 223
Keratometer (ophthalmometer), 61, 62*f*, 241, 241*f*
care of, 241
Keratometry, 61, 79
contact lens prescription determination and, 218
procedure for, 63–65*b*
recording measurements and, 65*b*
Keratotomy, radial (RK), 48
Ketoconazole, 179
Ketorolac, 179
Kinetic perimetry, 111, 111–114, 112*f*
advantages and disadvantages of, 114
arc perimeter, 114
Autoplot, 114
examiner-related factors affecting accuracy of, 124
Goldmann, 113–114, 113*f*
tangent screen test, 112–113, 112*f*
Koeppe lens, 91, 237, 237*f*
care of, 237–238, 238*b*

Lacerations, corneal, 33
Lacrimal apparatus, 16, 17*f*
abnormalities of, 32–33
Lacrimal gland, 16, 17*f*
Lacrimal instruments (lacrimal set), 206–207, 206*f*
Lacrimal needle (cannula), 206–207, 206*f*
Lacrimal probes, 206*f*, 207, 207*t*, 208
Lacrimal sac, 16, 17*f*
inflammation of (dacryocystitis), 16, 32–33, 33*f*
Lacrimal-system probing, 208–209
Lagophthalmos, 30
Laser-assisted in situ keratomileusis (LASIK), 48
Lasers/laser therapy, 246–247
care of equipment and, 247
in office setting, 2, 3*f*
for refractive correction, 48
Latanoprost, for glaucoma, 178
Lateral canthus, 14, 15*f*
Lateral geniculate body, 21, 22*f*
Lateral rectus muscle, 13, 13*f*
Legal blindness, 159, 161
Lens care
for contact lenses, 223–224
Acanthamoeba infection and, 191, 191*f*, 230
cleaning and, 223, 224, 224*f*
disinfection and, 223, 224
lubrication and, 223, 224
storage and, 224
for eyeglass lenses, 138–140
for ophthalmic (diagnostic) lenses, 236–238
standard guidelines for, 236
Lens clock, Geneva. *See* Geneva lens clock
Lens disinfection, 223, 224
allergic reactions and, 227–228
Lenses
concave (negative/minus), 43, 44*f*
corrective, 48*t*
passage of light rays through, 44, 44*f*, 45
spherical, 48*t*, 49
contact. *See* Contact lenses
convex (positive/plus), 43, 44, 44*f*
corrective, 48*t*
passage of light rays through, 44, 44*f*
spherical, 49, 49*t*
corrective. *See* Corrective lenses
curved, refractive properties of, 43, 43*f*
eyeglass. *See* Corrective lenses
ophthalmic (diagnostic). *See* Ophthalmic lenses
Lens of eye. *See* Crystalline lens
Lens materials, 129–131
refractive indexes of, 129–130
Lensmeters, 57, 60*f*, 241, 241*f*. *See also* Lensometry
care of, 241
types of, 57–58
Lensometry, 51, 57–61, 79. *See also* Lensmeters
elements of, 58–59
for multifocal lenses, 60–61, 61*b*
for prisms, 61, 62*b*
procedure for
basic, 58–59*b*
for multifocal lenses, 61*b*
for prisms, 62*b*
transposition in, 56
Lens overwear syndrome, 228
Pseudomonas aeruginosa infection and, 189, 230
Lens (vergence) power, 45
focal length relationship and, 45, 45*f*
measuring, in lensometry, 58–59*b*, 59
Lens proteins, age affecting, 36
Lens sterilization, 237–238, 238*b*
Lens zonules, 20
Lesions, definition of, 33
Letter-matching tests, for acuity testing in children, 164
Leukemia, 256
Levator palpebrae superioris muscle, 14–15, 15*f*
Levobunalol, for glaucoma, 177
Levocabastine, 180
Levostin. *See* Levocabastine
LGV. *See* Lymphogranuloma venereum
Lid-lesion surgery, 207–208, 208*f*
Lid margin
collecting specimen from, 197, 197*f*
infection of, 30, 31*f*
lashes on, 14, 15*f*
meibomian glands on, 14, 14*f*
infection of, 14, 29–30, 31*f*
Lidocaine, 177, 203
for lacrimal-system probing, 208
for lid-lesion surgery, 208
Lids. *See* Eyelids
Light. *See also* Light rays
perception of, low vision testing and, 162*b*
pupillary reaction to, testing, 70, 82, 83*b*
visible, 42, 42*f*
Light rays. *See also* Light
parallel, 43–44, 44*f*
refraction of, 42–43, 42*f*, 43*t*
Limbus, 18
Lodoxamide, 180
for giant papillary conjunctivitis, 230
Lopidine. *See* Apraclonidine
Loss of vision. *See* Visual loss
Loteprednol etabonate, 179
Lower canaliculus, 16, 17*f*
Lower punctum, 16, 17*f*
Low vision. *See also* Visual impairment
acuity testing in patients with, 78, 161, 162*b*
Lubricants, 180
for contact lenses, 223, 224
Lumigan. *See* Bimatoprost
Lupus erythematosus, systemic, ocular manifestations of, 251, 251*f*
Lyme disease, ocular manifestations of, 189
Lymphogranuloma venereum (LGV), 189

MacKay-Marg tonometer, 86
Macula, 20, 20*f*
Macular degeneration
age-related, 37
visual acuity affected by, 21
Malignant neoplasms, 28
of eyelid, 30, 31*f*
metastatic, 255–256, 256*f*
ocular manifestations of, 255–256, 256*f*
Manifest refraction, 52
Mannitol, for glaucoma, 178
Manual lensmeter, 57, 60*f*
Manual refractors (Phoroptor), 54, 55*f*, 240, 240*f*
Mapping, visual field, 108–110, 109*f*, 110*f*
standard chart for, 109, 109*f*

Masks
in infection control, 194, 194*t*, 258
for office surgery, 211
Mast cell stabilizers, 180
Medial canthus, 14, 15*f*
Medial rectus muscle, 13, 13*f*
Media opacities, 98
vision tests for patients with, 98–99
Medical assistant, ophthalmic. *See* Ophthalmic medical assistant
Medical eye examination. *See* Eye examination
Medical eye specialist. *See* Ophthalmologist
Medical history, 73. *See also* History, ophthalmic and medical
family, 74
Medical instruments. *See* Instruments
Medical records, patient's right to privacy and, 6
Medications, 171. *See also* Drugs
Meibomian glands, 14
infection of (internal hordeolum), 14, 30, 31*f*
Meridians, 47
in astigmatism, 47
horizontal and vertical, in visual field mapping, 108, 109*f*
radial, in visual field mapping, 108, 109*f*
of spherocylinders, 50, 50*f*
Metabolism/metabolic disorders, 27
ocular manifestations of, 252
Metastasis, 28
ocular, 255–256, 256*f*
Methazolamide, for glaucoma, 178
Metipranolol, for glaucoma, 177
Miconazole, 179
Microorganisms (microbes), 187–199. *See also specific type and* Infection/infectious diseases
infection control and, 193–197
specimen collection for identification of, 197, 197*f*
transmission of, 192–193
types of, 188–191
Migraine, ocular manifestations of, 253
Minor surgery, 201–215. *See also* Office surgery
Minus (concave/negative) lenses, 43, 44*f*
corrective, 48*t*
passage of light rays through, 44, 44*f*, 45
spherical, 48*t*, 49
Minus-cylinder technique, in lensometry, 58–59*b*
Miotics, 177
Mires, adjusting, in lensometry, 58*b*
Moist heat, for sterilization, 195, 195*f*
Molds, 191, 191*f*
Monocular distance IPD, 132, 132*t*
procedure for measuring, 134*b*
Moraxella species
catarrhalis, 189*t*
lacunata, 189*t*
Motility examination, 70, 79–82
MS. *See* Multiple sclerosis
Mucinous fluid, in tear film, 16
Mucopurulent discharge, in bacterial conjunctivitis, 30
Multifocal lenses, 49, 49*f*, 128–129, 128*f*, 129*f*
lensometry technique for, 60–61, 61*b*
progressive-add, 60–61, 60*f*, 128–129, 129*f*
segment placement and, 139–140, 140*f*
Multiple sclerosis (MS), 256
Murine, 180
Muscle balance (alignment of eyes), assessment of, 70, 79–82
Myasthenia gravis, ocular manifestations of, 250, 250*f*
Mycobacterium tuberculosis, airborne transmission of, 192
Mydfrin. *See* Phenylephrine
Mydriacyl. *See* Tropicamide
Mydriasis, 173
Mydriatics, 173–175
Myopia (nearsightedness), 46, 46*f*
prescription for, 56
retinoscopic reflex in, 53–54, 53*f*, 54

Naphcon-A. *See* Phenaramine
Nasal lacrimal obstruction, congenital, lacrimal-system probing for, 208
Nasal step, 120, 122*f*
Nasolacrimal duct, 16, 17*f*
blockage of, dacryocystitis caused by, 16, 32–33, 33*f*
Nausea
change in base curve causing, 135
fluorescein causing, 102
Nd:YAG laser, 246*f*, 247
Near acuity test, 78, 78*f*
for elderly persons, 166
procedure for, 79*b*
Near add, in multifocal lenses, 128, 128*f*
Nearsightedness (myopia), 46, 46*f*
prescription for, 56
retinoscopic reflex in, 53–54, 53*f*, 54
Near visual acuity, 78
testing, 78, 78*f*, 79*b*
Nedocromil sodium, 180
Needle holders, 205, 205*f*, 207*t*
Needles
contaminated, handling of, 194*t*, 196
on instrument tray, 211
suture, 203–204, 204*f*, 207*t*
on instrument tray, 211
Negative (concave/minus) lenses, 43, 44*f*
corrective, 48*t*
passage of light rays through, 44, 44*f*, 45
spherical, 48*t*, 49
Neisseria gonorrhoeae, 188, 188*f*, 189*f*, 189*t*
Neodymium:yttrium-aluminum-garnet (Nd:YAG) laser, 246*f*, 247
Neomycin, 178
Neonatal conjunctivitis, 30, 188–189, 189*f*
Neoplasms/neoplastic disorders, 27–28, 255–256, 256*f*. *See also* Cancer
Neosynephrine. *See* Phenylephrine
Neovascularization
of iris, 36
retinal, in diabetes, 252
Neptazane. *See* Methazolamide
Nervous system, 250
Neuritis, optic, 37
in multiple sclerosis, 256
Neutralization. *See* Lensometry
Neutralization point, in retinoscopy, 53, 53*f*
Nevi, of bulbar conjunctiva, 32
Night vision, rods in, 20
No light perception, low vision testing and, 162*b*
Nonabsorbable suture materials, 204
Nonsteroidal anti-inflammatory drugs (NSAIDs), 179
Nontoothed tying forceps, 205
NSAIDs. *See* Nonsteroidal anti-inflammatory drugs
Nurse, ophthalmic, 3
Nystagmus, 29
Nystatin, 179

Objective refractors/retinoscopes, 52, 52–54
automated, 57
Objective/subjective refractors, automated, 57
Oblique muscles, superior and inferior, 13, 13*f*
Occlusion/occluded blood vessel, 27
Occlusive dressing, after chalazion surgery, 207
"Occupational Exposure to Bloodborne Pathogens," OSHA regulation, 193
Ocucoat, 180
Ocufen. *See* Flurbiprofen
OcuHist. *See* Phenaramine

Ocular alignment and motility examination, 70, 79–82
Ocular herpes simplex, 33–34, 34*f*, 190, 190*f*, 255
Ocular histoplasmosis, 191, 255
Ocular history, 73. *See also* History, ophthalmic and medical
  family, 74
Ocular infections, 26, 187–199, 254–255
  bacterial, 26, 188, 188–189, 188*f*, 189*f*, 189*t*
  fungal, 26, 191, 191*f*
  protozoan, 190, 191*f*
  specimen collection for microorganism identification and, 197, 197*f*
  transmission of, 192–193
  viral, 26, 189–191, 190*f*
    herpes simplex causing, 33–34, 34*f*, 190, 190*f*, 255
Ocularist, 3
Ocular media, 98
  opacities of, vision tests for patients with, 98–99
Ocular motility, testing, 70, 79–82
Ocular pain
  as emergency, 148
  as urgent situation, 148
Ocular surgery, in office, 201–215. *See also* Office surgery
Oculi uterque (OU), in optical prescriptions, 181*t*
Oculomotor nerve palsy, ptosis caused by, 30
Oculus dexter (OD), in optical prescriptions, 56
Oculus sinister (OS), in optical prescriptions, 56
Ocupress. *See* Carteolol
OD (oculus dexter), in optical prescriptions, 56
Office surgery, 201–215. *See also specific procedure*
  anesthesia administration and, 202–203, 203*f*
  assistant's tasks during procedure and, 212, 212*f*
  for chalazion, 207, 208*f*
  dressings and patches and, 209, 209*b*
  first experience with, 209–210
  lacrimal-system probing, 208–209
  lid-lesion, 207–208, 208*f*
  materials and instruments for, 203–207. *See also* Instruments
  patient assistance and, 202, 203*f*
  patient dizziness/faintness and, 210
  patient questions and, 202
  preparing patients for, 202, 203*f*, 210, 211, 211*f*
Office waiting periods, 158
Ofloxacin, 178
Ointments, for topical drug administration, 172
  applying, 174*b*
  maintaining sterility of, 196
Olopatadine, 180
Opacities
  lens, 20. *See also* Cataracts
    vision tests for patients with, 98–99
  media, vision tests for patients with, 98–99
Opaque, definition of, 42
Opcon-A. *See* Phenaramine
Open-angle glaucoma, primary, 35, 35*f*
Ophthaine. *See* Proparacaine
Ophthalmia neonatorum, 30
Ophthalmic assistant, certified, 4. *See also* Ophthalmic medical assistant
Ophthalmic care, providers of, 2–4
Ophthalmic dispenser, 3
Ophthalmic emergencies, 147–148, 149–153
  triaging patients with, 147–148
Ophthalmic lenses
  care of, 236–238
    for lenses that contact eye, 237–238, 238*b*
    for lenses that do not contact eye, 236–237, 237*b*
    standard guidelines for, 236
  corrective, 48–52, 48*t*. *See also* Corrective lenses
  for gonioscopy, 91, 91*f*
Ophthalmic medical assistant, 4
  first experience with surgery and, 209–210
  ill, hygienic practices in infection control and, 197, 258
  professional growth and, 4, 5, 5*f*
  responsibilities of, 4
    ethical, 5–7
    during office surgery. *See also* Office surgery
      anesthesia administration and, 202–203, 203*f*
      assisting, 210–213
      patient preparation and, 202, 203*f*, 210, 211, 211*f*
      postsurgical dressing and patching and, 209, 209*b*
      during procedure and, 212, 212*f*
Ophthalmic medical personnel, 4. *See also* Ophthalmic medical assistant
Ophthalmic medical technologist, certified, 4
Ophthalmic migraine, 253
Ophthalmic pharmacology, 171–185. *See also* Drugs
Ophthalmic photographer, 3
Ophthalmic photography, 101–103
  external, 101
  fundus, 101–103, 102*f*
  slit-lamp, 101, 101*f*
  specular microscopy and, 99, 101, 101*f*
Ophthalmic registered nurse, 3
Ophthalmic technician, certified, 4
Ophthalmic ultrasonography (biometry), 103–104, 103*f*, 104*f*
Ophthalmologist, 2
Ophthalmology
  advances in, 2
  definition of, 2
Ophthalmometer (keratometer), 61, 62*f*, 241, 241*f*
  care of, 241
Ophthalmopathy, thyroid, 252, 252*f*
Ophthalmoscope, 2, 2*f*
  direct, 91, 92*f*
  examination with in glaucoma, 34
  indirect, 91–92, 92*f*
Ophthalmoscopy, 71, 91–92, 92*f*
  direct, 91, 92*f*
  in glaucoma, 34
  indirect, 91–92, 92*f*
Ophthetic. *See* Proparacaine
Optical centers, 131, 131*f*
  checking, 139, 140*b*
  distance between, 132
    measuring, 139, 140*b*
    prismatic effect and, 132, 133*f*
  lensmeter for verification of position of, 61
Optical lenses. *See* Ophthalmic lenses
Optical prescriptions, 181–182, 181*f*
  abbreviations and symbols used in, 181, 181*t*
  interpretation of, 55–56, 181–182
  transposition of, 56
Optical system, eye as, 12, 12*f*
Optic chiasm, 21, 22*f*
Optic disc (optic nerve head), 20, 20*f*
Optician, 3, 127
Opticianry, 127–144. *See also* Corrective lenses
Optic nerve, 12, 12*f*, 21, 21*f*
  damage to/lesions of, field defects caused by, 120, 123*f*
Optic neuritis, 37
  in multiple sclerosis, 256
Optic radiations, 21, 22*f*
Opticrom. *See* Cromolyn
Optics
  definition of, 42
  principles of, 42–45
Optic tract, 21, 22*f*
OptiPranolol. *See* Metipranolol
Optometrist, 3
Optotypes, Snellen, 75, 75*f*
Oral drug delivery, 173

Orbicularis oculi muscle, 14, 15*f*
Orbit, 12, 13*f*
  abnormalities of, 28–29
  trauma to, 29
Orbital cellulitis, 28
Organic solvents, chemical burns of eye caused by, 147, 150
Orthophoric patient, interpupillary distance in, 132
Orthoptist, 3
OS (oculus sinister), in optical prescriptions, 56
OSHA (United States Department of Labor, Occupational Safety and Health Administration), regulations of for prevention of infection transmission, 193
Osmitrol. *See* Mannitol
Osmotics, for corneal edema, 180
OU (oculi uterque), in optical prescriptions, 181*t*
Overwearing syndrome, 228
  Pseudomonas aeruginosa infection and, 189, 230
Oxygen, lack of (hypoxia), 27

Pachymeter (pachometer), 100, 100*f*
Pachymetry (pachometry), 99, 100, 100*f*
Pain, ocular
  as emergency, 148
  as urgent situation, 148
Palpation, in external eye examination, 89
Palpebral conjunctiva, 15, 15*f*
Palpebral fissure, 14, 15*f*
Palsy (paralysis), extraocular muscle, 29
PAM. *See* Potential acuity meter
Panretinal viewing (condensing) lenses, 236, 236*f*
  care of, 236–237, 237*b*
Pantoscopic angle, of eyeglass frame, 137–138, 138*f*
Papilledema, 37
Papilloma, eyelid, surgical removal of, 207–208, 208*f*
Papoose board, for examining infant, 162
Papules, conjunctival, contact lens wear and, 230
Paracentral scotoma, 120, 122*f*
Parallax, IPD measuring errors and, 132–134
Parallel light rays, 43–44, 44*f*
Paralysis (palsy), extraocular muscle, 29
Paraxial rays, 44, 44*f*
Patanol. *See* Olopatadine
Patches, postsurgical, 209, 209*b*
Pathogens. *See also* Microorganisms; Infection/infectious diseases
  bloodborne, universal precautions in protection against, 193, 257–258
Pathologic change, definition of, 26
Patient-assistant interaction, 146, 158
  with visually impaired/blind patient, 159–161, 161*f*
Patient-doctor relationship, professional behavior by assistant and, 7–8
Patient fall, guidelines for handling, 152
Patients
  assisting, 160–161, 161*f*
    office surgery and, 202, 203*f*
  children, 161–165
  comfort of, eyeglass frames affecting, 138
  consideration of as individuals, 158
  disruptive, 159
  elderly, 165–166
  fainting
    assisting, 152, 152*f*
    office surgery and, 210
  families and, 158
  fatigued, perimetry affected by, 124
  greeting, 146
    visually impaired/blind patients and, 160
  infants, 161–165
  interaction of with assistants, 146, 158
    with visually impaired/blind patient, 159–161, 161*f*
  perimetry, accuracy affected by factors related to, 123–124
  physically disabled, 166–167, 167*f*
  positioning
    infants and young children and, 162–163, 162*f*
    for office surgery, 202, 203*f*
  preparing for office surgery, 202, 203*f*, 210, 211, 211*f*
  questions about office surgery and, 202
  referred, 149
  scheduling appointments for, 148–149
    for diabetic patient, 168
    triage procedure and, 147–148
    waiting periods and, 158
  screening, 146–149
    appointment scheduling and, 148–149
    procedure for, 147–148
  with special considerations, 157–170
  visually impaired/blind. *See* Blindness; Visual impairment
  young children, 161–165
PCF. *See* Pharyngoconjunctival fever
Pediatric ophthalmologists, 3
Pemirolast potassium, 180
Peptostreptococcus, 189*t*
Perimeter
  accuracy of affected by factors related to, 123
  arc, 114
  Goldmann, 86–88, 87*f*, 113–114, 113*f*
Perimetry, 107–126
  defects shown by, 117–120. *See also* Visual field defects
    focal, 118–119, 118*f*, 119*f*
    general, 117–118, 117*f*
    in glaucoma, 35, 120, 122*f*, 123*f*
    hemianopic, 119, 120*f*, 121*f*
    in optic nerve damage/lesions, 120, 123*f*
  explaining procedure to patients and, 123–124
  factors affecting accuracy of, 120–124
    device-related, 123
    environment-related, 121
    examiner-related, 124
    patient-related, 123–124
  kinetic, 111, 111–114, 112*f*
  principles and techniques of, 107–126
  purposes of, 111
  static, 111, 114–117
  types of, 111–117
  visual field mapping and, 108–110, 111*f*
Periocular injections, 173
Peripheral vision, testing. *See* Visual fields, examination of
Perkins tonometer, 86
Personal protective equipment, in infection control, 194, 194*t*, 212
Pharmacology. *See also* Drugs
  definition of, 171
  ophthalmic, 171–185
Pharyngoconjunctival fever (PCF), 191
Phenaramine, 180
Phenol, for disinfection, 194
Phenylephrine, 175. *See also* Mydriatics
Phoria, 29
Phoroptor (manual refractor), 54, 55*f*, 240, 240*f*
  care of, 240–241
Photochromic lenses, 130–131
Photocoagulation, for retinal detachment, 37
Photographer, ophthalmic, 3
Photography, ophthalmic, 101–103
  of corneal endothelium, 101, 101*f*
  external, 101

Photography, ophthalmic, *(continued)*
fundus, 101–103, 102*f*
slit-lamp, 101, 101*f*
specular microscopy and, 99, 101, 101*f*
Photophobia
tinted contact lenses for, 222
as urgent situation, 148
Photoreceptors, 20, 21*f*
Photorefractive keratectomy (PRK), 48
Physical abuse, eye trauma and, 147
Physically disabled patients, 166–167, 167*f*
Physical optics, 42
Physiologic blind spot, 21, 108, 108*f*, 109
Physostigmine, 177
Pigment epithelium, 20, 21*f*
Pilocarpine, 177
Pimaricin, 179
Pinguecula, 32, 32*f*
Pinhole, super, 98
Pinhole acuity test, 77–78, 77*f*
procedure for, 77*b*
Pinhole occluder, 77–78, 77*b*, 77*f*
"Pink eye." *See* Conjunctivitis; Pharyngoconjunctival fever
Placido disk, in corneal topography, 100
Plane (flat) sides, of prism, 43
Planned- (programmed-/frequent-) replacement lenses, 221
Plano (flat) mirror effect, 53
Plastic lenses, 130
cleaning, 139
refractive index of, 130
ultraviolet coating for, 131
Pledget, for anesthesia administration, 203, 203*f*
Plus (convex/positive) lenses, 43, 44*f*
corrective, 48*t*
passage of light rays through, 44, 44*f*
spherical, 49, 49*t*
Plus-cylinder technique, in lensometry, 58–59*b*
PMMA (polymethylmethacrylate) contact lenses, 219, 220
insertion and removal of, 226, 227*b*, 228*b*
PMMA plastic, refractive index of, 43*t*
Pneumatonometer, 86
Pneumatoretinopexy, for retinal detachment, 37
Polarized lenses, 131
Polycarbonate
refractive index of, 130
for safety lenses, 130
Polymethylmethacrylate (PMMA), refractive index of, 43*t*
Polymethylmethacrylate (PMMA) contact lenses, 219, 220
insertion and removal of, 226, 227*b*, 228*b*
Polymyxin B, in combination products, 178
Pontocaine. *See* Tetracaine
Positive (convex/plus) lenses, 43, 44*f*
corrective, 48*t*
passage of light rays through, 44, 44*f*
spherical, 49, 49*t*
Posterior chamber, 19, 19*f*
Posterior segment, 16. *See also* Retina; Vitreous
examination of. *See* Ophthalmoscopy
Postsurgical dressing and patching, 209, 209*b*
Potential acuity meter (PAM), 98, 98*f*, 246, 246*f*
Potential visual status, tests to determine, 98–99
Power of lens, 45
focal length relationship and, 45, 45*f*
measuring, in lensometry, 58–59*b*, 59
Prednisolone, 179
in combination products, 178
Prednisone, 179
Prepping, 202, 203*f*, 210, 211, 211*f*
Presbyopia, 20, 36, 47–48
perimetry accuracy affected by, 124
Prescriptions, 181–182, 181*f*
abbreviations and symbols used in, 181, 181*t*
for contact lenses vs eyeglasses, 218, 219
interpretation of, 55–56, 181–182
transposition of, 56
Preservatives
in contact lens solutions, adverse reactions to, 224, 227–228
in infection control, 196
in lubricants, sensitivity/allergy to, 180
in topical drug solutions, 172
in topical drug suspensions, 172
Pressure patches, 209, 209*b*
after chalazion surgery, 207
Primary angle-closure glaucoma, 35, 35*f*
mydriatics simulating attack of, 175
Primary open-angle glaucoma, 35, 35*f*
Principal axis of lens, 44, 44*f*
Principal meridians, in astigmatism, 47
Principal (axial) ray, 44, 44*f*
Prism and alternate cover test, 80*f*, 81
Prismatic effect, 132, 133*f*
Prism diopters, 51, 52*f*
Prisms
corrective, 48*t*, 51–52, 51*f*, 52*f*
definition of, 43
lensometry technique for, 61, 62*b*
passage of light through, 43, 43*f*
procedure for measuring power and orientation of, 62*b*
Privacy rights, patient's, 6
PRK. *See* Photorefractive keratectomy
Probes, lacrimal, 206*f*, 207, 207*t*
Professional behavior, 7–8
Professional development, 4, 5, 5*f*
Prognosis, informing patient about, as physician responsibility, 6
Programmed- (planned-/frequent-) replacement lenses, 221
Progressive-addition multifocal lenses, 60–61, 60*f*, 128–129, 129*f*
segment placement and, 139–140, 140*f*
Projector, for visual acuity charts, 75, 75*f*, 242, 243*f*
care of, 242–243
Proparacaine, 177, 202–203
plus fluorescein, 177
Propine. *See* Dipivefrin
Propionibacterium acnes, 189*t*
Proptosis (exophthalmos), 28, 28*f*
assessment of (exophthalmometry), 89, 94, 94*f*
in thyroid disorders, 252, 252*f*
Prostaglandin analogs, for glaucoma, 178
Prostheses, ocularist in fitting for, 3
Protective equipment, personal, for infection control, 194, 194*t*, 212
Protective eyewear, 130, 130*f*
for infection control, 194, 212
Proteus mirabilis, 189*t*
Protozoa/protozoan infections, 191, 191*f*
Pseudoisochromatic color plates, for color vision testing, 92,93*f*
Pseudomonas aeruginosa, 189, 189*t*, 230
Pseudophakia, 36
Pterygium, 32, 32*f*
Ptosis, 15, 30, 31*f*
in myasthenia gravis, 250, 250*f*
perimetry accuracy affected by, 124
Punctum (puncta), 16, 17*f*
Punctum dilator, 206, 206*f*, 208
Pupillary reaction, direct and consensual, 82
Pupils, 12, 12*f*
cycloplegics affecting, 175
examination of, 70, 82, 83*b*
miotics affecting, 177

mydriatics affecting, 173–175
size of, perimetry accuracy affected by, 124

Radial keratotomy (RK), 48
Radial meridians, in visual field mapping, 108, 109*f*
Reading distance, assessment of visual acuity at, 78, 78*f*, 79*b*
Reading glasses, 49
Rectus muscles, superior/medial/inferior/lateral, 13, 13*f*
Red eye
decongestants for, 180
as urgent situation, 148
Referred patients, 149
Refinement, 52, 54, 55*f*
Refraction, 45–48
clinical, 52–55, 79. *See also* Refractometry; Refractors
automated, 56–57, 57*f*
components of, 52–55
contact lens prescription determination and, 218
cycloplegic, 52
manifest, 52
manual (Phoroptor), 54, 55*f*
by concave lens, 44, 44*f*, 45
by convex lens, 44, 44*f*
by curved lens, 42–43, 42*f*, 43*t*
cycloplegic, 52, 175
by cylinder, 50, 50*f*
definition of, 52
by prism, 43, 43*f*, 51–52, 51*f*, 52*f*
by spherical lens, 49*f*, 59
by spherocylinder, 50–51, 51*f*
Refractive errors, 41
changes in, lensometry to determine, 57
contact lens prescription determination and, 218
correcting. *See* Contact lenses; Corrective lenses; Refractive surgery
focal defects caused by, 118
measuring. *See* Refractometry
types of, 46–48
Refractive index, 43, 43*t*
of lens materials, 129–130
Refractive power, of prism, 51–52, 52*f*
Refractive states of eye, 45–48
Refractive surgery, 48
Refractometry, 52–55, 79
contact lens prescription determination and, 218
objective (retinoscopy), 52, 52–54
automated, 57
subjective (refinement), 52, 54, 55*f*
automated, 57
Refractors
automated, 56–57, 57*f*
manual (Phoroptor), 54, 55*f*, 240, 240*f*
care of, 240–241
Refresh, 180
Regular astigmatism, 47, 47*f*
Reichert (American Optical) Phoroptor, care of, 240–241
Relative defect, 119, 119*f*
Reservoir, of microorganisms, 192
Respiratory emergency, first aid for, 182*b*
Respiratory system, 250
Retina, 12, 12*f*, 20–21, 20*f*
abnormalities of, 37
hypertensive changes in, 253, 254*f*
leukemia causing changes in, 256, 256*f*
Retinal artery, central, 20
embolus causing occlusion of, 253, 253*f*
Retinal detachment, 37
Retinal neovascularization, in diabetes, 252
Retinal pigment epithelium, 20, 21*f*
Retinal vasculitis, in systemic lupus erythematosus, 251, 251*f*
Retinitis
cytomegalovirus (CMV), 190, 254, 254*f*
pigmentosa, 37
Retinopathy, diabetic, 37, 167, 252, 252*f*
Retinoscope, 53, 53*f*, 240, 240*f*
care of, 240
Retinoscopic reflex, 53–54, 53*f*
Retinoscopy (objective refractometry), 52, 52–54
automated, 57
Retrobulbar injections, 173
Retrobulbar visual pathway, 21, 22*f*
injury to, 37
Retroscopic tilt, 138
Retrovirus, HIV as, 190
Reverse cutting needle, 204, 204*f*
RGP (rigid gas-permeable) contact lenses, 219, 220, 220*f*. *See also* Contact lenses
advantages and disadvantages of, 220
daily-wear, 221
extended-wear, 221
insertion and removal of, 226, 227*b*, 228*b*
for keratoconus, 223
storage of, 224
Rheumatoid arthritis, ocular manifestations of, 250, 251*f*
Right to privacy, patient's, 6
Rigid gas-permeable (RGP) contact lenses, 219, 220, 220*f*. *See also* Contact lenses
advantages and disadvantages of, 220
daily-wear, 221
extended-wear, 221
insertion and removal of, 226, 227*b*, 228*b*
for keratoconus, 223
storage of, 224
Rimexolone, 179
RK. *See* Radial keratotomy
Rods, 20, 21*f*
Rose bengal dye, 93, 176. *See also* Dyes
Round-top segments, 128, 128*f*
Routine situations, triaging patients with, 148
Rubeosis iridis, 36

Safety standards, for corrective lenses, 130
Saline (salt) solutions, homemade, *Acanthamoeba* infection and, 191, 230
Sarcoidosis, ocular manifestations of, 250, 251*f*
Scalpels/scalpel blades, 206, 206*f*, 207*t*
on instrument tray, 211
Scheduling patient appointments, 148–149
for patients with diabetes, 168
triage procedure and, 147–148
waiting periods and, 158
Schiøtz indentation tonometry, 88–89, 88*f*
Schiøtz tonometer, 88–89, 88*f*, 244, 245*f*
care of, 244–245
Schirmer test, 89, 93, 93*f*
Schlemm, canal of, 18, 18*f*
School-age children, visual acuity and ability testing in, 164
tips for, 165
Scintillations, in migraine, 253
Scissors, surgical, 205, 205*f*, 207*t*
Sclera, 18
abnormalities of, 33–34
Scleral buckle, for retinal detachment, 37
Scleritis, 34
in rheumatoid arthritis, 250, 251*f*
Scopolamine, 176
Scotoma, 112, 113*f*, 118, 119*f*
absolute, 112, 113*f*, 119, 119*f*
altitudinal, 120, 122*f*
arcuate, 120
Bjerrum, 120, 122*f*
central, 120, 123*f*
deep, 112, 113*f*, 119*f*
paracentral, 120, 122*f*
relative, 118, 119*f*
shallow, 112

Scratch-resistant coating, 131
Screening patients, 146–149
Scrubbing, 210–211. *See also* Hand washing
Secondary glaucoma, 35–36
Segment, multifocal lens, 49, 128, 128*f*
  round-top, 128, 128*f*
Segment height, 139–140, 140*f*
Seizures, first aid for, 182*b*
Sensitivity reactions. *See also* Allergic response/allergies
  contact lens preservatives/disinfectants causing, 227–228
Serratia marcescens, 189*t*
Sharps
  counting, 211, 212
  disposing of, 194*t*, 196, 212
  on instrument tray, 211
Sharps container, 194*t*, 196, 212, 258
Shields, postsurgical, 209, 209*b*
Shingles (zoster), 190, 255
Signs, definition of, 28
Single lines, focusing, in lensometry, 58*b*, 59*b*
Single-vision lenses, 128
Sinuses, orbital fracture pushing eye contents into, 29
Sjögren's syndrome, ocular manifestations of, 250–251
SLE. *See* Systemic lupus erythematosus
Slit lamp (biomicroscope), 71, 90, 90*f*, 242, 242*f*. *See also* Biomicroscopy
  care of, 242
  in tonometry, 86–87*b*, 87*f*, 243, 243*f*
Slit-lamp photography, 101, 101*f*
Snellen acuity test, 74. *See also* Snellen chart
Snellen chart, 74–76, 75*f*
  for children who know alphabet and numbers, 164
  for elderly persons, 166
  pinhole occluder used with, 77–78, 77*b*, 77*f*
  procedure for acuity testing with, 76*b*
Snellen optotypes, 75, 75*f*
Soft (hydrophilic) contact lenses, 218, 219–220, 220–221, 220*f*. *See also* Contact lenses
  daily-wear, 221
  disposable, 221
  extended-wear, 221
  insertion and removal of, 225–226, 225*b*, 226*b*
  planned- (programmed-/frequent) replacement, 221
  storage of, 224
  therapeutic, 223
Solution–lens interaction, 230–231
Solutions. *See also* Eyedrops
  for topical drug administration, 172
Spatula suture needle, 204*f*
Specimen collection, for microorganism identification, 197, 197*f*
Spectacle blur, minimization of with RGP lenses, 220
Specular microscopy/photography, 99, 101, 101*f*
Spheres/spherical lenses, 48*t*, 49, 49*f*
  measuring power of, 58–59*b*
Spherocylinders/spherocylindrical lenses, 48*t*, 50–51, 50*f*, 51*f*
  corrective, prescription for, 56
Sphincter muscle of iris, 18, 19*f*
  cycloplegics affecting, 175
  miotics affecting, 177
Spores, bacterial, 188
Sports activities, protective eyewear and, 130, 130*f*
Staining, in bacteria identification, 188
Standard precautions, 187, 193–194, 194*t*
Staphylococcus species, 188
  aureus, 188, 188*f*, 189*t*
  epidermidis, 189*t*
Static perimetry, 111, 114–117
  advantages and disadvantages of, 116–117
  automated, 115, 115*f*
  computerized, 115–116, 116*f*
  suprathreshold, 114
  threshold, 115, 115*f*
Steep defect, 118*f*, 119
Stereopsis, 29
  loss of, 79
  Titmus test of, 81–82, 82*f*
Sterile drapes, for office surgery, 211
Sterile gloves, for office surgery, 210–211
Sterile instruments, aseptic technique for handling of, 195–196
Sterile operating field (sterile field), 210
Sterilization, 195, 258
  lens, 237–238, 238*b*
Steroids, 179
  in combination preparations with antibiotics, 178
Storage, of contact lenses, 224
Strabismic amblyopia. *See* Amblyopia
Strabismus, 14, 29, 29*f*
  testing for (ocular alignment and motility examination), 70, 79–82
Streptococcus species
  pneumoniae, 189*t*
  pyogenes, 189*t*
  viridans group, 189*t*
Stroke, ocular manifestations of, 253, 253*f*
Stye (external hordeolum), 14, 29–30, 31*f*
Subconjunctival hemorrhages, 16, 32, 32*f*
Subconjunctival injections, 173
Subcutaneous injections, 173
Subjective refractors, 52, 54, 55*f*
  automated, 57
Sugar, blood levels of, monitoring in diabetes, 167, 167*f*
Sulfacetamide, in combination products, 178
Sulfonamides, 178
Superior oblique muscle, 13, 13*f*
Superior rectus muscle, 13, 13*f*
Super pinhole, 98
Suppression, Worth four-dot test for, 81, 81*f*
Suprathreshold static perimetry, 114
Surfactant cleaners, for contact lenses, 224
Surgical assisting skills, 210–213
Surgical materials and instruments, 203–207. *See also* Instruments
  care of, 212–213, 258
  disposition of after procedure, 212–213, 258
  passing to surgeon, 212, 212*f*
  preparation of instrument tray and, 211–212, 211*f*
Surgical scissors, 205, 205*f*, 207*t*
Suspensions. *See also* Eyedrops
  for topical drug administration, 172
Suture needles, 203–204, 204*f*, 207*t*
  on instrument tray, 211
Sutures, 203–204, 204*f*, 207*t*
  on instrument tray, 212
Swinging-light test, for direct and consensual pupillary reaction, 82
Symptoms, definition of, 28
Synapses, in visual pathway, 21
Syndrome, definition of, 28
Syphilis, ocular manifestations of, 189, 255
Syringe, in lacrimal set, 206, 206*f*
Systemic diseases, ocular manifestations of, 249–256
Systemic drug delivery, 173
Systemic lupus erythematosus (SLE), ocular manifestations of, 251, 251*f*

Tangent screen test, 112–113, 112*f*
Taper point suture needle, 204, 204*f*
Target slides, 242, 243*f*
  care of, 242
Tarsus (tarsal plate), 14, 15*f*
Tear film, 16

Tearing (epiphora)
  contact lenses causing, 229
  lacrimal-system probing for, 208–209
Tear output tests, 89, 93, 93*f*
Tear pump, 218
Tears
  artificial, 180
  HIV isolated from, 190
  as protective barrier, 192
Tears Naturale, 180
Tears Plus, 180
Teller Acuity Cards, for acuity testing in children and infants, 164
Temporal (giant cell) arteritis, ocular manifestations of, 253
Tetracaine, 177, 202–203
Therapeutic contact lenses, 223
Therapeutic medications, 177–180
Thermal trauma, 28
Thimerosal, allergic reaction caused by, 228
Threshold static perimetry, 115, 115*f*
  computerized, 115–116, 116*f*
Thyroid disorders, ocular manifestations of, 251–252, 252*f*
Thyroid ophthalmopathy, 252, 252*f*
Timolol, for glaucoma, 177
Timoptic. *See* Timolol
Tinted contact lenses, 222, 222*f*
Tints, lens, 130–131
Tissue forceps, 205
Titmus stereopsis test, 81–82, 82*f*
Tobramycin, 178
Toddlers, visual acuity and ability testing in, 164
  tips for, 164–165
Tonometers, 34, 84, 86
  disinfection of, 196
  Goldmann (applanation), 86–88, 87*f*
    care of, 243–244
  Schiøtz (indentation), 88–89, 88*f*, 244, 245*f*
    care of, 244–245
Tonometry, 70, 84, 85–89
  applanation, 85, 86–88, 87*f*
    indentation tonometry compared with, 89
  Goldmann, 86–88, 86–87*b*, 87*f*
  indentation, 85, 88–89, 88*f*
    applanation tonometry compared with, 89
  principles of, 85–86
Tono-Pen, 86, 88
Toothed tissue forceps, 205
Topical drugs, 172, 172–173
  administration of, 173, 174*b*, 175*f*
  anesthetics, 177
  for conjunctivitis, 30
  miotics as, 177
Topography, corneal, 100, 100*f*
Toric contact lenses, 222
Toric cornea, 36
Toric lenses, 50, 50*f*. *See also* Spherocylinders/spherocylindrical lenses
Toxins, disorders caused by, 28
Toxoplasma gondii, 191
Toxoplasmosis, 191, 255
Trabecular meshwork, 18, 18*f*
Trachoma, 189
Transitional zone, of multifocal lenses, 128–129, 129*f*
Translucent, definition of, 42
Transparent, definition of, 42
Transposition of prescriptions, 56
Trauma, 28, 147, 150
  chemical, 28, 147, 149–150
  corneal, 33
  orbital, 29
  physical abuse and, 147
Travatan. *See* Travoprost
Travoprost, for glaucoma, 178
Tremors, first aid for, 182*b*
Treponema pallidum, 189, 255
Triage (patient screening), 146–149
  appointment scheduling and, 148–149
  procedure for, 147–148
Trial frame, 54, 54*f*
Trial lens set, 54, 55*f*
Triamcinolone, 179
Trichiasis, 14, 30
Trifluorothymidine, 179
Trifocals, 49, 49*f*, 128, 128*f*
  double-D segment, 129, 129*f*
  D segment, 128, 129*f*
  executive, 128, 128*f*
  measuring power of, 61*b*
  prescription for, 56
  round-top, 128, 128*f*
  segment placement and, 139, 140*f*
Trimethoprim, in combination products, 178
Triple lines, focusing, in lensometry, 58*b*, 59*b*
Tropia, 29
Tropicamide, 176
Trusopt. *See* Dorzolamide
Tuberculosis, airborne transmission of, 192
Tumbling E distance acuity chart, 75, 75*f*, 164, 164*f*
  difficulties with use of, 164–165
Tying forceps, 205

Ulcers, corneal, 18, 33
  contact lenses causing, 221, 230
  extended-wear lenses and, 221
  herpetic, 33–34, 34*f*
  in rheumatoid arthritis, 250, 251*f*
Ultrasonic pachymeter, 100
Ultrasonography, ophthalmic (biometry), 103–104, 103*f*, 104*f*
Ultraviolet coating, 131
United States Department of Labor, Occupational Safety and Health Administration (OSHA), regulations of for prevention of infection transmission, 193
Universal precautions, 193, 257–258
Upper canaliculus, 16, 17*f*
Upper punctum, 16, 17*f*
Upward gaze, extraocular muscles in, 13
Urgent situations, 148
  triaging patients with, 148
Uveal tract (uvea), 18–19, 19*f*. *See also* Choroid; Ciliary body; Iris
  abnormalities of, 36
Uveitis
  in sarcoidosis, 250, 251*f*
  in syphilis, 255

Valacyclovir, 179
Valtrex. *See* Valacyclovir
Varicella-zoster virus (VZV), 190, 255
  airborne transmission of, 192
  ocular manifestations of infection with, 190, 255
Vascular diseases, ocular manifestations of, 252–253, 253*f*, 254*f*
Vasculitis, retinal, in systemic lupus erythematosus, 251, 251*f*
Vasocon, 180
Vectors, in disease transmission, 192
Vehicle, in topical drug solution, 172
Vergence (lens) power, 45
  focal length relationship and, 45, 45*f*
  measuring, in lensometry, 58–59*b*, 59
Vernal conjunctivitis, 30
Vertex distance, 131, 134–135, 135*f*
Vertical meridians, in visual field mapping, 108, 109*f*
Vidarabine, 179
Vira-A. *See* Vidarabine
Viroptic. *See* Trifluorothymidine
Viruses/viral infections, 26, 189–191, 190*f*
  conjunctivitis, 30, 191
  drugs for treatment of, 178, 179, 190
Visine, 180
Vision
  age-related changes in, 165–166
  anatomy of eye and, 11–24
  double. *See* Double vision *or* Diplopia

Vision, *(continued)*
eye examination in evaluation of. *See* Eye examination
island of, 108, 110, 111*f*. *See also* Visual fields
defects of, 112–113, 113*f*, 117–120
normal, 117*f*
loss of. *See* Visual loss
Vision correction, contact lenses vs eyeglasses for, 219
Visual acuity, 74
macular injury/degeneration affecting, 21
testing. *See* Visual acuity examination
Visual acuity examination, 70, 74–79
in children, 163–165
charts used for, 164, 164*f*
for distance vision, 74–77
procedure for performing, 76*b*
in elderly persons, 166
in infants, 163, 163*b*
for near vision, 78, 78*f*
procedures following, 78–79
in school-age children, 164
tips for, 165
in toddlers, 164
tips for, 164–165
for visually impaired patient, 78, 161, 162*b*
Visual cortex, 21, 22*f*
Visual field defects, 21, 112–113, 113*f*, 117–120
focal, 118–119, 118*f*, 119*f*
general, 117–118, 117*f*
in glaucoma, 35, 120, 122*f*, 123*f*
hemianopic, 119, 120*f*, 121*f*
in optic nerve damage/lesions, 120, 123*f*
Visual fields
anatomic basis of, 108, 108*f*
contracted/constricted, 117–118, 117*f*
examination of, 70, 83–84, 84*b*, 107–126. *See also* Perimetry
Amsler grid testing in, 83, 84, 85*b*, 85*f*
confrontation testing in, 83, 84, 84*b*, 84*f*, 111
in glaucoma, 34, 35
mapping of, 108–110, 109*f*, 110*f*
orientation for plotting and, 110, 111*f*
standard chart for, 109, 109*f*
normal, 110, 110*f*, 117*f*
Visual function testing, by orthoptist, 3
Visual impairment. *See also* Blindness; Visual loss
acuity testing and, 78, 161, 162*b*
assisting patients and, 160–161, 161*f*
history-taking and, 160
patient greeting and, 160
patient interaction and, 159–160
Visual loss. *See also* Blindness; Visual impairment
in giant cell (temporal) arteritis, 253
in migraine, temporary, 253
subacute, as urgent situation, 148
sudden, as emergency, 147
Visual pathway, 21, 22*f*
abnormalities of, 37
Visual potential tests, 98–99
Vitreous detachment, 37
Vitreous floaters, 20, 36–37
as urgent situation, 148
Vitreous (vitreous body), 12, 12*f*, 20
abnormalities of, 36–37
Voltaren. *See* Diclofenac
VZV. *See* Varicella-zoster virus

Waiting periods, 158
Warping, of corneal curvature, improperly fitted contact lenses causing, 229
Water
boiling, for disinfection, 194
refractive index of, 43*t*
Wavelength, 42
Wetting/cushioning solutions, for contact lenses, 223, 224
Wheelchairs, patients in, 166–167, 167*f*
With motion movement, of retinoscopic reflex, 53, 53*f*, 54
"Working distance," adjusting for, 54
Worth four-dot test, 81, 81*f*

Xalatan. *See* Latanoprost
Xanthoma, eyelid, surgical removal of, 207–208, 208*f*
Xylocaine. *See* Lidocaine

Yeasts, 191, 191*f*

Zonules, 20
Zoster (shingles), 190, 255
Zovirax. *See* Acyclovir